W9-BWX-308

ROBERTS' PRACTICAL GUIDE TO COMMON MEDICAL EMERGENCIES

INFOCUS

ROBERTS' PRACTICAL GUIDE TO COMMON MEDICAL EMERGENCIES

James R. Roberts, MD

Professor and Vice Chairman, Emergency Medicine
Medical College of Pennsylvania
Chairman, Department of Emergency Medicine
Director, Division of Toxicology
Mercy Catholic Medical Center, Philadelphia, PA

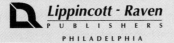
Lippincott - Raven
PUBLISHERS
PHILADELPHIA

Publisher: Michael Randers-Pehrson
Acquisitions Editor: Elizabeth Greenspan
Developmental Editor: Lisa Hoffman
Manufacturing Manager: Dennis Teston
Production Manager: Larry Bernstein
Art Director/Compositor: Kathleen Giarrano
Printer: Quebecor, Kingsport

Copyright ©1996, by Lippincott-Raven Publishers. All rights reserved. This book is protected by copyright. No part of it may be reproduced, stored in a retrieval system, or transmitted in any form or by any means—electronic, mechanical, photocopy, recording or otherwise—without the prior written consent of the publisher, except for brief quotations embodied in critical articles and reviews. For information, write **Lippincott-Raven Publishers, 227 East Washington Square, Philadelphia, PA 19106-3780.**

Materials appearing in this book prepared by individuals as part of their official duties as U.S. Government employees are not covered by the above-mentioned copyright.

Printed in the United States of America

9 8 7 6 5 4 3 2 1

Library of Congress Cataloging-in-Publication Data

Roberts, James R., 1946-
        Roberts' practical guide to common medical emergencies / James R. Roberts.
            p.   cm.
        At head of title: InFocus.
        Includes bibliographical references.
        Distinctive title: InFocus.
        ISBN 0-397-51838-2
        1. Medical emergencies.   I. Title
        [DNLM: 1. Emergency Medicine—methods. 2. Emergencies. WB 105 R645r 1996]
RC86.7.R586   1996
616.02 5—dc21
DNLM/DLC
for Library of Congress   96-40889
                                                                                              CIP

Care has been taken to confirm the accuracy of the information presented and to describe generally accepted practices. However, the authors, editors, and publisher are not responsible for errors or omissions or for any consequences from application of the information in this book and make no warranty, express or implied, with respect to the contents of the publication. This material is the opinion of the author based on his experience and clinical practice. It is not meant to strictly define standard of care, and similar clinical situations may require an alternative approach.

The authors, editors, and publisher have exerted every effort to ensure that drug selection and dosage set forth in this text are in accordance with current recommendations and practice at the time of publication. However, in view of ongoing research, changes in government regulations, and the constant flow of information relating to drug therapy and drug reactions, the reader is urged to check the package insert for each drug for any change in indications and dosage and for added warnings and precautions. This is particularly important when the recommended agent is a new or infrequently employed drug.

Some drugs and medical devices in this publication have Food and Drug Administration (FDA) clearance for limited use in restricted research settings. It is the responsibility of the health care provider to ascertain the FDA status of each drug or device planned for use in his clinical practice.

DEDICATION

To Lydia, Matthew, and Martha

AKNOWLEDGMENTS

In no particular order, I would like to acknowledge the gargantuan efforts of Michael Randers-Pehrson, Lisa Hoffman, Rose Bacher, and Kathleen Giarrano in bringing this book to print. Without their help, I would still be missing deadlines, and this project probably never would have been started and clearly never would have been completed.

The original concept for InFocus came from Jerris Hedges, MD, who has been an inspiration and mentor to countless emergency physicians. Throughout the years, my inspiration to continue the columns has come from many kind readers, residents, and colleagues. At the risk of omitting some of them, I would particularly like to acknowledge a few physicians who have challenged and supported my efforts and have advanced medical education on many fronts. They certainly know a lot more about most of the topics than I do: Lewis Goldfrank, MD; David Wagner, MD; Robert McNamara, MD; George Schwartz, MD; Mel Otten, MD; William Barsan, MD; Earl Siegel, PharmD; Richard Bukata, MD; Jerome Hoffman, MD; Dan Tandberg, MD; Dennis Price, MD; and Michael Greenberg, MD.

The author and publisher wish to thank Parke-Davis for an educational grant toward the production costs of this book.

J. R. R.

CONTENTS

PREFACE

In 1979, emergency medicine was still in its infancy, and Emergency Medicine News was a scarcely read newspaper circulated to a small cadre of interested physicians. I had been involved with the publication since its inception as a member of the editorial board under the direction of David Wagner, MD, but as Dave became immersed in the machinations of the board certification process, he reluctantly turned the editorial responsibilities over to me. Concurrently, Dr. Jerris Hedges, who had originally created the InFocus column, likewise found a plethora of other academic pursuits to fill his time, so I began writing the columns for what was to be only a few years.

Some 17 years later, I find myself still meeting last-minute deadlines and struggling to come up with ideas. I hope the topics are as interesting to the readers of the newspaper — now numbering about 23,000 — as they are to me.

Most of my ideas come from my clinical practice and interactions with ever-challenging residents, and most of my thoughts are merely repetitions of a more learned colleague's ideas or erudite hindsight based on my own many misstatements and clinical foibles. The column tries to put everyday emergency medicine practice into some usable form by espousing a common sense and practical approach that is based on experience but is at least somewhat supported by that literary morass we call the "medical literature." Because many of the columns have been well received by readers, Lippincott-Raven Publishers, under the leadership of Michael Randers-Pehrson and Lisa Hoffman, have consented to collate some of my favorite columns into a readable form.

J. R. R.

SECTION I

PUNCTURE WOUNDS

STEPPING ON A NAIL

Puncture wounds of the foot can have disastrous complications for patients and for physicians who are often sued for poor outcomes

Most people who step on a nail shrug it off as an unfortunate minor inconvenience or perhaps call their doctor to arrange a tetanus booster, and then think no more of it. Hardly a day goes by, however, that such a patient does not show up in the emergency department. Depending on which physician is on duty, the exact same patient may get either a 10-second exam and a few quick words of advice on home care or a rather invasive surgical debridement, radiographs, and antibiotics. There is, in essence, no standard of care for this entity.

In this discussion of this universal injury, I will focus on the emergency department treatment, morbidity, and a review of the sparse data that appear in the medical literature. One thing is crystal clear: stepping on a nail may result in significant, even disastrous, complications for the patient, and life-long disability and the need for amputation are well-documented. Because most emergency physicians do not routinely have long-term follow-up, most have no idea of the potential for such complications. Most emergency physicians also have no idea how often their colleagues get sued because of complications from stepping on a nail.

PUNCTURE WOUNDS OF THE FOOT

Fitzgerald RH, Cowan JDE

Orthopedic Clinics of North America 1975;6(4):965

This frequently quoted 20-year-old article is still one of the best reviews in the medical literature on the problem of puncture wounds of the foot. It appeared in a symposium on infectious diseases and orthopedics, but it contains vitally important information and timely advice for the emergency physician. The authors note that puncture wounds of the foot frequently have incomplete medical histories on the emergency department record and hastily performed or otherwise ineffective wound care. Discharge instructions are similarly poorly documented. Importantly, puncture wounds do have a rather high rate of serious complications (certainly higher than seen with lacerations), even when wound care is textbook-perfect with proper attention to every detail.

The authors present a retrospective review of 887 patients with puncture wounds to the feet, mostly children who stepped on a nail (98%) during the warm months (May to October). The majority of clinical histories recorded on the chart did not adequately address the location of the puncture, the depth of penetration, or information documenting the patient's footwear. Most patients were seen within 24 hours post-injury. Twenty-six patients (3%) demonstrated a retained foreign body at the puncture site, the majority being a small piece of tennis shoe or a fragment of sock. Other foreign bodies included rust, gravel, grass, straw, or specks of dirt. Of those 774 patients treated in the emergency department within 24 hours following the injury, 65 (8.4%) returned with cellulitis. Of those patients who waited one to seven days after injury to come to the hospital, 57 percent developed cellulitis or other localized soft tissue infections. Five patients with soft tissue infection who did not improve with antibiotics did improve after an unsuspected or previously missed foreign body was found and removed during surgical exploration.

> FOREIGN BODIES SUCH AS SHOE AND SOCK FRAGMENTS, GRAVEL, GRASS, AND RUST CAN CAUSE INFECTION IN PATIENTS WHO STEP ON NAILS

Many patients were given prophylactic antibiotics, usually penicillin or a semi-synthetic penicillin. Probably the most important point in this review is that osteomyelitis developed in the bones of the feet in 16 patients. The mean time interval between the puncture wound and the osteomyelitis diagnosis was 10 days, although one patient presented 16 months after the injury, having experienced intermittent drainage from the wound for 10 months. The location of the osteomyelitis included the os calcis (7), navicular (1), cuneiforms (1), and a metatarsal or phalanx (7). Of even greater interest is the fact that all 16 patients had received antibiotics for their puncture wounds prior to the development of osteomyelitis. *Pseudomonas* was isolated from 13 of 16 patients, making this organism the most common cause of osteomyelitis. Surgical debridement was required to cure the bony infection in all patients; none resolved with only the administration of antibiotics.

The authors stress that puncture wounds are often considered trivial injuries, but major complications can occur. The general infection rate quoted in the literature is five to 10 percent. *Pseudomonas* osteomyelitis has been noted previously and is the most serious well known complication in both children and adults who step on a nail. The authors stress that puncture wounds of the feet should be carefully cleaned with an antiseptic solution, and debrided and probed (no specific details given). Other standard post-operative instructions include elevation and a caution to return if symptoms persist. The authors note that under normal circumstances, there is little indication for the use

of antibiotics if patients are seen within 24 hours. Antibiotics are definitely indicated in patients who present with established infection. In this series, prophylactic antibiotics did not alter the subsequent infection rate.

Although cellulitis or other localized soft tissue infections are probably the most common infectious complications (usually secondary to staphylococcus) following puncture wounds, osteomyelitis is well known and the most feared sequela.

In summary, serious complications occurred in 29 of 887 patients (4%). *Pseudomonas* osteomyelitis was the most common serious complication, and it was uniformly refractory to medical management, requiring surgical intervention. The authors indicate that antibiotics are not routinely required following puncture wounds to the feet, but antibiotics should be given to patients who present with cellulitis or an established infection. An anti-staphylococcal drug is preferred for soft tissue infection, but the clinician should be aware of the possible development of *Pseudomonas* osteomyelitis.

PSEUDOMONAS ARTHRITIS FOLLOWING PUNCTURE WOUND OF THE FOOT

Chusid MJ, et al *Journal of Pediatrics* 1979;94(3):249

This is a report of four children who developed septic arthritis of the foot after stepping on a nail. Interestingly, all patients received oral antibiotics within 72 hours of the injury, but increasing pain and swelling of the foot noted one to two weeks later prompted hospital admission and investigation for osteomyelitis. Physical findings included swelling, erythema, and painful motion. Fever was never noted throughout the patient's course, and regional adenopathy did not develop. The diagnosis was not suggested by the CBC (normal leucocyte count and differential in all cases), but the sedimentation rate was abnormal (range 27 to 84 mm/hr) in all patients. The diagnosis was suggested by a widened joint space on plain radiographs in three, but a bone scan was required to confirm a joint infection in one child. No organisms were seen on gram stain of aspirated fluid, but cultures did yield *P. aeruginosa* in all cases. Blood cultures showed no growth. Surgical treatment consisted of joint aspiration, rather than operative debridement.

All patients were treated with a parenteral aminoglyco-side and a semi-synthetic penicillin. The average length of hospitalization was 22.5 days. The authors note that *Pseudomonas* is the most common etiology of osteomyelitis following puncture wounds of the feet. The specific differentiation between osteomyelitis and septic arthritis has not been made in most clinical reports because clinically the two cannot be distinguished. *P. aeruginosa* has an interesting propensity to infect cartilage, making the bones of young children particularly at risk. The authors suggest using diagnostic and therapeutic aspiration of the joint under fluoroscopic control, but not to withhold wider surgical treatment should conservative therapy be ineffective in a reasonable period of time.

Two of the four patients developed ankylosis of the infected joints, and one had persistent pain. It is speculated that initial antibiotics may have contributed to the development of the resistant organism or selected out *Pseudomonas*. Clearly, prophylactic antibiotics do not prevent this unusual complication.

COMMENT: During my review of this topic, I was amazed that I could not find a single prospective study addressing the ED treatment of this common entity. In essence, there is no standard of care, only suggested

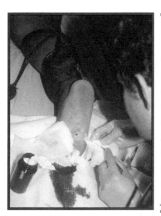

To examine a puncture wound of the foot properly, have the patient lie prone on a stretcher, get a good light and an ischemic tourniquet, and then set aside a few minutes. Examining the patient in a wheelchair in the hall is an amateur move that invites trouble. See color plate in center well.

approaches based on bias, retrospective observations, and unproved theories. This is not merely a controversial issue, it's a real dilemma for the clinician. I am amazed by the very poor science — or total lack thereof — that goes into dogmatic treatment protocols and review articles. One thing you can be sure of, however, is that some "expert" colleague will find fault with your care should the patient be unfortunate enough to develop complications from stepping on

HISTORICAL INFORMATION IN PATIENTS SUSTAINING A PLANTAR PUNCTURE WOUND

- *Type and condition of the penetrating object*
- *Footwear at the time of injury*
- *Location of puncture*
- *Estimated depth of puncture*
- *Possibility of a retained foreign body*
- *Elapsed time since injury*
- *Whether the injury occurred indoors or outdoors*
- *Significant past medical history (diabetes, peripheral vascular disease)*

Source: Emergency Medicine Clinics of North America, "Soft Tissue Emergencies," CD Chisholm and JM Howell, eds., W.B. Saunders Co., Philadelphia, Vol. 10, No. 4, November 1992.

a nail. Except for obvious screw-ups, I think most horrendous complications are the luck of the draw, and would occur no matter what initial therapy was prescribed.

Where most EPs drop the ball is failure to recognize a potential disaster brewing two to three weeks after the puncture. Patients present with persistent pain but otherwise look well. Therapy at this critical juncture is too often opting for a change in antibiotic or a different pain pill and a "few more days to see what happens."

Retrospective reviews of puncture wounds reveal a number of interesting facts that should be emphasized. Certainly, most individuals who step on a nail never experience a single problem afterward. Asymptomatic people do not usually come to the ED, so those with infections or other morbidity skew retrospective studies in favor of sicker patients and project a higher complication rate. The literature quotes an infection rate following stepping on a nail at approximately five to 10 percent, even when patients are treated within 24 hours. Generally, the most common complication is simple cellulitis or deeper soft tissue infection. Although these symptoms are bothersome, they are usually easily treated, with little long-term morbidity. The sparse available data indicate that a bone or joint infection occurs in up to two percent of patients post-puncture wound. It is impossible to make the distinction between deep soft tissue infection, abscess, septic arthritis, and osteomyelitis on clinical grounds. The actual distinction is not always necessary because complications and treatment are quite similar, although some authors suggest joint aspiration as the initial therapy for an infected joint. It is often stated that inadequate primary care is the main cause of late complications and that some specific regimen in the emergency department will magically lower the complication rate to near zero. This assumption has never been proven and, in fact, to my knowledge has never even been studied prospectively.

How then does one approach such patients? Obviously a reasonable history should be obtained, including tetanus prophylaxis status, underlying health, the circumstances of the wound, and a description of the offending object. Some historical facts can never be obtained, however. You should assume that the entire length of an exposed nail penetrated the foot; human reflexes are not quick enough to keep the entire weight of the body off a nail. If the nail has a half centimeter of exposed length, it won't hit the bone. If it protrudes four inches, you can be assured that it went in all the way and hit the bone. Wounds over the forefoot, especially the metatarsal heads, are at higher risk for complications. In this area, the joints can be punctured, tendons are vulnerable, and tough fibrous tissue can harbor a slow-growing infection. The table points out essential historical data to be obtained.

Every puncture has the potential to harbor a foreign body (FB), and retained material is the major cause of infectious trouble. What is clear is that a retained foreign body is commonplace; they're found in three to four percent of initial wounds and in many more infected wounds. Importantly, a FB will guarantee an infection. In my mind, every infected puncture wound or relapse of infection should be considered to contain a FB that must be found and removed if one expects a cure.

It is not uncommon to find pieces of rubber sneaker or material from socks within the puncture wound. No amount of even the most potent antibiotic will stave off an infection if foreign material is left in the wound. One study demonstrated that post-puncture wound infections that did not respond to intravenous antibiotics were associated with retained foreign material 60 percent of the time (*J Bone and Joint Surg* 1975;57A:535). Be careful, however, because you will not find a tiny piece of rubber sneaker or thread of sock if you bend

down and examine patients in the hallway who are sitting in a wheelchair. Patients should be placed prone on a stretcher, and the non-hurried clinician should examine the clean foot closely under a bright light in a relaxed environment. You won't find most FBs with an x-ray; it requires your eyes, some patience, and some effort. Deep FBs can rarely be found on probing or inspection, and they can even be missed at surgery. Fortunately most

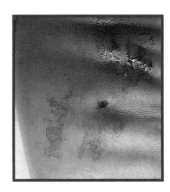

In this case, material from a sock was imbedded in a relatively superficial wound. The overlying skin was debrided, and the patient did well without antibiotics. See color plate in center well.

FBs can be confirmed with a CT/ultrasound/MRI, but you have to be smart enough to know that infection equals FB and to order these studies in a timely manner, hopefully before your antibiotics fail for the third or fourth time. Antibiotics may temporarily "cure" an infection if a foreign body is present, so if you see a relapse after initial success, a foreign body is likely.

Superficial soft tissue infections are obvious to anyone, usually occur during the first few days, and are usually from staphylococcus. They are easily cured with antibiotics and minimal debridement, and they don't recur unless there is a retained FB. Bone/joint infections are destructive processes that develop insidiously over weeks or months. They can look deceptively benign on external examination, and frequently appear normal on x-rays and laboratory values despite extensive involvement of bones, cartilage, or soft tissue. These infections are caused by *Pseudomonas* 90 percent of the time. Antibiotics alone will often not cure *Pseudomonas* osteomyelitis of the foot. Fungal bone infections have been reported (*J Trauma* 1976;16:993). The organisms found in infected puncture wounds come from a variety of sources. Bacteria may be on the penetrating nail itself, may be normal flora on the skin, or may be contained in an imbedded foreign body. Studies have demonstrated that *Pseudomonas* is not normal skin flora in healthy people (*J Pediatr* 1977;1:161). One investigator demonstrated positive *Pseudomonas* cultures in biopsies taken from the soles of sneakers in five of six children with proven

Pseudomonas osteomyelitis (*J Ped* 1985;106:607). This suggests that *Pseudomonas* may be normal flora in the soles of rubber shoes. The growth of this organism can be fostered by the warm, moist, and dark environment that occurs in all children's sneakers, particularly during the summer months. I know of no other situation where *Pseudomonas* is so frequently associated with bone infections.

It's difficult to convince a patient (or a jury) that antibiotics at the time of puncture will not prevent an infection. The literature is quite clear that prophylactic antibiotics have no magic to prevent infection following puncture, and their routine use is usually discouraged. Broad-spectrum antibiotics may be harmful if they select out resistant organisms (*Ped* 1971;47:598) and many patients with disastrous complications have been immediately treated with very potent antibiotics. Much has been promulgated about the use of ciprofloxacin as prophylaxis against *Pseudomonas* osteomyelitis. Many EPs now prescribe it routinely on the first visit. Again, there are absolutely no data supporting its use, either prophylactically or therapeutically for acute osteomyelitis. In the report of Miron et al (*Isr J Med Sci* 1993; 29:194), three children who had been treated with surgical incision plus intravenous anti-pseudomonal agents developed *Pseudomonas* osteochondritis. They all required extensive surgical debridement to be cured, so even parenteral anti-pseudomonal antibiotics have their limitations.

I could find no data that delineate criteria for ordering an x-ray. Some physicians order x-rays on every puncture wound while some never do. Because much foreign material is radiolucent, a normal x-ray does not invariably rule out a foreign body. A small fracture could be detected. If the patient presents with an infection or cannot describe the puncturing object, I will get an x-ray (but in 20 years of practice I have yet to find it of any value, not even a single case!) Importantly, don't expect a plain film to help you diagnose early osteomyelitis or a wooden FB.

Authors are quick to emphasize that initial wound care should be complete, but few describe exact proper therapy in detail, particularly how aggressive one needs to be with debridement or irrigation. Most authors state that

you should determine the depth of penetration because therapy often depends on how far into the foot the nail protruded. I know of no accurate way to determine the depth of a puncture by physical exam, and except for selected cases, you are usually guessing. Basing invasive therapy on a guess never made sense to me.

It is important to realize that a puncture wound cannot realistically be irrigated because the puncture tract and skin immediately close the wound. Likewise, a puncture wound cannot be probed in order to gain any useful information unless it is surgically widened. You can examine (or probe) the entrance wound, but you can't deeply probe a puncture tract. Therefore, textbooks or articles that say "irrigate and probe the wound" and leave it at that are a cop-out; such statements are not helpful to the clinician. To my thinking, forcing saline under pressure into a closed puncture tract will not irrigate anything, but will only further disperse contamination and foreign matter.

Some authors recommend routinely excising a small plug of tissue at the puncture site, thereby facilitating irrigation and probing. Whether this should be done for all puncture wounds or only those visibly contaminated is unclear, and there is little consensus in the literature to clear

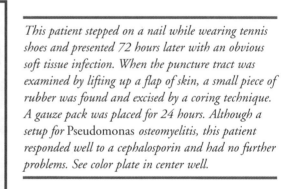

This patient stepped on a nail while wearing tennis shoes and presented 72 hours later with an obvious soft tissue infection. When the puncture tract was examined by lifting up a flap of skin, a small piece of rubber was found and excised by a coring technique. A gauze pack was placed for 24 hours. Although a setup for Pseudomonas *osteomyelitis, this patient responded well to a cephalosporin and had no further problems. See color plate in center well.*

up the controversy. Excising tissue clearly increases discomfort and disability, and in order to be completely effective, the entire tract must be removed, so excising a core of a few millimeters deep seems to make little sense, unless the excision is actual debridement of visible foreign matter. Tissue coring is a procedure that has never been shown to reduce the incidence of serious sequelae, even though some staunchly support it. Excising a plug may alter superficial post-puncture cellulitis, but it can hardly be expected to prevent bone infection. Most authors confuse routine tissue coring with removing a superficial plug of tissue that harbors foreign material.

Krych and Lavery (*Clin Pod Med and Surg* 1990; 7(4):725) recommend a surgical treatment protocol based on a scoring system that has never been tested or validated, and it's a bit unrealistic. If the wound is necrotic, has obvious foreign matter, an x-ray shows a fracture, or the puncture is through the dermis, they recommend excision of the puncture tract, exploration, copious lavage, aerobic and anaerobic cultures, a drain, and immobilization.

Antibiotics against staph/strep are considered at 72 hours, but not prophylactically. The podiatry literature seems very aggressive with this coring prophylactic technique (see also *J Foot Surg* 1990;29:147), but to my analysis, the procedure is based purely on theory and likely puts a lot of big holes in a lot of feet needlessly. I have tried to follow puncture tracts into soft tissue to no avail, and taking a culture of a fresh wound seems ridiculous.

Stepping on a Nail: Some Rational Guidelines

Emergency physicians are often sued because of complications following puncture wounds, and then find themselves frustrated by contradictions in the literature

In the previous chapter, I described the clinical issues involved in the evaluation and treatment of patients who step on a nail. I emphasized that there are no prospective scientific data comparing initial treatment protocols, and even though some authors steadfastly adhere to their own dogmatic treatment plans, we don't know what's best to do. In essence, there is no standard of care, and recommendations range from benign neglect to attacking the sole of the foot with scalpels and drains. What we do know, however, is that a small percentage of unfortunate patients will develop disastrous complications from a puncture wound of the foot. Bones and tissue can be lost, and pain and disability can be chronic. Emergency physicians can easily wind up in court trying to defend their actions and be frustrated by controversy and contradictions in the literature, and the emotional yet nonsensical ramblings of a plaintiff's expert.

Aside from common sense rules, the initial therapy of a puncture wound probably does little to change the ultimate course, and one can find "experts" to support almost anything. However, if pain and swelling persist for a few weeks to months, a whole new set of guidelines are needed that consider retained foreign bodies (FBs) and smoldering osteomyelitis. Above all, clinicians must realize that puncture wounds of the foot are a disaster waiting to happen. The prudent clinician will approach even the most benign-appearing puncture wound with great respect and a great appreciation for Murphy's Law. The wise doctor will spend a little extra time and effort educating patients and documenting the chart. Now I will review some strategies for avoiding lawsuits in the management of puncture wounds of the foot, and will offer what I believe is a rational approach (although as unproven as any other) to patients who hobble into your emergency department.

Watch Your Step: Avoiding Lawsuits for Management of Plantar Puncture Wound

Gonzalez S, et al *Emergency Legal Briefings* 1993;4(12)

I came across this informative medical/legal brochure while preparing this column, and I review it here because it emphasizes some salient points. The authors (two attorneys and one physician/attorney) discuss four scenarios that pitted physician against patient in medical malpractice cases because of complications from stepping on a nail. This series is published by American Health Consultants, Inc.

In this classic example of how to get sued, a man stepped on an anchor bolt and suffered a puncture wound through the rubber sole of his shoe. The wound was cleaned and bandaged but not probed or debrided. The chart contained an incomplete history and sketchy physical exam. A plain x-ray was taken and showed no foreign body. Over the next month, the patient had inflammation and infection and underwent an amputation of his fourth metatarsal because of osteomyelitis. No foreign body was found during the initial surgical debridement, but because of a recurrent infection, a second operation was required, and at this time a fragment of rubber was identified and removed from the wound. In this case a foreign body was missed by three emergency physicians and one surgeon. The patient sued and claimed the physicians failed to detect and remove a foreign body, and it was this foreign body that caused chronic infection, bone loss, and significant wound morbidity. Interestingly, the wife also sued for loss of consortium (love, sex, companionship, comfort, solace). The emergency physicians lost the case, but the first surgeon who missed the foreign body (FB) was not found negligent. (Figure that one out!)

This case raises one major important point: infection, especially a recurrent or delayed one, means FB until proven otherwise. It is extremely easy to miss a foreign body, and such a mistake is a common occurrence in malpractice cases involving disasters from wound infections. Rubber, plastic, aluminum, and wood do not show on a plain radiograph, and the only way to find these objects is to inspect the wound carefully or use ultrasound/CT/MRI. In this case, a puncture through a rubber shoe is a red flag that mandates a careful search for a FB. Unfortunately, puncture wounds can rarely be fully explored unless you create an unacceptable surgical incision. Kneeling down to examine the bottom of the foot while the patient is still in the wheelchair is definitely not the way to look for a FB. Wound evaluation must be done with the patient lying prone, with a good light, and enough time to examine the area adequately. Once the patient returns with an infection, I have a firm rule: Unless proven otherwise, there is a foreign body causing the infection, and it's my job to find it. I'm right most of the time. Retained foreign bodies are every physician's nightmare, and they pay the mortgage on that summer home for many malpractice lawyers.

Finally, this case was treated by more than one EP on the initial visit, probably a casualty of the change of shift where both physicians wrongly assumed that the other had paid attention to the details. A mandatory wound check at 48-72 hours would have probably caught this case in time to prevent a disaster. Having different emergency physicians provide follow-up is another way to delay more definitve therapy. These wounds often appear benign or minimally infected so the natural inclination for the first-time evaluator is to "wait a bit longer" or make a useless change in antibiotics, pain medication, or local care.

The next case discusses a 60-year-old man who stepped on a nail, and did not receive a tetanus shot in the ED, despite the physician knowing of the lack of prior tetanus immunization. A short five days after the puncture wound, the patient developed tetanus and subsequently died. The physician obviously lost this case. Tetanus immune globulin should be given in addition to the vaccine if tetanus prophylaxis is in question. We give so many tetanus shots needlessly, it's almost unheard of for any patient to get out of the ED without too many tetanus shots. You will probably never see a case of tetanus in your career, but this disease is still around and totally preventable. This is a case of bad luck and of overlooking a small but obviously important detail. Even my 12-year-old knows you get a tetanus shot when you step on a nail!

Another classic case involved a 38-year-old man who stepped on a nail while wearing a rubber soled boot and presented with a seemingly benign puncture wound. An x-ray was negative, and the patient received a tetanus shot, ceftriaxone and a cephalexin prescription, and Tylenol Codeine No. 3. He was advised to elevate the foot and to see his doctor "if he got worse." Five days later, the patient was seen by an orthopedic surgeon and was admitted for the treatment of a deep foot abscess. He ultimately developed *Pseudomonas* osteomyelitis and claimed partial disability for life.

This patient claimed that he should have been treated with ciprofloxacin because *Pseudomonas* was cultured at surgery. The plaintiff also claimed that the wound was not probed to determine its depth nor irrigated or debrided. Had this been done, the possibility of infection and subsequent osteomyelitis would have been reduced. The physician claimed that the minor nature of the small puncture wound negated extensive initial surgical therapy. The physician also failed to document the size of the penetrating foreign body. An expert witness was produced who testified that the standard of care required debridement of the wound, probing of the wound to look for contamination, and irrigation to guard against infection.

The emergency physician's attorney argued that this was not a high-risk wound because there was no necrotic or devitalized tissue, that ciprofloxacin was not standard of care, and that it was the patient's fault because he did not follow up when signs of infection were evident. The plaintiff stated that he did not understand the need for follow-up. The chart's instructions for follow-up were vague. The jury found for the EP in this particular case, and said the patient was negligent for not contacting his family doctor when infection was obvious. The jury was able to be convinced, but the authors note that a different outcome could easily have occurred with a different jury. (This EP lucked out.)

In the final case, a 30-year-old man presented for treatment of a puncture wound of the foot. The wound was cleaned, a tetanus shot administered, and no antibiotics were prescribed. Follow-up instructions were vague. An abscess formed in this case, and the physician was unable to convince the jury about the lack of benefit of prophylactic antibiotics and the uselessness of cultures at the time of injury. The authors of this article stress that the decision not to administer antibiotics should be documented because nearly all cases of liability associated with puncture wounds involve infection. The authors stressed the need for specific and detailed discharge instructions with a specific follow-up examination scheduled. "As needed" follow-up is generally not sufficient because it is well known that patients have difficulty separating infection from the normal healing process. They may stay at home while a significant infection is brewing, yet they consider this pain and swelling to be normal healing. In essence, patients cannot be relied upon to diagnose their own wound infections even if they have printed or verbal instructions so a definite follow-up visit should be arranged.

The authors admit that punctures to the foot present a difficult problem for emergency physicians, and they also point out that there are no good scientific studies to guide the practitioner. As with any malpractice case, maintaining a good rapport with the patient and providing an adequate explanation goes a long way in preventing a lawsuit. Basics should be attended to: An adequate history and physical are essential, and documentation should be complete. In complicated or infected wounds, especially in high-risk patients, follow-up should be routine, specifically mandated and documented, and not left to the patients discretion.

Reading an article such as this is a frustrating and maddening endeavor. Because there is no consensus on how to treat a puncture wound, it seems unfair to be sued for a conservative approach. Clearly the facts mean little, and

your defense and outcome is based mainly on the finesse of the lawyers and expert witnesses. Just try to convince a jury that some off-the-wall, totally unproven treatment protocol that appears in a medical journal is garbage; it's a hard sell. If you have not read articles such as this, if you have not been an expert witness, or you have not been personally sued, you'll have a hard time understanding the issues. The bottom line is this: Be very careful with patients with puncture wounds of the feet. Pay attention to the details. I cannot overemphasize the potential for disastrous complications, but with a little bit of knowledge and common sense, both you and your patient should fair well.

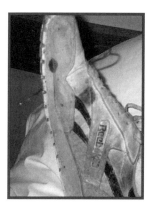

This patient stepped on a wire while wearing sneakers. Despite aggressive coring, a drain, and anti-staphylococcal antibiotics, he developed a deep soft tissue infection that required prolonged IV antibiotics. Long-term sequelae did not occur, but pseudomonal osteomyelitis, especially in this high-risk area of the foot, is a potential complication. See color plate in center well.

SUMMARY: To guide the clinician through the puncture wound morass, I have constructed a guide to therapy that seems reasonable based on my analysis of the literature. It is vitally important to make a distinction between initial therapy and caring for patients who present late.

1. Take an adequate history. Determine whether the offending nail was actually seen or examined by the patient and if the nail remained intact. It is not uncommon for a long nail to puncture the foot deep enough to inoculate bone. Some patients can give you a hint about length of the nail or depth of penetration, but it's often a guess. If the patient unequivocally states that the nail was intact, note this on the chart. If the patient cannot tell you what the object was or if he recognizes that the nail may have broken, radiographs are prudent. Always assume that the entire length of the nail penetrated the foot. Be especially wary of punctures in the area of the metatarsal heads, a high-risk area.

2. Take time to examine the patient. This does not mean bending down for a quick look at a foot after it's taken out

of a basin of Betadine. The only way to examine a puncture wound on the bottom of the foot properly is to have the patient lie on a stretcher, get a bright light, clean the skin, and carefully examine the puncture site. You will be surprised how often a little thread of material or a piece of rubber is seen poking out from under the surface. If there is a flap of skin over the puncture, lift it up with a needle and trim it away to visualize the tract opening.

3. Test neurological function distally (looking for digital nerve injury) and have the patient actively flex and

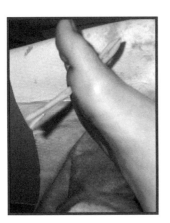

When treating a through-and-through puncture wound, it is difficult to get adequate debridement or irrigation. An option is to place a small Penrose drain through the puncture track. It should be left in place for only 24-36 hours. See color plate in center well.

extend the toes. Nerve injury or pain on toe flexion/extension indicates that the deeper structures (e.g., tendons and ligaments) may have been violated. Likewise, passive extension of the toes should not cause pain over the puncture site unless deep structures have been injured.

4. I do not always routinely order x-rays on every patient who steps on a nail, but I do get plain films frequently. If the patient stepped on a clean short new nail in the basement and it's still intact, x-rays are excessive. If the injury occurred while running through a field and the offending object is not located, an x-ray should be obtained. Note that many foreign bodies are radiolucent, and you won't see plastic, rubber, cloth, or wood. Specific criteria for ordering x-rays and their positive yield have not been studied.

5. It is axiomatic that puncture wounds cannot be cleaned and attempting to irrigate a tract is ridiculous. You should evaluate the opening of the tract for visible foreign matter, but probing a closed puncture tract yields nothing except a false sense of security. If you probe the wound, you should do so via a generous incision over the puncture site.

6. My approach to surgical treatment has changed over the past few years, precipitated partly because of my review of the literature and partly because of medicolegal con-

cerns. As previously mentioned, many textbooks stress the need for aggressive initial treatment, but that is based only on theory. There are no data to prove that (beyond removing obvious foreign matter) invasive procedures alter subsequent morbidity. Under proper light and with a blood pressure cuff around the calf to stop arterial flow, I will tease away the skin edges of the puncture wound (unroof it) with a needle or iris scissors and pull the wound apart to inspect the tract visually. (Any surgeon will agree that you cannot adequately assess soft tissue unless the field is bloodless, so the ischemic tourniquet is an absolute requirement.) If the wound opening contains no foreign body, it's locally irrigated and a dressing is applied, and no further cutting is done. If you see distinct foreign material at the site or if you are concerned about deep contamination (often a gut feeling or wild guess), anesthetize the skin with 1% lidocaine (this hurts!) and excise a 3 mm plug of skin with a number 11 blade. I have no firm rules about how deep to go; each case is different and based on findings as you progress. A nerve block of the foot can be done if you are adept, but I always have trouble getting complete anesthesia. After spreading the puncture track with a hemostat looking for a foreign body, I will try to irrigate the track, being well aware that it is often only a gesture at best. A small piece of gauze can be inserted as a drain to be removed in 24 hours. This is a two-person procedure, where an assistant irrigates the wound while I spread it open. Don't irrigate the wound unless the fluid will flow out!

I do not stick the irrigating catheter in the depths of the puncture track itself because this generally creates a false passage, ballooning up the tissue and disseminating the infected material throughout the foot. I do not excise deep tissue unless there is some extenuating circumstance.

7. My follow-up care includes non-weight-bearing for a day (partly due to my invasiveness) with elevation, soaking two to three times a day in hot water, and firm instructions for any patient who had debridement to return for follow-up in 48 hours. An "as needed" follow-up is acceptable in diabetics, those with a removed FB, or for those with any sign of infection. If a plug of tissue was removed or a drain placed, a 48-hour follow-up is mandatory.

I specifically address the topic of delayed osteomyelitis with patients and inform them that if, after two to three weeks postinjury they have continued aching or discomfort in the foot, they must seek medical attention, armed with the history of having a previous puncture wound. They should be told of the possibility of osteomyelitis.

8. I do not routinely prescribe antibiotics. For the diabetic or immunocompromised host, I will consider a cephalosporin for three to four days. Remember that antibiotics can delay or mask serious infection and can potentially select out resistant strains. There are no data to suggest that prophylactic ciprofloxacin is effective in preventing *Pseudomonas* infections, and the literature contains examples where IV antipseudomonal antibiotics failed to prevent osteomyelitis.

1. This is an instance where the emergency physician can easily get into trouble. If the patient presents with an obvious soft tissue infection following a puncture wound, I would assume a foreign body and definitely do an x-ray, some debridement, and treat with an antistaphylococcal antibiotic. Always weigh outpatient vs. inpatient therapy. If this is a simple soft tissue infection, it should respond immediately and not recur. Diabetics, the immunocompromised, or those with peripheral vascular disease should usually be admitted unless infection is miniscule. If infection does not respond in 24-48 hours, admission is certainly mandated. If a patient presents three to four weeks post-injury with pain or swelling of the foot or a recurrence of an obvious infection that initially responded,

assume a deep infection and proceed carefully. Don't blow this off as a benign inflammatory process; it's probably a retained FB or osteomyelitis.

At this juncture, I usually order a plain x-ray, a CBC, and a sedimentation rate, but my decision to pursue osteomyelitis or a FB is rarely altered by the results. Consider a bone scan or MRI within the next few days, and get the patient to a surgeon! It is a common pitfall (and may be disastrous) to treat such patients conservatively for weeks while an osteomyelitis is smoldering. Most early cases of osteomyelitis have a normal x-ray and normal CBC. Remember, feet with early osteomyelitis look deceivingly benign.

2. It is paramount that the above procedures and discharge instructions be well-documented on the chart. Clearly document your thinking about x-rays, antibiotics, and surgical care.

3. When I asked my colleagues to name the most common serious infection postpuncture wound, few had ever heard of *Pseudomonas* osteomyelitis. (This question will be on your board examination.) Probably the most serious pitfall in dealing with a puncture wound is the failure to appreciate the significance or serious potential of persistent pain in the foot two to four weeks post stepping on a nail.

For an excellent overview of controversies and treatment recommendations, see Chisholm and Schlesser, Ann Emerg Med 1989;18:1352-1357, and Chudnofsky and Sebastian, *Emerg Med Clin North Am* 1992;10(4):801-822.

SECTION II

ACETAMINOPHEN TOXICITY

THE FINER POINTS OF ACETAMINOPHEN TOXICITY

The use of acetaminophen by those with active alcoholic liver disease may be harmful, even in therapeutic doses

The evaluation and treatment of patients with intentional acetaminophen (APAP) ingestion is second nature to most emergency physicians. Diagnostic and therapeutic protocols have been refined to the point where there is little controversy concerning the approach to the routine overdose. Some overdoses, however, tend to be obscure, unknown, unintentional — even fatal — so significant APAP toxicity can occasionally be missed, misdiagnosed, or ignored completely. Because acetaminophen is widely available over the counter, and it is frequently combined with a variety of analgesics and muscle relaxants, EPs should be cognizant of uncommon or unusual presentations and toxicities. The ED is the ideal place to raise the issue of APAP toxicity. Because even a massive APAP overdose can be asymptomatic for 24 hours, it is possible for significant hepatic and failure to develop insidiously on the second or third hospital day because the patient was admitted for another reason and APAP toxicity was not addressed in the ED. This chapter will begin a series of discussions on some of the finer points of acetaminophen toxicity that are uncommon but should be familiar to all clinicians. My first discussion will focus on those specific instances in which acetaminophen may be harmful in therapeutic doses, with serum levels significantly lower than those identified as toxic by the standard treatment nomogram. Of major concern is the use of APAP by individuals with active alcoholic liver disease.

ACETAMINOPHEN HEPATOTOXICITY IN ALCOHOLICS: A THERAPEUTIC MISADVENTURE

Seeff LB, et al *Ann Intern Med* 1986;104(3):399

This informative article is a report of six chronic alcoholics who developed severe hepatotoxicity from the therapeutic (nonsuicidal) use of relatively moderate doses of acetaminophen. It also reviews 19 additional cases that were reported in the literature as of 1986. The authors note that APAP is commonly prescribed to patients who are subject to gastritis because this compound lacks the gastric mucosal irritation seen with aspirin and nonsteroidal, anti-inflammatory drugs (NSAIDs). A subgroup of patients who would be prime candidates to use APAP as an analgesic are alcoholics. Although APAP is generally safe, patients with active liver disease may be at increased risk for potentially lethal side effects from therapeutic doses that are well tolerated by the general population. Because acetaminophen is such a popular analgesic and because alcoholism is so ubiquitous, a largely unappreciated therapeutic misadventure may be more common than previously expected.

The authors describe in detail the cases of six patients who experienced a relatively similar phenomenon. All patients were chronic alcoholics who developed minor painful conditions, such as headache, toothache, or muscle trauma, for which they took acetaminophen as an analgesic. They ingested APAP over a few days to weeks, and did not take the drug to harm themselves intentionally. The magnitude of the APAP use was 2-6 grams per day. Patients became symptomatic but were initially suspected of having a worsening of their alcoholic liver disease. The association of the clinical deterioration with APAP was made when the history of APAP use was uncovered and laboratory testing was inconsistent with alcohol-induced hepatic dysfunction. Other causes of hepatotoxicity, such as viral hepatitis, were ruled out. Some cases were complicated by hepatic encephalopathy and ascites, coagulation problems, and renal failure.

The authors also comment on 19 other patients whose case histories were reported in the literature. In each case, the scenario was similar. Patients were chronic alcoholics who had a decompensation, were admitted to the hospital, and were initially thought to have an exacerbation of alcoholic liver disease. The laboratory evaluation of hepatic injury was not consistent with the profile generally seen with ethanol-induced liver disease. Although all patients in this report survived, the literature review identified a mortality rate in similar cases of about 20 percent.

Although the amount of acetaminophen ingested is generally difficult to calculate with certainty, in each case hepatotoxicity developed following the use of near-therapeutic doses. Importantly, acetaminophen use was frequently not identified at the time of admission, and APAP levels were rarely ordered. In almost every case, the drug was used as an analgesic. Gastrointestinal complaints, such as nausea and vomiting and abdominal pain, were common upon admission. Almost all patients were jaundiced, had tender or nontender hepatomegaly, and manifested other stigmata of chronic liver disease.

Biochemical abnormalities included severe hypo-

DIFFERENTIATING HEPATOTOXICITY

Finding	Alcoholic with APAP Insult to Liver	Recent Suicide Ingestions of APAP	Alcoholic Hepatitis
AST (SGOT)	• Markedly increased (greater than 500IU/L) • Usually greater than twice ALT level	Initially normal, then markedly increased in 36+ hours	• Slightly to moderatel elevated, usually less than 300-400 IU/ml • Usually greater than twice ALT level
ALT (SGPT)	Increased, but less than AST	Initially normal, then markedly increased in 36+ hours	• Slight to moderate increase
Prothrombin Time	Increased, more than 20-30 seconds	Initially normal, then markedly increased in 36+ hours	Slight to moderate increase, usually less than 20 seconds
APAP Serum	Therapeutic to moderately elevated • May be absent if remote use	Increased, toxic level determined from nomogram	Negative
History	Therapeutic use of APAP, 3-10 grams/day	Large ingestion, toxic greater than 150 mg/kg (10g)	Not used

Source: Arch Intern Med 1991;151:1189.

glycemia, markedly prolonged prothrombin time, elevated AST/SGOT and ALT/SGPT levels and metabolic acidosis. In all instances the ALT/SGPT values were lower than corresponding AST/SGOT values. Bilirubin levels were also elevated, sometimes markedly. The treatment consisted of general supportive care, vitamin K, fresh frozen plasma, and correction of hypoglycemia, dehydration, and electrolyte abnormalities. Importantly, *N*-acetylcysteine (NAC) was administered to only three patients, presumably because the diagnosis was delayed.

The authors specifically comment on the extreme elevation of AST/SGOT values and note that these high levels, ranging from 1960 to 30,000 IU/L, are not consistent with the diagnosis of alcoholic hepatitis. AST/SGOT values rarely exceed 300 IU/L when alcohol is the only hepatic toxin involved. In addition, the aminotransferase values declined rapidly, and often within two to three days they were within the normal or slightly elevated range. Although it is possible that some cases were complicated by concurrent acute viral hepatitis, serological tests were not confirmatory when they were ordered.

The exact reason for toxicity from such small doses of acetaminophen is unknown, but the authors cite the mechanism that is commonly attributed to this process, the potentiation of acetaminophen hepatotoxicity by ethanol. The authors concluded by cautioning physicians to educate alcoholics about the potential dangers of even therapeutic doses of acetaminophen in the setting of active liver disease. They advise including specific questioning about the use of acetaminophen in patients thought to have symptoms only of alcoholic liver disease.

COMMENT: The potential for therapeutic doses of APAP to produce significant liver toxicity in alcoholics has been known for many years. The condition is largely unappreciated but potentially lethal. When evaluating chronic alcoholics who present with decompensation, vague GI symptoms, and increasing hepatic dysfunction, most clinicians would automatically indict ethanol and not consider APAP as the culprit. I suspect many cases are subclinical or are admitted to the hospital and resolve with supportive care, and an analgesic etiology is never even considered. Even if the compulsive internist considers the diagnosis on the second or third hospital day when the biochemical profile is confusing, one way to confirm the

diagnosis has been lost if the emergency physician had not ordered an APAP level upon admission.

Having seen two fatal cases of hepatotoxicity secondary to clandestine acetaminophen use in alcoholics (one intentional and the other probably accidental), I have been ordering APAP levels routinely on almost any patient admitted with liver disease.

The ultimate diagnosis is largely a clinical one. It is difficult to make a definitive diagnosis because the APAP level following chronic or repeated ingestion is of little diagnostic significance and difficult to interpret. If the drug had been stopped a few days earlier, levels may be entirely negative. Liver injury does not occur for a few days following an acute single overdose and patients may be well on their way to hepatic necrosis when the APAP level is undetectable, therapeutic, or deceivingly low. With chronic ingestion, serum levels seem inconsequential to the uninitiated clinician.

The critical issue is that even moderate doses of acetaminophen, known to be safe in other patients, have been implicated as a potent toxin in patients with active liver disease. Patients reported in the literature have ingested only a few grams per day, and both physician and patient may not consider this to be excessive. Although acetaminophen use should always be included in the history, patients may not consider this a true drug and physicians may not respect its potential toxicity even if the patient mentions it.

Patients in these reports ingested the equivalent of only 10-12 regular strength or 6-8 extra strength acetaminophen pills per day, well within the guidelines listed on the bottle. Patients with a severe backache, toothache, or headache, especially if their judgment is somewhat clouded by alcohol use or encephalopathy, can quickly reach excessive levels of use and not give it a second thought.

The APAP level is of only minimal diagnostic significance, but the liver profile is the best tip-off for this retrospective diagnosis. Alcohol, viral hepatitis, and APAP toxicity can all raise hepatic enzymes, prolong prothrombin time, and induce hyperbilirubinemia. Severe liver disease of any type can cause hypoglycemia and a metabolic acidosis so these abnormalities are nonspecific. Emergency physicians are not called upon to interpret liver enzymes on a daily basis, even if they are ordered in the ED.

I suspect that most of us would attribute the findings

> PATIENTS ON ISONIAZID FOR TB MAY SUFFER SIGNIFICANT HEPATOTOXICITY WITH EVEN MODERATE DOSES OF APAP

commonly seen with occult acetaminophen overdose to viral hepatitis or alcoholic liver disease. ALT/SGPT is found primarily in the liver, but AST/SGOT is present in many tissues, including the heart, muscles, and kidney. These enzymes are elevated to some extent in almost any liver pathology with acute hepatocellular injury, but the highest levels are found in conditions that cause acute and

DRUGS THAT CAN INDUCE P450 MIXED FUNCTION OXIDASE SYSTEM

Anticonvulsants	TB Drugs	Other
Phenobarbital	Isoniazid	Ethanol
Phenytoin	Rifampicin	
Carbamazepine		
Primidone		

Source: James R. Roberts, MD

extensive hepatic necrosis, the most common being severe viral hepatitis, toxin-induced liver disease, or prolonged cardiovascular collapse (shock liver).

The absolute level of the enzymes correlates poorly with the severity of liver injury or its prognosis, but it is important to note that isolated alcoholic hepatitis generally produces only modest increases in transaminases. Should the liver enzymes be reported while the patient is still in the ED and the AST/SGOT and ALT/SGPT exceed the 400-500 IU/L range, a toxin other than alcohol should be considered. There are few things other than APAP that give you an AST/SGOT of 10,000. Both enzymes usually parallel each other, but it has been noted that with alcohol or toxin-induced hepatic necrosis, the AST:ALT ratio is usually greater than 2. Bilirubin levels are not specific. Alcoholics can bump their prothrombin time to the 16-20 second range, but usually not much higher. It would not be common for alcohol-induced liver injury to produce prothrombin times in the 60-80 second range, but this would be a common finding in APAP-induced hepatic necrosis.

Kumar et al (*Arch Intern Med* 1991;151:1189) recently emphasized how easy it is to miss APAP hepatotoxicity in chronic alcoholics. They identified six patients in a two-year period who had marked elevations of aminotransferases and a markedly prolonged prothrombin time, where an exacerbation of alcohol-induced hepatotoxicity was initially diagnosed. The correct diagnosis was missed by the attending internist and house staff until a consultant suggested APAP as the etiology. All patients had been taking acetaminophen for therapeutic reasons. The diagnosis was missed because of failure to ask about APAP use, inappropriate reliance on APAP levels, and lack of knowledge to interpret properly liver enzyme elevations in alcoholic disease vs. toxic hepatitis. Interestingly, even when an APAP level was drawn on admission, it was dismissed as unimportant because levels were in the therapeutic range. These authors also comment that AST/SGOT elevations greater than 1000 IU/L and prothrombin times greater than 20-25 seconds are not usually seen with alcoholic hepatitis, so finding these laboratory values in the alcoholic should immediately suggest APAP toxicity.

The mechanism thought to explain the phenomenon of APAP-induced hepatic necrosis in the alcoholic is well accepted, and can be used to understand why minor doses of APAP further injure the alcoholic's liver. About 90 percent of APAP is conjugated in the liver, producing benign substances (glucuronide or sulfate conjugates) that are excreted in the kidney. About 10 percent of APAP is metabolized by the cytochrome mixed function oxidase pathway (P-450 system) in the liver to produce a reactive intermediate metabolite called NAPQI. This toxic substance is rendered nontoxic when it is conjugated with glutathione, a substance normally found in abundance in healthy livers.

In a massive overdose, excessive acetaminophen metabolites overwhelm the protection offered by glutathione in the healthy liver, and excess NAPQI causes hepatic necrosis. The problem with alcoholics is twofold. First, the P-450 system is enhanced or induced by chronic alcohol ingestion, and the production of the toxic metabolite is accelerated. In addition, alcoholics tend to be depleted of the normally protective glutathione. The combination of the revved-up production of a toxic metabolite and the decreased ability to detoxify the toxin provides a mechanism by which even minor (especially repeated) doses of acetaminophen can destroy an already compromised liver.

The implications of this phenomenon in the ED are unclear. From a diagnostic standpoint, it seems reasonable to question carefully all alcoholics who present to the ED with complaints of pain requiring analgesics or with evidence of liver failure about their acetaminophen use.

Those with active hepatitis should be carefully advised about APAP use. Those with deterioration should be evaluated for APAP toxicity even if the drug was used therapeutically. Because the quantitative APAP serum test is relatively inexpensive and straightforward, patients with liver dysfunction should have an acetaminophen level sent routinely. The problems of interpreting this level have been mentioned. Obviously, LFTs, prothrombin times, and bilirubin levels should be evaluated as soon as possible.

In my mind, any alcoholic who has liver dysfunction and any level of acetaminophen whatsoever in the blood should be considered a candidate for NAC therapy. NAC should be administered as soon as possible. If the biochemical picture and historical data are consistent with APAP toxicity. The theory is that there is still more toxic metabolite to be made from circulating APAP. It's not clear, however, if NAC would be helpful in this circumstance, and the best treatment regimen is unknown. Undoubtedly, many patients who come to the ED in poor shape are past the time when NAC would be protective. Most would empirically still treat such patients with the standard protocol for an acute ingestion. If APAP has been taken chronically, but the serum level is not detectable, the use of NAC is even more confusing. I personally would administer the standard protocol anyway.

There are some data suggesting a role for NAC for the treatment of hepatic failure even if APAP is no longer present. Another difficult question arises when one deals with alcoholics who deliberately overdose on acetaminophen with a single ingestion. Some toxicologists have recommended lowering the nomogram treatment levels to approximately 50 percent of those used as the threshold for treating patients without preexisting liver disease. This issue has not been studied with any rigor and the implications of the nomogram for making therapeutic decisions on patients with active liver disease is unsettled. To my thinking, it appears reasonable to use NAC therapy liberally in the presence of acute liver disease and current acetaminophen overdose, but it's anyone guess what the threshold for therapy should be. Finally, it seems logical to extend these thoughts to patients with active viral hepatitis, but I could find no data on this.

It is difficult to make firm recommendations on the therapeutic use of APAP in the face of alcoholic liver disease. Acetaminophen is probably the safest analgesic to use under these circumstances. Alcoholics, and probably any other patient with acute liver inflammation (such as viral hepatitis), should be cautioned about excessive APAP use.

Exactly how much APAP is "too much," is unclear. Those with chronic stable liver disease, such as cirrhosis, have been shown to tolerate up to 4 grams of APAP daily for five days without any problems. Most of the morbidity and mortality associated with APAP seem to be in those patients with active hepatic inflammation.

ACETAMINOPHEN HEPATOTOXICITY: POTENTIATION BY ISONIAZID

Crippin JS *Am J Gastroenterol* 1993;88(4):590

This is a single case report of a patient who developed significant hepatotoxicity that was thought to be related to an interaction between isoniazid (INH) and moderate doses of acetaminophen. The patient was a 21-year-old women who took 10 acetaminophen tablets (325 mg) over a 12-hour period for the treatment of dysmenorrhea. She

RELEVANT FEATURES IN 25 CHRONIC ALCOHOLICS WITH HEPATOTOXICITY FROM MODERATE DOSES OF ACETAMINOPHEN

Feature	Number (Median)
Men	16
Women	9
Age, years	23-59 (38)
Drug dose, g/24 h	2.6-16.5 (6.4)
Total bilirubin, mg/dL	1.3-23.9 (7.3)
Prothrombin time, s prolonged	1-63 (16.0)
Aspartate aminotransferase, IU/L	1960-29,700 (6888)
Alanine aminotransferase, IU/L	12-12,500 (2480)
Mortality, %	20

Source: Ann Intern Med 1986;104:399-404.

was on chronic INH therapy for tuberculosis prophylaxis. Prior tests revealed normal AST/ALT hepatic enzymes while on isoniazid. She was taking no other medications, was not considered to be an alcoholic, and had no signs of chronic liver disease. Because of gastrointestinal complaints and a history of acetaminophen ingestion, liver functions were evaluated and an APAP level was sent.

Six and a half hours postingestion, the level was 104 µg/ml, a level considered to be nontoxic according to the standard nomogram. While awaiting laboratory tests, she received a single 140 mg/kg loading dose NAC, but this therapy was discontinued when the APAP level was available. NAC therapy was never reinstituted. In 24 hours, she had a marked elevation of her liver enzymes (AST 22,000 IU/L; ALT 10,000 IU/L), with a marked elevation of bilirubin and prothrombin time. Viral hepatitis tests were negative. Over the next eight days, her liver function returned to normal.

The author incriminates acetaminophen as the culprit for hepatotoxicity in this patient. INH is a known inducer of the P-450 enzyme system. An association between chronic INH use and acetaminophen hepatic necrosis has been previously reported. While this single case report does not prove a direct cause and effect, the author repeats previous cautions that patients on INH therapy should be warned against the excessive use of acetaminophen.

COMMENT: This article is similar to the previous one that associates moderate doses of APAP with significant liver toxicity in a small subset of patients at high risk. INH is commonly used as prophylaxis for or to treat patients with TB, and its use is rapidly increasing with the emergence of AIDS-related microbacterium infections. While no human studies have been performed and there are only occasional case reports, acetaminophen hepatotoxicity has been potentiated in rats pretreated with INH. Elevated transaminase levels are seen in 10-20 percent of patients treated with INH, and its liver toxicity is well described.

Generally, enzyme elevations occur within the first few months of therapy and subside when INH is withdrawn. Advanced INH-induced hepatitis carries a mortality rate of about 10 percent. The author of this study believes that INH hepatitis was not responsible for the clinical picture in their patient. It is unclear whether INH was stopped and why maintenance NAC therapy was not instituted. It would make sense to me to reinstitute NAC under such circumstances.

INH is not thought to decrease protective glutathione levels in the liver so the mechanisms of toxicity are postulated to be similar to that of ethanol induction of the enzyme system that creates an excess of the toxic metabolite. Although a direct cause-and-effect relationship has not been proven, other reports echo the authors concerns (*Ann Intern Med* 1990;113:799, *Ann Intern Med* 1991;114:431).

The issue of microsomal induction is quite complicated and poorly understood. Numerous drugs used as anticonvulsants and for TB are known to induce the P-450 system. Chronic ethanol use, however, is the most potent inducer. Experimental animals fed ethanol for only three weeks manifest a significantly lower LD 50 for APAP. The table lists some other medications that induce the P-450 system and concomitant use of these agents theoretically puts patients at risk for APAP toxicity. Except for ethanol, the others have been poorly studied and their contribution is largely theoretical.

ACETAMINOPHEN OVERDOSE: LABORATORY EVALUATION AND GASTRIC DECONTAMINATION ISSUES

Emergency physicians should order an acetaminophen level on all drug overdoses; the test costs only a few dollars and could save a life

Alcoholics are at much higher risk for liver necrosis when they ingest doses of acetaminophen (APAP) that would be considered nontoxic to normal individuals. The explanation for this phenomenon centers around the alcoholic's enhanced metabolism of APAP to its toxic metabolite, a decrease in liver stores of the naturally protective substance glutathione, and a toxic insult to an already damaged liver.

Treating patients with active liver disease (such as alcoholic hepatitis) with the N-acetylcysteine (NAC) antidote when serum APAP levels are at a level that would normally be considered nontoxic on the acetaminophen poisoning nomogram is recommended. The exact cutoff is not known; about 50-60 percent has been empirically suggested. In addition, patients taking antituberculous drugs, particularly isoniazid, also may be at increased risk for hepatotoxicity when they are exposed to acetaminophen in an amount that would normally be considered safe. The mechanism of INH synergism is similar to the alcoholic's dilemma: enhanced production of a toxic metabolite. Other important issues involved in the diagnosis and treatment of ED patients with possible exposure to APAP raises questions that also should be addressed by the emergency physician during the initial assessment.

VALUE OF RAPID SCREENING FOR ACETAMINOPHEN IN ALL PATIENTS WITH INTENTIONAL DRUG OVERDOSE

Ashbourne JF, et al *Ann Emerg Med* 1989;18(10):1035

Acetaminophen poisoning usually has no specific recognizable clinical manifestations during the first few hours following overdose, so the ED diagnosis is generally based on an index of suspicion gleaned from historical parameters. Because the overdose patient's history correlates with the actual substance ingested only about half the time if one considers all overdoses in general, it is certainly likely that many cases of acetaminophen ingestion would surely go unrecognized if the clinician relied only on the medical history. Because APAP toxicity can be successfully treated if identified early and because acetaminophen is universally available as an over-the-counter drug, many clinicians order a routine serum, acetaminophen level in their initial evaluation of all overdose patients.

Ashbourne et al were the first to study prospectively this rather common but unproven practice, and they attempted to determine the incidence of unrecognized but potentially toxic acetaminophen toxicity in patients who presented with any type of intentional drug overdose.

All adult patients who were treated in the EDs of two large urban county hospitals during a five-month period were eligible for inclusion in this study. Patients with isolated admitted substance abuse, such as alcohol intoxication or cocaine or heroin use, were excluded. After the history was taken, a screening APAP level was ordered on all patients diagnosed with drug overdose.

Physicians were required to complete a questionnaire indicating whether an APAP ingestion was suspected and to describe the basis for that suspicion. The physicians were also asked if they would have sent a screening APAP level in individual cases.

The authors analyzed data from 486 patients. About 75 percent of subjects with no suspected APAP ingestion had no serum APAP detected and were therefore believed to have a true negative history. About nine percent were suspected to have an APAP overdose and were, in fact, found to have an elevated serum level. These patients were true positives by history. About 15 percent had a history of APAP overdose, but were found to have an insignificant level and were considered false positives. Only 1.4 percent had no history or suspicion of APAP use, but had elevated APAP levels, rendering them true false negatives. Therefore, when routine acetaminophen levels were sent on 486 patients who presented with an undifferentiated overdose, the authors identified seven individuals who specifically denied APAP ingestion but were found to have elevated levels on routine screening.

Only one patient, however, had what was considered a potentially hepatotoxic APAP level (196 mg/L at 12 hours postingestion). None of the other six patients with a false negative history for APAP ingestion had significant serum levels, and none required treatment with NAC. Interestingly, 30 percent of the physicians indicated that despite a negative history, they would have routinely or automatically ordered an APAP level anyway. When the data were analyzed for false negative histories of patients treated by these physicians, the APAP screen was negative in all but one case. Overall, the sensitivity of the medical history was 86 percent.

> THE HEALTH CARE SYSTEM IS NOT GOING BANKRUPT BECAUSE EPS ARE ORDERING APAP LEVELS ON ALL ODS

Based on this study, the authors point out that approximately 25 percent of all overdose patients will ingest some acetaminophen. Only one of 70 patients who presents with intentional drug overdose, however, will have an unrecognized acetaminophen ingestion and only one in 500 who clandestinely ingests APAP will have an overdose serious enough to be potentially hepatotoxic. There were some language barriers in this study, and the authors state that the incidence of unrecognized APAP overdose may be even less in other institutions. There were no distinguishing characteristics in the seven patients with a false negative history that could lead the clinician to suspect APAP ingestion. The cost to the hospital per screening test was approximately $10 using an immunoassay technique, and turnaround time was about an hour.

The authors conclude that about one in every 500 overdose patients will have a potentially treatable acetaminophen overdose that cannot be identified by historical parameters. The authors suggest that it may be clinically justifiable to screen all patients with drug overdose for acetaminophen toxicity despite the fact that unrecognized serious overdose is uncommon. They were reluctant, however, to make firm recommendations.

COMMENT: All emergency physicians know the issues involved in this controversy. Acetaminophen is widely available, it usually produces minimal or no symptoms that would initially indicate its presence or subsequent toxicity, hepatotoxicity can be fatal, and a safe and effective antidote is available (but it must be given within 16 hours postoverdose). Routine APAP levels are not yet considered standard of care. Ordering the screening test is currently a clinical decision made on a case-by-case basis.

Clearly it would be unusual for the diligent clinician to miss a significant APAP overdose, but given these widely accepted axioms, I believe it is difficult to defend not ordering a routine APAP level on most patients with an intentional drug overdose. The test costs only a few dollars, and it should be readily available in all hospitals, so I don't see what the big deal is all about. Certainly the health care system in this country is not going bankrupt because emergency physicians are ordering APAP levels on all drug overdoses. I have not seen this point tested in the courts, but I am sure you would have a difficult time defending a hepatotoxic death should you be unfortunate enough to fall into the trap of trying to save a few dollars on such a complicated clinical interaction as a drug overdose.

My recommendation, therefore, is to order the test on most cases and be done with it. If you can be sure the history is stone cold accurate, then the test is certainly not needed, but numerous studies have proven that the history can be quite misleading and there is no way to determine accurately which histories can be trusted. I will agree that with this screening approach you will rarely find a patient who otherwise would have slipped through the cracks, but our hospital sees 500 overdose patients per year, and I would not like to have one death per year. The few thousand dollars in laboratory tests you would save per year would barely pay for some high-priced expert to review your malpractice case.

In my experience, acetaminophen overdose is not always clinically silent during the first few hours. Many patients have abdominal pain, become nauseated, or suffer from vomiting or other gastrointestinal disturbances within a short time after a massive ingestion. The presence of GI complaints are ubiquitous following drug overdose, but they should alert the clinician to the possible presence of APAP. I have not seen it reported, but I have been impressed with the early finding of diaphoresis after a large APAP ingestion.

Another advantage of ordering a routine APAP level is that it may point to another unsuspected ingestion, specif-ically another drug that is combined with APAP. What readily comes to mind is a recent patient who presented with a seizure, a bizarre tricyclic antidepressant-like cardio-gram, and in a coma, with a relatively high (but nontoxic) acetaminophen level. The tricyclic antidepressant analysis was negative. She had just been to another emergency department complaining of back pain, and from this data we correctly pieced together a propoxyphene (Darvocet) overdose. In this case, the acetaminophen was not a prob-lem, but the propoxyphene was life-threatening. Finding the APAP helped focus our clinical efforts.

Because acetaminophen is found in numerous pre-scription medications, finding an elevated APAP level can at least suggest that the patient's symptoms are due to a drug overdose, even though the acetaminophen itself is not the major concern. Unexpected acetaminophen toxi-city in a patient who presents with a known drug overdose is probably only a partial insight into the problem. I would be more concerned about the patient who has end-organ failure and an APAP ingestion is never considered. A familiar example is an alcoholic with known liver disease who presents with decompensation that is attributed to alcoholic hepatitis rather than a potential new and easily treated hepatotoxin. I am in favor of liberally ordering APAP levels on all patients with liver dysfunction, even though the history of APAP ingestion is negative and there are other obvious reasons for liver fail-ure. A nice study, but one I have not yet seen conducted, would be to order a routine APAP level on all alcoholics seen in the ED. They are a subgroup clearly at high risk for APAP toxicity with rather minimal overdose or even thera-peutic use.

Some of my colleagues routinely order a salicylate level based on similar reasoning. It's clearly not the same, and I think this is rather silly because patients with significant salicylate ingestions are clearly symptomatic early in their course with a rather classic toxidrome. You would have to be a very poor clinician to miss the signs and symptoms of acute sal-icylate poisoning (chronic salicylate tox-icity is another issue).

Finally, another blood test which I believe should be routinely ordered on all overdose patients — when they hap-

RESULTS OF RAPID SCREENING FOR ACETAMINOPHEN

	Highland General Hospital	San Francisco General Hospital	Total
	No. (%)	No. (%)	(%)
True negatives	167 (79)	198 (72)	365 (75)
True positives	16 (8.6)	27 (9.8)	43 (8.8)
False positives	26 (12.3)	45 (16.4)	71 (14.6)
False negatives	2 (1)	5 (1.8)	7 (1.4)
Total cases	211	275	486 (100)

Sensitivity of the history = .86   Positive predictive value = .38
Specificity of the history = .84   Negative predictive value = .99

Source: Ann Emerg Med 1989;18:1035-1038.

pen to be women of childbearing age — is a pregnancy test. Because hospitalized patients receive numerous x-rays, drugs, and procedures that could put a developing fetus at risk, it's a good idea to know if they are pregnant in the ED before the radiologist calls you with an embarrassing incidental finding on your KUB.

This article has been the subject of much interpretation, and I find it amazing that clinicians use exactly the same data to both support and refute routine APAP screening. The authors themselves failed to take a firm stand — so does an accompanying editorial — but I for one see this as a very straightforward issue. I'm sure many patients get needless CBCs, clearly a worthless test when one is dealing with the initial evaluation of a drug overdose. No doubt a few other "routine" tests also were sent, costing 10 times more than one APAP level. Finally Sporer et al (*Am J Emerg Med* 1996;14:433) prospectively studied the practice of routine APAP and salicylate levels in 1820 adult overdoses. They found only eight patients (0.3%) with potentially hepatotoxic APAP levels with negative histories and therefore recommended routine APAP screening for all comers. All patients with potentially toxic salicylate levels were identified by the presence of symptoms (usually altered mental status) or an elevated anion gap. This prompted a conclusion that a routine salicylate test is not warranted if the history is negative and the mental status and anion gap are normal. This, of course, mandates an electrolyte panel.

EFFICACY OF CHARCOAL CATHARTIC VS. IPECAC IN REDUCING SERUM ACETAMINOPHEN IN A SIMULATED OVERDOSE

McNamara RM, et al *Ann Emerg Med* 1989;18(9):934

This random-assignment prospective crossover trial on human volunteers compared the effects of ipecac-induced emesis vs. activated charcoal plus sorbitol in reducing serum concentrations of acetaminophen in a simulated overdose model. Ten healthy volunteers were given 3 g of APAP followed by no intervention, 30 mL of syrup of ipecac, or 50 g of activated charcoal/70 percent sorbitol solution. Serial serum APAP levels were assessed for eight hours following ingestion. Subjects served as their own controls and were given the second regimen after a washout period.

All 10 subjects vomited following ipecac administration (in about 25 minutes), and none vomited after the activat-

ACTIVATED CHARCOAL IN A SIMULATED POISONING WITH ACETAMINOPHEN

Side Effect	No. Control	No. Charcoal
Diarrhea	8	10
Flatulence	6	4
Nausea	2	3
Headache	2	1
Belching	1	1
Drowsiness	0	2
Contipation	2	0
Light-headedness	1	0

Source: Ann Emerg Med *1993;22:1398-1402.*

ed charcoal. Two subjects experienced hyperemesis after the ipecac. A charcoal laden stool was noted in the mean time of 109 minutes after the charcoal-sorbitol therapy.

Serum APAP levels were converted to area under the curve to reflect total drug absorption over time. Both therapies significantly decreased the amount of acetaminophen absorbed when compared to controls. There were no significant differences observed between the two treatments, although there was a trend toward charcoal being more effective than ipecac in reducing the total amount of APAP absorbed into the systemic circulation. The authors conclude that charcoal-sorbitol is as effective as syrup of ipecac in reducing absorption of APAP in a simulated overdose model. The authors stress the obvious disadvantage of ipecac: the patient would subsequently be unable to tolerate the oral antidote, NAC.

COMMENT: This is one of many studies that evaluate the usefulness of gastric emptying procedures by comparing them to the administration of oral activated charcoal alone. Because APAP is readily bound to charcoal, it makes sense to administer charcoal over ipecac and negate the vomiting that will ensue. Because NAC is such a nauseating drug in itself — many patients who take it will vomit continuously — the additional stress of ipecac-induced emesis is something all patients can do without.

Most toxicologists consider ipecac a clinical dinosaur, and I can't remember the last time I used it. It's difficult to justify it at all, except perhaps in the prehospital phase or in pediatric patients. Ipecac lengthens the hospital ED stay, increases complications, and precludes the use many oral antidotes. In addition, many overdoses are complicated primarily by vomiting. Numerous authors have demonstrated the equal or superior efficacy of activated charcoal alone for gastric decontamination when compared to other gastric emptying procedures, and the use of ipecac or lavage has dropped dramatically.

If the clinician's first reflex in all drug ingestions is to order gastric emptying, that reflex is clearly a pathologic one by current standards. The dose of APAP administered in this report was not a massive one, but numerous well designed studies and at least three prospective clinical trials have championed the use of charcoal alone over routine gastric emptying (*Ann Emerg Med* 1985;14:562, 1981;10:528, and 1987;16:838 and *Arch Intern Med* 1984;144:48).

One should note, however, that there are some toxic drugs that are not bound by charcoal and therefore administering the black substance will have little benefit. In these cases, some other form of GI decontamination should be considered. Substances not absorbed by charcoal include lithium, iron, hydrocarbons, ethanol, many heavy metals, organophosphates, and acids/alkalis. The issue for APAP is, however, quite clear. When a patient presents with a known APAP overdose, you should opt for the charcoal alone, and eschew ipecac/lavage.

USE OF ACTIVATED CHARCOAL IN A SIMULATED POISONING WITH ACETAMINOPHEN: A NEW LOADING DOSE N-ACETYLCYSTEINE?

Chamberlain JM, et al *Ann Emerg Med* 1993;22(9):1398

There is some concern that oral activated charcoal will interfere with the bioavailability of NAC. Therefore, some clinicians have been reluctant to administer charcoal initially in a overdose and have opted for either gastric lavage or ipecac-induced emesis to provide gastric decontamination. It is clear that activated charcoal will bind some NAC, but the actual clinical effect of this adsorption or the optimal loading dose of NAC to overcome this phenomenon remains controversial. There have been suggestions simply to increase the dose of NAC to compensate for any absorbent effects of activated charcoal to maintain adequate serum levels of the protective NAC. The authors of this study investigated the ability of excess NAC to overcome the undesirable effects of activated charcoal on NAC bioavailability.

Ten healthy adult volunteers, serving as their own controls in a crossover experiment, participated in this study. Subjects were given 3 g of APAP followed in one hour by a normal loading dose of NAC (140 mg/kg). In the second phase, subjects ingested similar amounts of APAP, were administered 60 g activated charcoal one hour later, and were given a supranormal loading dose of NAC (235 mg/kg). The measures of outcome were serum NAC levels measured serially over six hours and the four-hour serum APAP level.

In short, giving oral charcoal does not negate the efficacy of NAC as an antidote if the initial dose of NAC is increased appropriately. The authors recommend, therefore, that charcoal be given initially to patients with APAP overdoses

ACTIVATED CHARCOAL IN A SIMULATED POISONING WITH ACETAMINOPHEN

Parameter	Control	Charcoal
N-acetylcysteine area under curve (µg/min/mL)	4,247±935.8	5,849±1,857.8
Peak N-acetylcysteine (µg/mL)	28.5±10.5	28.7±6.2
Time to peak N-acetylcysteine (min)	60.3±18.5	78.9±16.8
Acetaminophen level (µg/mL)	19.4±4.0	12.4±6.6

Values are mean ± SD for area under the curve, peak level, and time to peak for serum N-acetylcysteine, and four-hour serum acetaminophen level.

Source: Ann Emerg Med *1993;22:1398-1402.*

regardless of the potential need for NAC therapy. Should further analysis indicate that NAC is required, the adequate bioavailability of the oral NAC can be ensured by increasing the loading dose to 235 mg/kg. The data also confirm previous studies demonstrating the efficacy of activated charcoal in preventing acetaminophen absorption. Interestingly, no subject vomited with the large dose of NAC, and no other significant side effects were noted.

COMMENT: There is ongoing controversy concerning the proper (scientific) administration of NAC to patients who have previously been given charcoal to reduce APAP adsorption. Clearly charcoal is preferred over ipecac for gastric decontamination because charcoal is as efficacious in reducing acetaminophen adsorption as ipecac does not produce vomiting. It is known, however, that charcoal will decrease the bioavailability of NAC. Previous investigators have demonstrated a decrease up to 40 percent in area under the curve for NAC when large doses (100 g) of charcoal are given to volunteers (*Am J Emerg Med* 1987;5(6):483). It has long been suggested, therefore, that the dose of NAC be increased by 40 percent if charcoal has been given. Until this study, the projected increased dose was not tested clinically.

The issue is further complicated by the fact that the optimal dose of NAC required to prevent APAP toxicity is unknown. I find it fascinating that the standard loading dose of NAC is not increased when the amount of acetaminophen ingestion is increased, and the standard loading dose (140 mg/kg) seems to be appropriate for patients who ingest either one or four bottles of APAP. Curiously, there are no recommendations that base NAC dosing on APAP levels; treatment is an all-or-nothing phenomenon. Obviously, the loading dose of NAC must be an overdose in

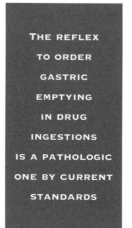

THE REFLEX TO ORDER GASTRIC EMPTYING IN DRUG INGESTIONS IS A PATHOLOGIC ONE BY CURRENT STANDARDS

itself in the vast majority of cases. Otherwise, it does seem somewhat irrational to use the same NAC dose for a patient whose level barely reaches the toxic line on the nomogram and the patient who has astronomical APAP levels. I think the whole charcoal/NAC issue is quite overstated.

There is certainly no rationale to withhold charcoal in APAP overdose because of the fear that it will preclude adequate NAC therapy. Oral charcoal will treat possible co-ingestions, and its ability to bind APAP will probably keep many patients from even entering a treatment protocol because toxic serum levels will never be reached.

The following approach appears scientifically valid and clinically reasonable: administer charcoal to all patients with APAP overdose to decrease absorption. If the APAP level is above the treatment line of the standard nomogram, administer NAC, but increase the initial amount given. You can either increase the loading dose (to 235 mg/kg) or simply repeat the standard (140 mg/kg) loading dose at four hours instead of the administering standard 70 mg/kg maintenance dose. Maintenance NAC therapy after the initial loading dose(s) will be unchanged. Although it has not been scientifically evaluated, I would suggest a similar scenario be used should the patient have a four-hour level above 1,000 mg/L. This would be considered a massive overdose, and it just seems logical to increase the amount of the antidote.

Repeating the loading dose rather than increasing the first dose may circumvent some of the vomiting problems associated with large NAC volumes, although it's interesting that no patient in this study experienced emesis with NAC. Some of the vomiting associated with NAC may be related to underlying early APAP GI toxicity. I have been routinely giving 20 mg IV metaclopramide (Raglan) prior to NAC, and this seems to decrease subsequent vomiting.

ACETAMINOPHEN TOXICITY: ISSUES FOR CHILDREN AND PREGNANT WOMEN

Acetaminophen toxicity in children rarely comes to mind unless the child is evaluated for a known ingestion

Ordering a serum acetaminophen (APAP) level should be somewhat routine in all overdose cases because it's cost effective in the long run. Routine screening is certainly not standard of care, but APAP is widely available, it is usually an initially silent overdose, has potential for significant morbidity or mortality, and effective treatment is available if the diagnosis is confirmed. But two subsets of patients — children and pregnant women — require special consideration with regard to APAP exposure.

REPEATED ACETAMINOPHEN OVERDOSING: CAUSING HEPATOTOXICITY IN CHILDREN

Henretig FJM, et al *Clin Pediatr* 1989;28(11):525

The authors of this study, pediatricians from Children's Hospital in Philadelphia, note that because acetaminophen is currently the antipyretic of choice for infants and young children, the incidence of overdose has risen accordingly. Fortunately, there have been relatively few cases of serious APAP toxicity in children, so clinical experience with this age group is somewhat sparse. Serious toxicity can occur in young children, however, and the authors report two such cases and review appropriate literature.

In the first case, an 11-month-old girl was initially seen for lethargy, vomiting, anorexia, and abnormal liver function. These symptoms developed three days after a fever and otitis media that was treated with amoxicillin and a decongestant. Acetaminophen was also prescribed as an antipyretic, and the dose suggested was one 65 mg suppository every four hours.

The child presented in a lethargic irritable state with persistent vomiting. Her neurological examination and hepatic dysfunction suggested Reye's syndrome. Liver function was markedly abnormal and findings included an elevated serum ammonia level and high transaminase levels. A urine drug screen was positive for the prescribed acetaminophen and phenylpropanolamine. Numerous studies for viral infections and hepatitis, as well as Wilson's disease, were normal. An APAP level obtained 36 hours after admission was nondetectable. Through some rather intense detective work, however, the clinicians uncovered a prescription error where the child had received suppositories of 650 mg strength rather than the prescribed strength. The box was mislabeled by the pharmacist as containing 65 mg suppositories. The child had received the adult strength suppository every four hours for eight doses. When blood was analyzed from a prior day, the acetaminophen level was in the high toxic range. With intensive supportive care, the child recovered.

In another case, a 22-month-old girl was admitted for evaluation of obtundation, liver failure, and elevated ammonia levels. She had been seen four days previously at a local emergency department where she had a clinical scenario suggestive of chicken pox. The child became increasingly ill and eventually became comatose. Her examination was consistent with resolving chicken pox and laboratory evaluation revealed hypoglycemia and liver/renal failure. The serum acetaminophen level was only mildly elevated (32 mg/L). Investigation revealed a similar scenario as seen in the first case: the child had received numerous 650 mg acetaminophen suppositories (total APAP dose of 6.5 grams) over the preceding three days. This child also recov-ered after a rocky course.

The authors note that chronic APAP toxicity has been described previously in the pediatric population, but the entity may not be well appreciated. APAP is used universally for fever control and when given in repeated doses it is almost impossible to interpret the significance of serum levels unless they are markedly elevated. It is emphasized that in both cases presented here the levels were clearly nontoxic if one were to use the nomogram. The nomogram cannot be used, however, to evaluate multiple ingestions, and the serum level has little relation to toxicity in chronic ingestions. Because Reye's syndrome is a well known entity that can mimic APAP-induced liver failure, it is not uncommon for such children to be misdiagnosed initially. Fatal cases of hepatic and renal failure following excessive acetaminophen therapy in children have been documented, but if a child recovers with only supportive therapy, the diagnosis may never be suspected.

SPONTANEOUS ABORTIONS AND STILLBIRTHS BY TRIMESTER AND ACETAMINOPHEN LEVEL

	First Trimester OD		Second Trimester OD		Third Trimester OD	
	Toxic	Nontoxic	Toxic	Nontoxic	Toxic	Nontoxic
Number	4	2	0	2	1	0
Mean age, years	22.5	26	27.5	20		
Range	17-31	19-33	19-36			
Mean time to NAC	14.3	12.3	11.5	12		
Range	12-17	10.5-14	4-19			
Maternal outcome						
AST >1000 U/L	2	0		0	1	
AST >45 & 1000 U/L	1	0	0		0	
Mean peak AST	6375				6237	
Range	846->14,000					
Deaths	1	0		1	0	

NAC=N-acetylcysteine; AST=aspartate aminotransferase. Toxic values are acetaminophen level above nomogram line at 4-24 hours post-ingestion. Mean peak AST includes patients with AST >45 U/L only.

Source: Obstet Gynecol 1989;74:247-53.

The authors note that APAP toxicity in children is generally due to repeated moderate acetaminophen overdosing rather than a single massive ingestion. Because serum levels are generally not impressive, clinicians may not make the causal association even if they think to order a level. Repeated overdose may be due to a prescription error, poor instructions by the physician, by parental error, or by child abuse.

The authors emphasize that merely doubling the recommended therapeutic dose of acetaminophen for several days could put children at risk for serious hepatotoxicity. Because APAP suppositories are available over-the-counter in various strengths — 120, 325, 650 mg — it would not be difficult for an inadvertent overdose error to be compounded many times. The authors calculate that the toxic threshold for children is in the range of 150 mg/kg per day over two to four days. With current safe dosing recommendations, up to 90 mg/kg per day could be administered to children if they are treated around the clock as commonly prescribed, so the chance for toxicity from minimal dosing errors is substantial.

COMMENT: It would be extremely easy for any busy emergency physician to overlook APAP toxicity in a septic-appearing child, and it's a diagnosis that rarely comes to mind unless the child is evaluated for a known ingestion. Like salicylate poisoning in a child, APAP toxicity is usually the result of repeated exposures, so the course, symptoms, and laboratory profile will be very different from the well-described acute overdose. Chronic salicylate poisoning is a classic example: a child with a viral syndrome is repeatedly given too much aspirin. The symptoms of chronic overdose — tachypnea, fever, vomiting, irritability — are similar to many viral illnesses, and the laboratory reports a salicylate level in a range usually thought to be nontoxic or therapeutic so the diagnosis is totally missed.

The cases presented here were both totally misdiagnosed initially by the referring hospital and were only picked up after some nifty investigative work at a specialized treatment center. Many emergency physicians would not even include APAP poisoning in a differential diagnosis of liver dysfunction in a child. Most would, as did the clinicians in this study, likely suspect viral hepatitis or Reye's syndrome because the abnormality developed after

afebrile illness. The one child who had chicken pox was a seemingly classic example of Reye's syndrome.

Children generally tolerate a single acetaminophen overdose quite well, and they are thought to be at less risk than adults for the same mg/kg single ingestion. It's difficult to find any reports of serious APAP toxicity following single childhood overdoses. In one multicenter report of 417 children age five or less with APAP overdose, only three children were found to have elevated liver enzymes, and all recovered uneventfully (*Am J Dis Child* 1984;138(5):428).

There are a few interesting points to make concerning APAP toxicity in children. First, they may be at higher risk for recurrent ingestions than adults. Also, an interesting finding in this report was severe hypoglycemia due to the liver insult. This is a common scenario in children. Obviously it's important to look for other causes of coma in the ED, even in the face of a "classic infection" or obvious liver failure. It should also be noted that the treatment nomogram developed for a single one-time ingestion is applicable for children as well as adults, but the data are based on pills and not on the liquid form commonly available to children. Who knows how to evaluate levels from suppositories?

There are numerous preparations of acetaminophen available, and one can certainly not just ask the parents vague questions about dosing and strength. As shown nicely in this case, it's best to get the actual product and examine it carefully.

It's not difficult for patients to get the concentrated pediatric drops mixed up with the elixir. When the pharmacists makes the error, even looking at the package label would be deceiving. In one of the cases detailed here, the box was labeled as prescribed yet the contents were 10 times more potent than designated on the label.

This scenario is reminiscent of the alcoholic with liver disease who has a straightforward and seemingly logical reason to suffer decompensation, and one can easily be lead down the incorrect diagnostic path. As with the alcoholic who has APAP toxicity, the SGOT levels in these children were sky high (over 10,000 U/L) and probably too high for most cases of viral hepatitis or Reye's syndrome. If APAP poisoning is not suspected in the ED and only considered three to four days later when an astute clinician finds that all the parameters do not add up, the chance to implicate high acetaminophen levels has prob-

> IF AN APAP
> OD CAUSES
> FETAL DISTRESS,
> AN EMERGENCY
> DELIVERY MAY
> BE REQUIRED

ably been lost if the analysis was not ordered in the ED. Once again, think APAP toxicity in all cases of liver dysfunction, even in children.

ACETAMINOPHEN OVERDOSE DURING PREGNANCY

Riggs BS, et al *Obstet Gynecol* 1989;74(2):247

Because acetaminophen is thought to be safer than aspirin during pregnancy, it is routinely recommended as an analgesic/antipyretic agent for pregnant women. Because acetaminophen does cross the placenta, with the potential to produce fetal injury, the authors of this study investigated the use of oral NAC for the treatment of acetaminophen poisoning during pregnancy. The report analyzes data obtained on 113 women who overdosed on APAP during various stages of their pregnancy. It is one of the few reports that specifically addresses APAP toxicity in this subgroup of patients.

In a study sponsored by the Food and Drug Administration, the Rocky Mountain Poison Center conducted a telephone mediated protocol to collect data. Subjects included pregnant women exposed to APAP or treated with NAC. NAC treatment criteria in pregnancy are the same for any nonpregnant patient with potential hepatotoxicity and was based on the standard Rumack-Matthew nomogram. The treatment protocol for NAC was also standard: 140 mg/kg as a loading dose followed by 17 maintenance doses of 70 mg/kg every four hours. Complete follow-up and appropriate laboratory data were available in only 60 of the cases. Of those 60 patients, 24 had an APAP level in the toxic range as defined by the nomogram. There were approximately 20 patients in each trimester of pregnancy.

Spontaneous abortion occurred subsequent to the overdose in six of 19 patients who ingested APAP during the first trimester. Eight of 19 women opted for an elective abortion, and only five of the 19 subjects delivered a normal term infant. Spontaneous abortions and still births occurred in a small number of patients who had APAP ingestions during the second and third trimester. In one instance a mother in her third trimester (33 weeks) was given NAC within 12 hours of ingestion of a toxic APAP overdose, and also received the full standard NAC regimen. She experienced moderate hepatotoxicity and survived, but the fetus died within two days of the overdose. Autopsy showed fetal liver necrosis and a toxic fetal APAP level. In this case, properly used NAC failed to save the baby.

There were two variables that were significantly predictive of pregnancy outcome. There was a statistically increased probability of fetal death if the administration of NAC was delayed or if the mother took the overdose early in pregnancy.

Because of the small number of patients, specific statistics or recommendations were not forthcoming. In this study, there were 42 live births and nine fetal deaths with a fetal mortality rate of approximately 18 percent. However, an exact cause-and-effect relationship to the overdose

MATERNAL AND FETAL PLASMA N-ACETYLCYSTEINE LEVELS ($\mu g/mL$)

Time (min)	End-Infusion	30	60	120	180	240
Ewe 1	893	1526	1757	503	204	121
Fetus 1	<2	<2	<5	7	6	<5
Ewe 2	631	603	236	54	214	121
Fetus 2	<2	<2	<2	<5	<2	<5
Ewe 3	619	513	332	30	<5	<5
Fetus 3	<5	<2	<5	<5	<2	<5
Ewe 4	2512	502	291	642	101	17
Fetus 4	<2	25	17	<5	10	<5

Limit of detection was 2 µg/mL. Limit of quantification was 4 µg/mL. Results reported as <2 mean that no NAC was detected. Results reported as <5 mean that NAC was detected but was too low to quantify.

Source: Ann Emerg Med *1991;20:1069-72.*

was not certain in all cases. It was difficult to control for other variables, such as prenatal care, or other maternal risk factors.

The authors conclude that the NAC is not teratogenic. They suggest that pregnant patients who are found to have hepatotoxic APAP levels should be immediately treated with NAC. The final conclusion is vague and merely suggests that early treatment with NAC will improve outcome by lessening the incidence of spontaneous abortion and intrauterine death.

COMMENT: It is extremely difficult to find hard data on acetaminophen overdose during pregnancy, and I am almost sorry I chose this topic because the data are so sparse and vague. It is generally assumed that there is no downside to treating APAP overdose in pregnancy with NAC, but the kinetics of acetaminophen metabolism and the placental transfer of NAC and APAP, toxic metabolites, and fetal metabolism are vague and confusing. Reports are few but cases of APAP causing fetal demise — with maternal survival — are well referenced. On the other hand, some women with significant APAP toxicity have delivered normal babies. Why fetal death occurs is not known, but autopsies show extensive liver/renal injury in the fetus classically associated with APAP poisoning.

A short course on APAP pharmacokinetics/metabolism will help explain the clinical issues raised in this column. In the adult (pregnant or otherwise), APAP is cleared by four known mechanisms. About one to two percent is excreted unchanged in the urine. Up to 95 percent is normally conjugated in the liver, with sulfation and glucuronidation, to a nontoxic product that is excreted in the urine. Children and the fetus rely on sulfation to a great extent and glucuronidation predominates after age 10-12. About five to 10 percent of APAP is metabolized through the P-450 system in the liver to a toxic metabolite (NAPQI). This toxin is rapidly detoxified by endogenous glutathione and excreted as a nontoxic metabolite in the urine. NAC is a glutathione precursor that is an efficient antidote when the normally protective endogenous glutathione is depleted, such as occurs in an overdose. Pregnant women demonstrate the same basic metabolism as other adults. The fetus and children have similar basic clearance rates for APAP except that sulfation predominates over glucuronidation.

Acetaminophen does cross the placenta, and it is metabolized in the fetal liver. Presumably some of it is transformed to the toxic metabolite as early as the 14th week of gestation. Some NAC may cross the placenta and may offer some protection from hepatotoxicity following a maternal overdose, but the kinetics and specifics are unclear.

In one impressive study of NAC transport across the placenta in pregnant sheep, it was found that little maternal NAC gets to the fetal circulation (*Ann Emerg Med* 1991;20:1069). These data suggest that the fetal liver is not protected from APAP toxicity by maternal NAC administration.

It is certain that a maternal APAP overdose can kill the fetus, even if the mother survives. Currently it is impossible to predict clinically or measure the amount of toxic metabolite produced by the fetus and other variables such as conjugation ability, or fetal glutathione levels and depletions. Susceptibility of the fetal liver to APAP injury remains largely a mystery. It is intuitive that pregnant women should be treated with NAC as soon as possible to limit the effect of toxic metabolite formation, but saving the mother from toxicity does not guarantee that the fetus will also be safe. It is not known how well maternal NAC will protect the fetus, but protection is far from complete.

In the setting of APAP toxicity or overdose, fetal monitoring should be rapid and constant, and emergency delivery should be considered if signs of fetal distress develop. It may be reasonable to perform emergency delivery if the mother presents in a toxic state and too late for effective NAC therapy, but this recommendation is not based on firm evidence. In fact, major toxicology textbooks (Haddad and Winchester; Ellenhorn and Barceloux) state that delivery should not be undertaken because the fetus can be treated by treating the mother. This recommendation is not referenced, and from my reading, this may not be true. I am particularly concerned by animal studies that show that NAC does not cross the placenta.

APAP is not teratogenic so in early pregnancy there is no rationale to recommend therapeutic abortion if the pregnancy remains viable. There are no clear guidelines, however, on the indications for pregnancy termination, early delivery, or methods to evaluate fetal toxicity in the later stages of pregnancy other than to employ the common axiom that what's good for the mother is probably good for the fetus. I could find no firm recommendations from the OB/GYN literature, and most textbooks ignore the issue completely. I would be tempted to suggest delivery if the fetus is viable and if there were any sign of fetal distress and not rely on NAC to save the baby.

ACETAMINOPHEN TOXICITY: ODDS AND ENDS

Acetaminophen can cause acute renal failure, even in the absence of liver necrosis, and NAC may have some life-saving potential even when used late

In these discussions of the diagnosis and treatment of acetaminophen (APAP) toxicity in the emergency department. I have assumed that all emergency physicians are cognizant of the basics, and have attempted to concentrate only on those topics that are outside the standard protocols but of clinical importance in the ED.

It was noted that alcoholics with preexisting liver disease are at much higher risk for fulminant hepatotoxicity from doses of acetaminophen that may be considered safe in non-compromised individuals, and one should not automatically assume that an alcoholic who decompensates from a hepatic standpoint is suffering solely from the effects of excess alcohol. Even moderate therapeutic doses of acetaminophen can be deleterious to these individuals.

Individuals taking certain drugs that increase the metabolism of acetaminophen to its toxic metabolite, such as INH and other anti-TB drugs, also can put the patient at risk for hepatotoxicity from relatively modest doses of the analgesic. In a discussion of the initial approach to a known or unknown APAP overdose in the ED, I have recommended that it is cost-effective and clinically reasonable to order a routine serum acetaminophen level on all intentional ingestions because even potentially fatal toxicity does not declare itself initially and certainly the patient's history is often misleading.

Routine levels are not, however, standard of care, and decisions should be made on a case-by-case basis. You will likely practice a few years before routine APAP screening will save the patient from liver failure and you from the malpractice lawyer.

When faced with an APAP overdose, oral activated charcoal is a reasonable sole form of gastric decontamination, and you can safely forgo lavage or ipecac-induced emesis. If charcoal is given, the bioavailability of NAC can be assured by increasing the loading dose of the antidote by 30 to 40 percent, but the clinical importance of charcoal binding to NAC has probably been overstated.

In a discussion of poisoning or therapeutic misuse of APAP in children, it was pointed out that clandestine acetaminophen poisoning can simulate Reye's syndrome or sepsis in the neonate, but usually only following dosing errors and repeated administration. There is a surprisingly low safety margin when the drug is used around the clock for fever control, but children have excellent tolerance for a single overdose. During pregnancy it is clear that APAP poisoning can be deleterious and not only to the mother; it can cause fetal demise or spontaneous abortion. APAP is not teratogenic, but *the exact issues concerning emergency delivery are still unsettled and even timely treatment of the mother does not guarantee the well being of the fetus. Emergency delivery should be considered with any sign of fetal distress.*

In this chapter, I have chosen to review two unappreciated issues. The first is that acetaminophen can cause acute renal failure, even in the absence of liver necrosis. Although NAC is best given before liver injury occurs, this antidote may have some life-saving potential when used late in the course of hepatic failure. NAC may be indicated long after the time traditionally suggested as the window of opportunity for prevention of hepatotoxicity.

ACUTE RENAL FAILURE AFTER ACETAMINOPHEN INGESTION

Curry RW, et al *JAMA* 1982;247(7):1012

It is well known that APAP is a liver toxin, and APAP-induced acute hepatic failure is often accompanied by renal failure. But most physicians do not appreciate the fact that acetaminophen can be a potent renal toxin in the absence of serious hepatic injury. The authors of this report document the case of a 36-year-old woman who was hospitalized with abdominal pains, nausea, and vomiting. There was no history of acetaminophen overdose, but laboratory evaluation revealed minimal hepatic and renal dysfunction. Over 48 hours, progressive oliguria ensued and the patient finally admitted taking an overdose of acetaminophen (about 30 g) two days prior to admission.

Creatine levels reached 18 mg/dL, and BUN peaked at 90 mg/dL. When renal failure was maximum, the patient demonstrated relatively normal hepatic function. She was never jaundiced, and the prothrombin time was never significantly elevated. With supportive care and hemodialysis, the patient made a full recovery.

Although acute renal failure occurs in 20-30 percent of patients with severe hepatic necrosis, there have been numerous case reports of renal failure without evidence of hepatic injury following overdose of acetaminophen. It is, therefore, not unusual to see acute tubular necrosis in patients critically ill from liver failure, but renal failure as an isolated finding in acetaminophen overdose is not well appreciated. In fact, some older textbooks specifically state in error that there is no direct nephrotoxicity associated with acetaminophen.

A theoretical basis for the occurrence of direct renal injury can be postulated. There is a high concentration of the glutathione and cytochrome P-450 system in the kidney, and this system is required for drug detoxification in this organ as well as in the liver. It has been suggested that a toxic metabolite is produced locally in the kidney, causing an injury in this organ in the same way toxicity is produced in the hepatocyte. It is unclear, however, why severe renal injury would selectively occur without major hepatic damage.

COMMENT: Although it has not been well studied, numerous authors have described cases where acute renal failure has occurred following acetaminophen overdose where there has been no clinical or biochemical evidence of significant liver involvement. Gabriel (*Br Med J* 1982; 284:505) reported 10 such cases where the clinical picture resembled acute tubular necrosis. Patients with renal failure have not been subject to periods of hypotension or other toxins to explain the renal failure. Characteristically the renal failure is delayed a few days later than the liver insult, occurring on day 3-6 postingestion.

Most emergency physicians have little experience with

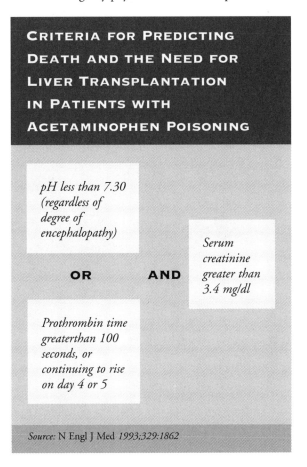

CRITERIA FOR PREDICTING DEATH AND THE NEED FOR LIVER TRANSPLANTATION IN PATIENTS WITH ACETAMINOPHEN POISONING

pH less than 7.30 (regardless of degree of encephalopathy)

OR

Prothrombin time greaterthan 100 seconds, or continuing to rise on day 4 or 5

AND

Serum creatinine greater than 3.4 mg/dl

Source: N Engl J Med 1993;329:1862

acetaminophen overdose causing fatal hepatotoxicity, and they may not appreciate the drug's toxic potential when they admit a relatively asymptomatic patient to the hospital. Because NAC is such an effective antidote, most fatal cases are entirely missed in the ED or present at a stage too late to be effectively treated, but certainly APAP should be on everyone's differential diagnosis of liver failure. I assume, however, that the majority of emergency physicians would not list acetaminophen as a cause of isolated renal failure.

We are all concerned about the renal effects of NSAIDs and prescribe them cautiously because of their antiprostaglandin effect and ability to decrease renal blood flow. Acetaminophen has clearly been implicated in renal failure, but most of us rarely consider the kidney as a target organ in APAP toxicity. Whether NAC would have antidotal effect in the development of renal failure is unclear, but if the theory of renal-based glutathione stores and cytochrome P-450 system is correct, it is likely that the antidote would be as effective in presenting renal failure as liver failure. Curiously, I could find no data to support this.

Combined hepatic and renal injury following acetaminophen use has been well described. Kaysen (*Arch Intern Med* 1985;145:2019) reports five patients who were receiving acetaminophen and developed liver failure. Interestingly, all patients were alcoholics and had received only moderate therapeutic doses of the drug. The three patients who survived all had features typical of acute tubular necrosis, and the authors suggest that the nephrotoxic effects of acetaminophen may be enhanced in alcoholic patients, as are the well described hepatotoxic effects.

As with other unusual pathology associated with acetaminophen use, it is the ED where the toxin should first be considered. Once the patient is admitted to the hospital and the acetaminophen is metabolized, one may lose the ability to correlate the clinical suspicion with acetaminophen levels. In addition, acetaminophen may be continued in the hospital for pain control or as an antipyretic, even though it was the toxin responsible for renal failure. Numbers are difficult to come by, but the incidence of renal failure from APAP without coexistent event liver failure is only about 1-2 percent. Fortunately most patients who are supported with dialysis will make a full recovery and resume normal renal function.

> **APAP SHOULD BE ON ALL DIFFERENTIAL DIAGNOSES FOR LIVER FAILURE**

IMPROVED OUTCOME OF PARACETAMOL-INDUCED FULMINANT HEPATIC FAILURE BY LATE ADMINISTRATION OF ACETYLCYSTEINE

Harrison PM, et al *Lancet* 1990;335:1572

This important article was one of the first reports to suggest that acetylcysteine may reduce mortality in patients with already established acetaminophen-induced fulminant hepatic failure. It is well accepted that while NAC was an excellent antidote, it must be given within 16-24 hours to be totally effective. Some clinicians have even suggested foregoing NAC therapy if treatment is delayed for more than 24-36 hours. The efficacy of NAC to prevent hepatic necrosis is well established, but an additional benefit in patients with well established hepatic failure is suggested by this report.

The authors retrospectively review a series of 100 consecutive patients admitted to their hospital's liver

OUTCOME OF PARACETAMOL-INDUCED FULMINANT HEPATIC FAILURE IN RELATION TO ACETYLCYSTEINE ADMINISTRATION

	n	Survivors	Deaths	Progress to grade III/IV coma	Dialysis treatment required
No antidote	57	24 (42%)*	33 (58%)*	43 (75%)*	38 (67%)
Early <10h	2	2 (100%)	0	0	0
Late >10h	41	26 (63%)*	15 (37%)*	21 (51%)*	21 (51%)

* $p<0.05$ between these groups.
** Anuria or oliguria with creatinine above 400 µmol/l.

Source: Lancet 1990;335:1572-3.

unit with established severe hepatic necrosis secondary to APAP overdose. All met standard criteria for fulminant hepatic failure. Many patients were already suffering from encephalopathy, coagulopathy, renal failure, acidosis, and other features indicating a poor prognosis. Although it was done retrospectively, patients were grouped according to the time that had elapsed between the overdose and the administration of acetylcysteine. This antidote was always given by an intravenous infusion that is not available in the United States.

The authors compared results in the patients treated late to those who were not treated at all because it was assumed that the window of opportunity to ameliorate liver necrosis had passed. NAC was administered 10 hours or more after the overdose in 41 patients; 57 patients were not given the antidote at all.

Significantly fewer patients with established hepatic failure who received NAC progressed to more serious stages of coma when compared to those who did not receive NAC (51% vs. 75%, respectively). The mortality rate was significantly lower in treated patients (37% vs. 58%). Treatment did not influence the maximum peak prothrombin times.

The authors conclude that the standard intravenous administration of NAC significantly improved survival in patients who had established fulminant hepatic failure secondary to acetaminophen toxicity. This benefit was seen when the antidote was given up to at least 36 hours postoverdose. No significant complications of NAC therapy were identified. Although NAC should be given as early as possible following an overdose, these authors believe that delayed therapy may be of value. The mechanism of protection with delayed administration of NAC is unknown, but the benefit is thought to be somehow mediated on the cellular level, through antioxidant properties, or by some other unknown mechanism.

COMMENT: Although this report is encouraging and lends credence to the contention that NAC should be used even if the diagnosis is considered at a late date or if the patient presents with established hepatic injury, a few caveats should be mentioned. First, the delay in treatment in these patients was never more than 36 hours postoverdose. Because the time of overdose may be difficult to establish, especially in a sick patient unwilling or unable

LABORATORY VALUES FOR A 36-YEAR-OLD WOMAN WITH ACUTE RENAL FAILURE

	Hospital Day			
	2	4	8	20
BUN, mg/dL	18	38	64	17
Creatinine, mg/dL	3.1	8.4	16.4	1.1
Calcium, mg/dL	8.2	-	8.8	9.5
Phosphorus, mg/dL	5.0	4.9	6.6	3.0
Uric acid, mg/dL	11.0	11.2	16.4	5.6
Bilirubin, mg/dL	0.8	0.8	0.3	0.2
Alkaline phosphatase, AAU	142	158	115	93
Lactic dehydrogenase, AAU	216	236	406	204
SGOT, AAU	>1200	602	43	28
SGOT, IU/L	2284	-	-	33
Prothrombin time, s	16/12	4/13	-	-
Partial thromboplastin time, s	27	-	-	-
Acetaminophen level, ug/mL	60	87	-	-

Source: JAMA *1982;247:1012-4.*

to communicate, the timing may have been off considerably. Also, at this point there may still be some unmetabolized APAP in the serum that is able to form more toxin. The authors did not describe analysis of this variable. Only intravenous NAC was used, a product that is not yet available in the United States.

Nevertheless, this report is encouraging and should prompt all physicians to consider NAC therapy at any time that hepatic failure secondary to APAP is recognized. Many times this would be a clinical diagnosis only because APAP levels may be negative once the diagnosis is finally considered.

Even with intensive care, fulminant hepatic failure secondary to APAP toxicity has a mortality rate of more than 50 percent (*Gastroenterology* 1988;94:1186). Several prognostic indicators have been found to identify those patients likely to experience a fatal outcome. Acidosis (pH less than 7.3) is highly predictive of death, as is a continuing rise in the prothrombin time on day 3 or 4, or a PT of greater than 100 seconds. A creatinine above 3.4 mg/dL is a poor prognostic indicator.

These prognostic factors, regardless of the grade of encephalopathy, have been used as indications for liver transplant in patients who are candidates for this procedure (*BMJ* 1990;301:964).

Harrison et al (*N Engl J Med* 1991;324 (26):1852) offer an attractive theory as to why NAC would benefit patients with fulminant hepatic failure. They studied the effects of NAC on oxygen transport and various hemodynamic parameters in 12 patients with APAP-induced hepatic failure and eight patients with acute liver failure from other causes. They administered intravenous NAC in a dose commonly used for APAP overdose.

In patients with APAP-induced liver failure, the NAC resulted in an increase in mean oxygen delivery and improvement in cardiac index and arterial pressure. Oxygen consumption was significantly increased, as was oxygen extraction. Similar effects were found in patients with liver failure from other causes. They conclude that NAC increases oxygen delivery and consumption on a cellular level, and this mechanism may enhance survival in patients with otherwise fatal hepatic failure. Because many critically ill patients have problems with oxygen delivery and extraction and suffer a progressive downhill course from multiple organ failures and coagulopathy, NAC offers an attractive therapy for other patients that has not been previously explored.

As a bottom line, the authors postulate that NAC improves micro-circulatory blood flow, possibly by stimulating the activity of endothelium relaxing factor. NAC also inhibits leukocyte chemotaxis, and may act as a free radical scavenger. Exactly how NAC can benefit critically ill patients with multiple organ dysfunction is still under investigation, but it is a promising therapy. The authors of this report suggest that NAC could benefit patients with multiple end organ failure from many other causes such as sepsis, burns, or preeclampsia.

For emergency physicians faced with such patients in the ED, it is reasonable to administer NAC to patients with advanced APAP hepato- or renal toxicity. Even if the liver failure is not caused by APAP, a benefit may be reaped. The same regimen of NAC should be used as previously described for preventing APAP toxicity.

There is no real downside to NAC, and even though the intravenous preparation is not available, it seems reasonable to substitute the oral form. The significant decrease in mortality in these few reports is quite encouraging. Finally, it is important to realize the poor prognostic value of markedly elevated creatine and prothrombin time or metabolic acidosis in patients with APAP toxicity. If a liver transplant is a viable option, patients in need of this procedure can be identified while there is still time to find a suitable donor.

> THERE IS NO DOWNSIDE TO NAC, AND THE ORAL FORM CAN BE SUBSTITUTED FOR THE UNAVAILABLE IV PREPARATION

SECTION III

OPHTHALMOLOGICAL DISORDERS

MYTHS AND MISCONCEPTIONS: AN EYE PATCH FOR SIMPLE CORNEAL ABRASIONS

If ever there were a sacred cow in emergency medicine, it is the axiom that all patients with corneal abrasions should receive an eye patch

Periodically I like to peruse the literature with the intent of finding true scientific data that invalidate commonly held myths and misconceptions in emergency medicine. Because medicine is not an exact science and because of the super-strong egos of many physicians, this is a relatively easy task. Numerous procedures and protocols are established and religiously adhered to that are based purely on tradition, anecdotal reports, personal belief, or seemingly logical parameters, but when studied rigorously, the dogma is found to be bogus. Yet these myths and misconceptions are continually handed down from housestaff to housestaff (or attending to attending) with such zeal and charismatic adherence that they quickly become ingrained as absolute truth. Even respected textbooks promulgate the erroneous concepts, often to the delight of malpractice lawyers. But one need not practice medicine for long to realize that yesterday's dogma can easily become today's heresy, and vice versa.

One of these is a commonly prescribed appliance: the eye patch for simple corneal abrasions. An eye patch is touted to hasten healing and relieve pain, and is considered standard of care for minor traumatic corneal injuries. For years I have followed this tradition, but when I tried to validate the dogma with scientific data, I could find no evidence that an eye patch was beneficial. In fact, the literature states that an eye patch is bothersome, unnecessary, and associated with potentially serious adverse side effects.

NO EYE PAD FOR CORNEAL ABRASIONS
Kirkpatrick J, et al *Eye* 1993;7:468

The purpose of this randomized clinical trial was to assess the healing rate and level of pain relief experienced by two groups of patients treated for a minor traumatic corneal abrasion. The authors questioned whether the established traditional treatment for a simple corneal abrasion — a topical antibiotic and an eye patch — offered benefit to patients with this common injury. Patients suffering a traumatic corneal abrasion of less than 20 hours duration were entered into this prospective study at an eye hospital in England. All 44 subjects were over age of 18, in relatively good health, and had no significant past ophthalmological problems. Injuries eligible for inclusion in the trial were simple corneal abrasions in the absence of co-existent significant ocular trauma. Patients with corneal foreign bodies or contact lens problems were excluded.

The size of the abrasion was initially measured with a slit lamp, and patients were then assigned to one of two treatment groups. The first group received an antibiotic ointment, homatropine drops, and a double eye patch. The second group also received antibiotic drops and pupillary dilation, but an eye patch was not used. Oral analgesics were permitted as needed for pain relief. Patients were rechecked at 24 hours to assess healing, and their level of discomfort was evaluated with a visual analogue pain scale. Patients were followed until complete healing

had occurred, and they also received a final evaluation one week later. The injuries were caused primarily by a fingernail (17/44) or a twig or leaf (11/44).

The rate of epithelial healing was rapid in both groups (1.5-2 days), but recovery was statistically better in patients who were not treated with an eye patch. There was no significant difference between the two groups with respect to pain scores; however, almost half of the eye patches were removed by the patients by the first revisit. The main reason given by the patients (20% removed it) was that the eye patch was just too uncomfortable. Ten patients also reported that their eye patch "fell off" while they were sleeping (although some may have voluntarily removed it). There were no significant complications in either group, and all abrasions were completely healed within three days. The authors conclude that there is a significant improvement in the rate of healing of corneal abrasions in patients treated with antibiotic ointment and mydriatic eye drops if an eye patch is not provided.

It has been traditionally taught that frequent eye blinking hinders epithelial attachment, retards corneal healing, and produces pain in the presence of a corneal abrasion. The theoretical purpose of a firm eye patch is to prevent blinking and therefore hasten healing. This tradition is questioned by the authors. A theoretical disadvantage of eye patching is that the patch will lower the partial pressure of oxygen in the corneal epithelium and the milieu produced by the patch may actually promote infection and retard epithelial migration and proliferation. The authors also believe that ointment, as opposed to drops, is a superior vehicle for antibiotics because ointment has a longer contact time and acts as a lubricant between the lid and the abraded surface.

The authors admit that the study was small and the corneal abrasions minor so patients were likely to do well with any intervention. Also, there may

PATIENTS WITH CORNEAL ABRASION RECEIVING EYE PATCHES

Patient Age	Patient Gender	Mode of Injury	Time Since Injury (hours)	Abrasion Size (mm)	Time to Heal (days)
57	M	Twig	20	8	2
30	M	Fingernail	21	14	-
29	F	Twig	5	3	3
20	M	Twig	16	2	-
25	M	Tool	2	0.4	1
63	M	Plastic	24	1	1
29	M	Nail	6	3	3
29	F	Dog	5	2	2
36	M	Fingernail	14	2	2
45	M	Fingernail	4	1	2
28	M	Fingernail	19	6	2
30	F	Fingernail	6	2	3
40	M	Fingernail	12	8	3
32	M	Twig	16	1	2
38	M	Stone	8	1	1
46	M	Cat	18	7	2
29	F	Fingernail	2	2	2
49	M	Twig	16	3	1
38	M	Fingernail	24	16	-
32	M	Fingernail	20	1	2

Source: Eye 1993;7:468.

have been some bias because the observers were not blinded to the use of an eye patch. In summary, the authors conclude that omission of an eye patch in patients with minor corneal abrasions is reasonable primary therapy that will lead to rapid corneal healing.

COMMENT: If there ever were a sacred cow in emergency medicine, it is the axiom that all patients with corneal abrasions should receive an eye patch. It is heresy to think otherwise, and the tradition is well ingrained. Because a soft tissue injury heals best when immobilized, it is reasonable to intuit that an injured eyeball will benefit from some sort of ophthalmologic splint. It is almost comical to see patients with minor eye injuries burdened with an elaborately placed double or triple eye patch, the face covered with multiple rolls of tape kept in place by sticky benzoin, and then vehemently ordered to keep the patch in place or risk severe pain and delayed healing. Of course, showering or hair washing must be prohibited.

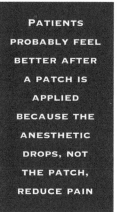

PATIENTS PROBABLY FEEL BETTER AFTER A PATCH IS APPLIED BECAUSE THE ANESTHETIC DROPS, NOT THE PATCH, REDUCE PAIN

It is generally believed that an eye patch offers a stable corneal environment that promotes epithelial healing. Even though an occlusive dressing may reduce corneal oxygenation and increase corneal temperature — and thereby slow healing and predispose a secondary infection — the eye patch is still omnipresent. If I were an aspiring *Pseudomonas* or tetanus organism, I would be delighted to be placed under an eye patch, just the right environment for me to grow to maturity.

There are practical as well as physiological reasons to avoid an eye patch. Not only is the patch annoying, it keeps patients out of the shower, and keeps them from driving or reading (and usually from working). From a physiological stance, antibiotics can't be instilled, normal blinking is interrupted, drainage and tearing is hampered, and the homeostasis of the cornea milieu is tampered with. Weissman (*Int Contact Lens Clin* 1980;5:41) was able to demonstrate a marked drop in oxygen tension in the corneal epithelium under a closed eye (155 mm Hg with the eye open compared to 55 mm Hg with the eye shut) so the disadvantage of patching from an oxygenation standpoint has real scientific validity.

When researching this subject, I noted that every emergency medicine textbook (even ophthalmologic handbooks) recommends ritual eye patching (even my own textbook promulgates this myth). Thirty years ago,

Jackson (*Br Med J* 1960;9:713) questioned the dogma and subsequently proved that an eye patch was basically worthless for the treatment of simple corneal abrasions. That study, along with others, was basically ignored. In a prospective alternate day study of 157 patients, Jackson could find no benefits of routine patching for corneal abrasions, and interestingly noted that the only complications he could demonstrate from an abrasion (an ulcer with hypopyon, conjunctivitis, and a recurrent abrasion) occurred in the patched patients. Despite this observation, the medical community has continued to ignore the facts, and we all routinely prescribe eye patches. I could not find a single study that supported routine eye patching for minor abrasions.

Hulbert (*Lancet* 1991;337(8742):643) likewise failed to demonstrate any advantage to an eye patch in patients with a minor corneal defect that was secondary to removal of a corneal foreign body. In a small random-assignment prospective controlled study following removal of a superficial corneal foreign body (FB), 16 subjects were managed with an eye patch and 14 were managed without one. Within 24 hours, all patients who were treated without a patch demonstrated healing of the corneal defect, but only 87 percent of those treated with an eye patch were completely healed. Three-quarters of the patients with an eye patch reported significant discomfort in the eye while only 28 percent of the controls complained of pain. Like others, this study also demonstrated faster corneal healing if an eye patch was avoided, but it also demonstrated a significant increase in pain and discomfort with the bulky dressing. Granted, it's a small study, but the findings are in agreement with others.

It should be emphasized that all the patients in these studies had minor superficial corneal abrasions that healed rapidly with either treatment, but these are the type of abrasions that are generally treated or followed by the emergency physician. Large or deep corneal abrasions, those with significant foreign bodies, or patients with underlying eye pathology should be expeditiously referred to an ophthalmologist for follow-up. If any abrasion persists for more than a few days, an ophthalmology visit is mandated. Also, if you can't use a slit lamp, don't even consider foreign body removal or providing your own follow-up. The issue of foreign bodies of the cornea is an individual clinical decision. Minor superficial foreign bodies can be removed from the cornea in the emergency department with relative ease and then treated as a simple corneal abrasion, but most EPs avoid drilling out rust rings or digging for deeply imbedded FBs.

I was recently reminded of how silly ritual eye patching can be. I observed an emergency medicine resident expending much time, effort, and energy to put an eye patch on an obstreperous 3-year-old who had a minor corneal abrasion. The child was comfortable until shackled by the patch, and he cried continuously once the patch was placed. It took three attempts to get the patch properly applied, and gauze mittens had to be wrapped on the child's hands to keep him from tearing it off. The child did manage to remove the patch at home soon after discharge so the mother, ritually advised about the magical healing powers of the patch by the physician, brought the child back for yet another battle to replace the patch. When the child removed the patch for the second time at home, the mother wisely gave up and let the child sleep. The only time he kept calm was when the patch was removed. On revisit 36 hours later, the abrasion was completely healed.

Although eye patches, as they are used in emergency medicine, are not likely to be detrimental to healing, the dressing is uncomfortable over-treatment. I also suspect that the obligatory single-dose antibiotic drops/ointment or mydriatic therapy are also excessive, and I would like to see a study that addressed the use of these commonly prescribed interventions. If antibiotics are so important, why don't we remove the patch to instill them on a regular basis? After all, the antibiotic effect of eye ointment can be measured in minutes.

There is no question that corneal abrasions are bothersome and irritating to the patient. Blinking and tearing are common, but they may actually be a helpful physiologic response that we short-circuit by applying a patch. Blinking tends to take away debris, and tearing provides soothing lubrication. Perhaps simple sunglasses would suffice.

Paying attention to details in your discharge instruc-

PATIENTS WITH CORNEAL ABRASION NOT RECEIVING EYE PATCHES

Patient Age	Patient Gender	Mode of Injury	Time Since Injury (hours)	Abrasion Size (mm)	Time to Heal (days)
18	F	Wire	6	3	1
51	M	Paper	1	5	-
52	F	Leaf	14	5	1
28	F	Fingernail	5	6	1
29	F	Fingernail	20	39	3
31	F	Twig	20	1	1
34	F	Leaf	12	1	2
24	M	Leaf	18	1	2
28	M	Bird	4	0.3	1
29	F	Glass	3	1	2
55	F	Paper	24	0.3	2
64	M	Fingernail	10	3	2
29	M	Wire	5	3	1
39	M	Twig	12	1	-
47	F	Twig	16	2	2
27	F	Fingernail	10	0.5	1
43	M	Wire	5	2	2
32	F	Nail	3	14	2
27	F	Toy	4	6	1
26	M	Fingernail	4	5	1
32	F	Fingernail	15	0.5	1
39	F	Paper	3	2	-
32	M	Fingernail	4	2	2
23	M	Fingernail	20	7	-

Source: Eye 1993;7:468.

tions can make you look like an ocular pro. I personally give patients with painful corneal abrasions a few narcotic tablets to take with them. I suggest that they avoid reading and television. I carefully document on the chart that driving is prohibited if they are patched because the dressing stops binocular vision, hinders depth perception, and greatly diminishes the visual field.

The skeptic might say that clinical experience proves that an eye patch reduces pain because, once applied, patients always feel much better. I would offer that an eye patch is usually placed after anesthetic drops are instilled, and it is the local anesthetic that actually reduces pain. I have heard colleagues state that an eye patch is used to keep the eyeball from moving, but because eyes move in tandem, the unaffected eye, with its normal to-and-fro activity, would also move the abraded eye under even the most carefully applied pressure patch.

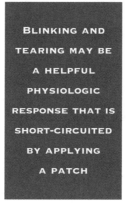

BLINKING AND TEARING MAY BE A HELPFUL PHYSIOLOGIC RESPONSE THAT IS SHORT-CIRCUITED BY APPLYING A PATCH

One need only to place an index finger over your closed eye lid and move the opposite eye to realize that no amount of patching will keep the injured eyeball from moving in concert with the unpatched eye (that's why reading and other visual activities aggravate symptoms in patched patients).

Although superficial corneal abrasions rarely become infected, it does make good bacteriological sense to consider that a warm dark patch, covering a moist injured area, is an ideal medium to foster bacterial growth. In short, I think it's time we stopped torturing our patients who seek care for minor corneal abrasions by prescribing annoying bulky eye patches that can foster infection and have never been proven either to relieve pain or promote healing. I admit that I have not seen significant complications from eye patching, but it's interesting to consider just how scientific (or unscientific) the procedure is.

CORNEAL ABRASIONS: POTENTIAL FOR SERIOUS MORBIDITY

Irritation and corneal abrasions are common in contact lens wearers, but disastrous complications can result if keratitis is missed

The vast majority of superficial corneal abrasions are bothersome, but they do not pose a threat to vision or cause long-term morbidity. There are, however, certain instances where a red flag should be raised. Disastrous complications can rapidly result from seemingly minor corneal injuries so it is absolutely essential for the emergency physician to be cognizant of these unusual but real concerns. Because extended-wear contact lenses are omnipresent, the require special consideration.

THE RELATIVE RISK OF ULCERATIVE KERATITIS AMONG USERS OF DAILY WEAR AND EXTENDED WEAR SOFT CONTACT LENSES

Schein O, et al *N Engl J Med* 1989;321:773

Approximately 20 million Americans wear contact lenses, and a good percentage of them show up in the emergency department with eye-related problems. Although soft extended-wear lenses are more patient-friendly than the old-fashioned hard lenses, their use has been associated with numerous adverse effects, the most serious being ulcerative keratitis. The authors of this study attempted to assess the risk of ulcerative keratitis in such individuals.

The report is a case-controlled retrospective evaluation of 99 patients who developed ulcerative keratitis associated with the use of soft contact lenses. A corneal ulcer at the time of enrollment was a prerequisite for inclusion. Controls consisted of individuals who wore soft contact lenses but were hospitalized for conditions unrelated to lens use. Study parameters included laboratory evaluation, lens care and hygiene issues, and various epidemiological data. The patients underwent corneal scraping or culture, and all were treated with ocular antibiotics. Patients who wore hard or rigid lenses were excluded.

About half of the patients had suppurative infiltrates of the visual axis, and most ulcers were less than 5 mm in diameter. All patients had infiltrates that had penetrated the corneal stroma. Bacterial cultures were positive in 70 percent of the cases, the most common organisms being *Pseudomonas aeruginosa,* staphylococci, and streptococci. Most of the patients were women, but this paralleled the epidemiological use of the contact lenses.

The relative risk of keratitis was almost fourfold greater in those subjects who used extended-wear lenses as compared to daily-wear lenses. When patients left lenses in their eyes overnight, as opposed to only daytime use, the risk was 10 to 15 times greater. The risk was incrementally related to the extent of overnight use. There was a trend toward a decreased risk of infection if proper lens hygiene was observed, although it did not reach statistical significance. The authors conclude that using extended-wear contact lenses, especially overnight, can be a risky prospect. They also estimated that for every consecutive day of lens use before proper cleaning was applied, the increased risk of keratitis was five percent. The authors were impressed by the alarming overall poor level of lens care that was noted in both patients and controls. Failure to pay attention to lens hygiene-related measures and proper cleaning of the lenses were significant risk factors for all individuals. The combination of trauma to the corneal epithelium from lens wear and the presence of pathogenic organisms were the proposed physiological basis for keratitis in these individuals.

COMMENT: Emergency physicians obviously do not prescribe or provide maintenance surveillance for patients who use contact lenses, but they must be cognizant of the

potential adverse complications from the use of these devices. The vast majority of injuries will be minor abrasions that will quickly resolve without sequelae. But the potential for serious complications is real. The bottom line is that if one sees a patient with eye complaints secondary to contact lens use, a red flag should be raised. At the minimum, these patients require careful slit lamp examination, ophthalmological follow-up, and no use of lenses until ophthalmological referral is obtained and an in-depth examination has been performed.

The vast majority of contact lenses usually cause only minor corneal abrasions that heal well by merely leaving lenses out for a few days. Ulcerative keratitis is, however, a significant complication that can't be missed. The following article describes just how serious complications can be.

CONTACT LENS ABRASION AND THE NON-OPHTHALMOLOGIST

Schein OD *Am J Emerg Med* 1993;11:606

This article is a case presentation and discussion of disastrous infectious complications resulting from corneal abrasions associated with contact lens wear. The author notes that there are more than 25 million contact lens wearers in the United States, and transient irritation or corneal abrasions are relatively common side effects. Because problems are so common, it would not be unusual for patients with contact lens-related pathology to present to an emergency department. The author of this paper believes that corneal abrasions from contact lenses represent a subset of injuries that should be respected for potential complications and carefully evaluated; these injuries should not be treated like abrasions from other causes. Three alarming cases are presented to emphasize this point.

In the first case, a 28-year-old woman who wore extended-wear soft contact lenses for three years developed pain in her left eye. At a local clinic, a corneal abrasion was diagnosed, and she was treated with a combination sulfaetamide and steroid eye drop and a pres-

ESTIMATED RELATIVE RISKS OF ULCERATIVE KERATITIS ACCORDING TO LENS TYPE AND LEVEL OF OVERNIGHT USE AS COMPARED WITH DAILY WEAR LENSES NOT WORN OVERNIGHT

Lens Type and Overnight Use	Case Patients vs. Population-Based Controls	Case Patients vs. Hospital-Based Controls
	Relative Risk (95% CI)	
Daily Wear		
No overnight use		1.00 1.00
Overnight use	8.96 (4.09-19.63)	9.55 (2.87-31.8)
Extended wear		
No overnight use	2.76 (1.06-7.20)	2.57 (0.7-9.51)
Overnight use	10.17 (5.29-19.55)	15.04 (5.21-43.43)

Source: N Engl J Med *1989;321:773-8.*

sure patch. She was told to remove the patch after 24 hours and then use ointment three times a day until symptoms were relieved. At 36 hours postinjury, she consulted an ophthalmologist because of increasing pain. Suppurative keratitis was diagnosed. Corneal perforation was noted with extensive inflammation, and corneal cultures confirmed a *Pseudomonas* infection. Significant loss of vision occurred as a result of scarring.

In the second case, a 19-year-old woman who had worn extended-wear soft contact lens for three years presented with a one-day history of eye pain. A large corneal abrasion was noted, sulfacetamide drops were given, a pressure patch was placed, and follow-up was arranged for three days later. At 24 hours, the patient returned with increasing symptoms and was reevaluated and repatched. Four days following the initial injury, suppurative keratitis was diagnosed and *Pseudomonas* was identified as the offending organism. After treatment, the visual acuity in the affected eye was 20/400.

In the third case, a 28-year-old female contact lens wearer presented with left eye pain and was found to have a small peripheral corneal abrasion. Sulfacetamide ointment and a pressure patch were prescribed. Within 24 hours, *Pseudomonas keratitis* was diagnosed, and visual loss occurred. In the latter two cases, malpractice issues were pursued.

Previous authors have reported *P keratitis* following pressure patching for the treatment of contact lens-associated corneal abrasions. Classically patients initially present with minor abrasions, without evidence of keratitis. Patients are usually prescribed an eye patch, but suppurative keratitis is diagnosed soon thereafter. The author emphasizes that abrasions associated with contact lens use appear to have a different physiology and complication rate from similarly appearing corneal abrasions caused by other trauma.

The author suggests that contact lens abrasion be treated with antibiotics effective against *Pseudomonas* (tobramycin, gentamicin or polymyxin, and bacitracin). It is noted that erythromycin and sulfa drugs, two commonly prescribed ointments for corneal abrasions, are inadequate therapy for *Pseudomonas*. Pressure patching of the lid is generally discouraged in this situation. Theoretically, patching favors replication of *Pseudomonas* by nurturing a protective environment. In addition, a patch inhibits routine blinking and tearing, the body's protective mechanisms against infection. These authors also note that a closed eye produces a dark, warm, hypoxic, and humid environment that particularly favors *Pseudomonas* proliferation. A well known caveat violated by one physician in this report is the prohibition of steroid-containing drops for the initial treatment of any corneal abrasion. Another mistake was suggesting "as needed" follow-up rather than specifying a timely repeat visit. The author of this report suggests routine 24-hour follow-up for patients with corneal abrasions from contact lens wear and the avoidance of a pressure patch.

COMMENT: If a previously healthy individual suffers vision loss or prolonged morbidity following a relatively superficial corneal abrasion, a lawsuit is almost guaranteed. Such a scenario would make any malpractice lawyer salivate profusely. Obviously, emergency physicians should

> IF A HEALTHY PERSON SUFFERS VISION LOSS OR PROLONGED MORBIDITY FOLLOWING A SUPERFICIAL CORNEAL ABRASION, A LAWSUIT IS ALMOST GUARANTEED

RELATIVE RISKS OF ULCERATIVE KERATITIS FOR EXTENDED WEAR LENSES AS COMPARED WITH DAILY WEAR LENSES NOT WORN OVERNIGHT, ACCORDING TO CONSECUTIVE DAYS WORN

	Relative Risk (95% CI)	
Days	*Case Patients vs. Population-Based Controls*	*Case Patients vs. Hospital-Based Controls*
1	*3.6 (1.3-9.7)*	*2.4 (0.7-9.0)*
2-7	*6.8 (3.3-14)*	*10.0 (3.1-31.9)*
8-14	*11.8 (4.7-30)*	*37.9 (3.4-423.2)*
>15	*14.5 (5.6-37.9)*	*45.0 (4.3-467.3)*

Source: N Engl J Med *1989;321:773-8.*

treat any eye injury with great respect, but this article points out the potential for a disaster from a relatively common and seemingly innocuous injury. I have seen multiple patients with abrasions from contact lens, but I have never seen *P keratitis*. The cases in this article are especially alarming because the rampant and destructive eye infections occurred so quickly, within one to two days following a relatively minor abrasion. Patching was felt to contribute to morbidity because it made life (and reproduction) simple for any *Pseudomonas* that happened to be in the vicinity.

Numerous authors have reported isolated cases with similarly disastrous results. Although *Pseudomonas* and other bacteria can be introduced with extended wear soft contact lenses, most of the time no infection will develop. A corneal abrasion, however, will allow the bacteria to penetrate an otherwise intact protective barrier of corneal epithelium. Like an eye patch, contact lenses themselves can provide an hypoxic environment that predisposes to infection when mechanical abrasion is present.

A number of caveats can help emergency physicians avoid the disastrous complications highlighted in this report. First, all patients with corneal abrasion should have mandatory and documented 24-36 hour follow-up, either in the emergency department or by an ophthalmologist. Follow-up is ideally continued until the abrasion has completely healed. Many EPs cavalierly follow abrasions, but they should not even consider this practice if they don't have access to (or know how to use) a slit lamp. If the injury presents on a Friday, it is almost axiomatic that follow-up occur in the ED. Some physicians have the rule that abrasions are followed daily until healing is complete, and I concur that this is prudent in most cases.

If your patient still has symptoms or a persistent abrasion after three to four days, it is certainly time to seek oph-

RELATIVE RISKS OF ULCERATIVE KERATITIS BASED ON LOGISTIC REGRESSION FOR SELECTED MEASURES

	Relative Risk (95% CI)	
Measure	Case Patients vs. Population-Based Controls	Case Patients vs. Hospital-Based Controls
Daily wear lenses not worn overnight	1.00	1.00
Daily wear lenses worn overnight	8.08 (2.72-24.01)	4.78 (0.80-28.75)
Extended wear lenses not worn overnight	1.17 (0.23-5.96)	1.84 (0.08-41.03)
Extended wear lenses worn overnight	5.15 (1.65-16.06)	16.84 (1.51-188.08)
Lens care index	0.86 (0.73-1.00)	0.87 (0.66-1.14)
Cigarette smoking	2.69 (1.24-5.81)	4.17 (0.82-21.09)

Source: N Engl J Med *1989;321:773-8.*

A DAMAGED AND PATCHED EYE IS AN INVITATION FOR TETANUS AND *PSEUDOMONAS* TO SET UP HOUSEKEEPING

thalmologic consultation. To the untrained emergency physician, a corneal ulcer can look much like a minor abrasion. Although many corneal abrasions will heal slowly without significant infection, I tend to get nervous after the second or third visit. The prohibition of steroid-containing drops is well referenced, as is the continuous use of anesthetic drops for the outpatient. Although sulfa or erythromycin ointments are standard first-line topicals for conjunctivitis, in the particular case of contact lens abrasion it seems reasonable to prescribe routinely anti-pseudomonas antibiotics. I prefer Polysporin (polymixin B and bacitracin) ointment as my routine ointment for all abrasions. Most authorities agree that ointment is preferable to drops. Ciprofloxacin drops are also commonly prescribed.

A short note on another disastrous infectious complication of corneal injury is in order. Pfahl and Ostler (*JAMA* 1988;260(4):553) address the risk of tetanus from corneal injuries. Most of his discussion is theoretical, but he notes the potential for the growth of *Clostridium tetani* following a corneal injury. The author states he is aware of three cases of tetanus (not reported or documented in the literature) from corneal injuries, and he recommends tetanus prophylaxis in a "dirty wound." Because all wounds are "tetanus prone," I think it's silly to hedge. I must admit that I frequently forget tetanus prophylaxis with corneal injuries, and many of my colleagues do not consider it, but it should be addressed. From a public health standpoint, routine tetanus immunizations in the ED can be supported, even if the incidence of corneal tetanus is infinitesimal.

Like *Pseudomonas* infections, a damaged and patched eye is an invitation for tetanus to set up housekeeping, but I could find only one old report documenting tetanus from a corneal injury (*Am J Ophthalmol* 1957;43: 772).

In a review of tetanus following ocular injuries, Benson et al (*J Emerg Med* 1993;11:677) were able to document only 38 cases reported in the medical literature. The vast majority of cases (33) occurred when there was perforation of the cornea or sclera. There were no cases of tetanus resulting from simple corneal abrasions. In an animal study, these authors introduced the tetanus organism into the eye of mice who had an experimentally produced abrasion, perforation, or penetration. Some of the nonimmunized animals who suffered a perforating injury did develop tetanus. None of the immunized animals developed tetanus. None of the nonimmunized animals that had only a corneal abrasion developed tetanus. This animal study would suggest that tetanus prophylaxis is certainly warranted following perforating or penetrating ocular injuries, but tetanus is very unlikely following an uncomplicated corneal abrasion.

Patients seen in the emergency department who have significant eye injuries are usually transferred immediately to an ophthalmologist, and it would be prudent to initiate tetanus prophylaxis prior to transfer. Tetanus is an extremely unusual complication, and prophylaxis could be inadvertently overlooked when the physician is confronted with a complicated eye injury. The ED is the perfect place to pay attention to this particular detail. I could not, however, find a single documented case of tetanus following a simple corneal abrasion.

OPHTHALMOLOGY TRIVIA: THE FIXED AND DILATED PUPIL

Fixed and dilated pupils can be caused by scopolamine patches, jimson weed, and phenylephrine nasal spray, all of which test the emergency physician's mettle

Although most corneal abrasions are nothing more than minor annoyances, various ophthalmological entities test the mettle of any emergency physician. The central theme for the following discussion is the approach to the patient who presents to the ED with a fixed and dilated pupil.

ANISOCORIA FROM SCOPOLAMINE PATCHES
McCrary JA, Webb NR *JAMA* 1982;248 (3):353

In 1982 this information was deemed important enough to appear in *JAMA*, but it is now well disseminated and should be universally known by emergency physicians. The authors report two cases of a unilaterally fixed and dilated pupil that were attributed to the topical effect of scopolamine that was inadvertently introduced into the eye of the patch user. Obviously one always considers central nervous system abnormalities, such as aneurysm or tumor, when faced with a unilaterally fixed and dilated pupil and often such a clinical presentation leads to an extensive and expensive investigation.

In the first case, a 33-year-old woman with a possible history of multiple sclerosis was hospitalized for the evaluation of a fixed and dilated pupil. She had no systemic complaints, her vision was normal, and there were no abnormalities of extraocular motility, visual fields, fundoscopic examination, or intraocular pressure. The left pupil was widely dilated, and showed no direct or consensual response to light. The dilated pupil failed to constrict following installation of 1% pilocarpine eye drops, but the unaffected pupil rapidly became pinpoint. The patient had been using a scopolamine patch for dizziness, and the offending topical delivery system was finally discovered behind the ear on the side of the dilated pupil. All local findings abated when the patch was removed, but it took more than three days for complete resolution.

In the second case, a 28-year-old woman was sent for ophthalmologic evaluation by a neurosurgeon when he noted that the left pupil was fixed and widely dilated. This patient also complained of headaches and occasional nausea. Examination of the eyes was normal except for the fixed and dilated pupil and, as in the other case, the abnormal pupil failed to constrict following the local installation of pilocarpine eye drops. A CT scan of the head was normal. Following an extensive evaluation, a scopolamine patch was eventually found behind the left ear. The patch was removed, and within a few days all the symptoms resolved.

In both cases, the patients did not tell the physicians about the use of the scopolamine patch and probably did not consider the scopolamine-impregnated patch to be a bona-fide drug because it was applied to the skin. There were no systemic symptoms of scopolamine toxicity in either case.

The authors note that failure of the pupil to constrict after the installation of pilocarpine eye drops is virtually diagnostic of three local conditions of the eye. They emphasize that neurological dilation of the pupil (from aneurysm, neoplasm, subdural hematoma, etc.) will never prohibit the eye from constricting following the intraocular installation of pilocarpine drops. Failure of pilocarpine to constrict a pupil localizes the problem to the parasympathetic synapse in the sphincter. The most common cause of a dilated pupil that is unresponsive to pilocarpine is pharmacologic blockade of pupillary constriction by atropine-like drugs. Rarer conditions, such as traumatic iridoplegia

> **PILOCARPINE SHOULD RAPIDLY PRODUCE PUPILLARY CONSTRICTION IN THE ABSENCE OF CHEMICAL BLOCKADE OF THE SPHINCTER**

If this fixed and dilated pupil is caused by the intraocular instillation of an anticholinergic medication (prototype is atropine), it will not constrict within 15-20 minutes after the local instillation of 1% pilocarpine eye drops. A pupil that is dilated because of a neurologic cause, such as cerebral herniation or a lesion of the oculomotor nerve, will constrict. Pilocarpine is a direct-acting cholinergic agent, like acetylcholine, that causes miosis by stimulating the neuromuscular junction of the sphincter of the eye. Pilocarpine will constrict a pupil that is dilated by an adrenergic agent. (See Thompson et al, Sur Ophthal 1976;21(2):45.) See color plate in center well.

and acute angle closure glaucoma, could produce similar findings. Surgery or trauma to the eye may also render the sphincter incapable of responding to pilocarpine, but this should be a chronic situation that is easily diagnosed. The reason pilocarpine is so diagnostic is that pupillary constriction depends on intact cholinergic receptor function in the pupillary sphincter, and this function is not affected by compression of the oculomotor nerve (III) or increased intracranial pressure. Pilocarpine is a potent parasympathomimetic agent that should rapidly produce pupillary constriction in the absence of chemical blockade of the sphincter. Importantly, pilocarpine will constrict a pupil that is dilated from Neo-Synephrine or epinephrine drops. These drops do not block parasympathetic receptors; rather they stimulate nerves that cause pupillary dilation.

This simple pilocarpine eye drop test was first described by Thompson et al (*Arch Ophthalmol* 1971;86:21). The test is so specific that failure of a dilated pupil to constrict within 30 minutes following the installation of 1% pilocarpine eye drops virtually rules out neurologic disease. In acute narrow angle glaucoma, the lack of pupillary constriction is due to iris sphincter ischemia secondary to the sudden onset of high intraocular pressure. When this intraocular pressure is decreased by acetazolamide and mannitol, the pupil will then constrict with local pilocarpine.

The authors believe that direct accidental contamination of the eye with scopolamine was the mechanism for the mydriasis in both patients. It was assumed that active medication contaminated the fingers when the patch was applied behind the ear, and the scopolamine was inadvertently placed in the eye by the patient's finger. A systemic effect was discounted because the problem occurred only in one eye.

COMMENT: Most emergency physicians are well aware of this phenomenon related to scopolamine patches, and it is one of the first etiologies to consider when patients present with an asymptomatic fixed and dilated pupil. Patches are used for motion sickness and could be used by a variety of patients, from the dizzy of vertiginous elderly to scuba divers. The pupillary dilation may be unilateral or bilateral, and it persists for two to four days. In most cases, no systemic symptoms will occur from ocular contamination by scopolamine. I treated, however, one elderly woman who became a bit forgetful and applied four patches during the day. She presented with an acute scopolamine-induced delirium (and bilateral dilated pupils).

Almost certainly, the dilated pupil is secondary to scopolamine locally contaminating the eye during patch application, but because the patch is always removed (sort of a reflex action that probably need not be done), the mechanism is not proven. Removing the patch or leaving it in place should have no effect on the pupil size. The manufacturer of the patch specifically recommends hand washing after applying or removing the patch. If the eye is contaminated when the patch is removed, or if an inquisitive child unknowingly gets hold of a discarded patch, the history becomes much more difficult to put together.

I find it interesting that one patient in this report underwent CT scanning and ophthalmological referral before anyone decided to look behind the ear for the scopolamine patch. Because they were so new in the early 1980s, it's difficult to believe the patients did not tell their physicians that they were used. As with eye drops, ointments, and over-the-counter preparations, patches are frequently not considered real medications by patients. Although it is reasonable for patients to fail to mention the use of a scopolamine patch, it's certainly embarrassing for the physician not to consider this as an etiology. One wonders about the completeness of the exam; they should at

capability of pilocarpine eye drops to distinguish between a local and distant etiology for pupillary dilation. Although patients with increased intracranial pressure severe enough to cause pupillary dilation (herniation) would not realistically be in the differential diagnosis of a walking, talking, and otherwise alert patient, the finding can easily lead the clinician on a wild goose chase looking for bizarre neurological problems. Therefore, one's ophthalmologic diagnostic armamentarium should always include the pilocarpine test.

One helpful hint that should be known by all clinicians is that the cap from eye drop dispensers are color coded. All medications that produce a dilated pupil have a red top, those that cause pupillary constriction have a green top, and antibiotics and other preparations have a clear, white, or other colored top.

ANISOCORIA FROM JIMSON WEED

Savitt DL, Roberts JR, Siegel EG
JAMA 1986;255(11):1439

The authors of this short report contribute an interesting addition to the differential diagnosis of a fixed and dilated pupil. They report the case of a 38-year-old man who presented to the ED with blurred vision and a fixed and dilated pupil. He had spent the morning trimming weeds with a mechanical weed trimmer. He was in good health, took no medication, and except for the blurred vision, he felt normal. Specifically there was no headache, nausea, or stiff neck. The exam was negative except for a fully dilated, nonreactive right pupil. The left pupil was normal. Pilocarpine drops had no effect on the involved eye. The patient recalled getting a piece of weed in his eye earlier that day during yard work, and from photographs he identified jimson weed (*Datura stramonium*) as a plant that grew in the area. A local anticholinergic effect, secondary to the belladonna alkaloids (atropine and scopolamine) found in this plant, was diagnosed, and the patient was discharged. Two days later he was normal.

To prove their clinical diagnosis, the authors instilled a jimson weed seed into the eye of a dog and also instilled drops of an extract made by boiling parts of the plant in

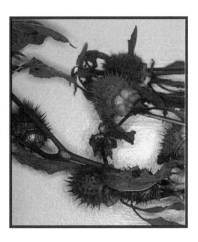

*The jimson weed plant (*Datura stramonium*) is ubiquitous in the United States. The seeds, leaf, and stem contain atropine/scopolamine alkaloids with potent anticholinergic effects. When ingested to get high, systemic anticholinergic effects can be seen, including bilateral dilated pupils. If parts of the plant inadvertently come in contact with the eye, a unilateral fixed and dilated pupil can result. See color plate in center well.*

least have looked for Battle's sign in the presence of a fixed and dilated pupil.

Instilling medication into the eye for a pharmacological effect is a well-known strategy in Munchausen's syndrome, and it is commonly used by the patient to simulate eye disease or intracranial pathology. Probably the most important message from this report is the diagnostic water. The animal demonstrated a fixed and dilated pupil in the treated eye, and the pupil did not constrict to 1% pilocarpine eye drops.

COMMENT: The jimson weed plant grows wild throughout the United States, and when ingested it is well known to cause classic systemic anticholinergic effects, including fixed and dilated pupils. Small doses are pleasurable and produce an LSD-like high. Large doses produce toxic delirium. Seeds can be eaten, or the plant can be boiled to make a tea. There would always be some systemic effects if both pupils were dilated due to plant ingestion, but a lack of systemic symptoms would be expected if the pupil were dilated from a local atropine-like effect. The seeds can be purchased through the mail for their euphoric or hallucinogenic effect. No part of the plant is a controlled substance. All portions of the plant, including the leaves and stems, contain atropine and scopolamine alkaloids.

This phenomenon has been reported by other authors, and although one cannot make the diagnosis of a local jimson weed effect by physical examination alone, the clinical scenario should suggest pharmacological mydriasis. As with scopolamine patches, this chemically dilated pupil will not constrict with local pilocarpine eye drops. I find it interesting that the emergency physicians in this article felt it unnecessary to contact an ophthalmologist and order a CT scan, where the ophthalmologist and neurosurgeon in the previous article felt compelled to do so. (Score one for us.)

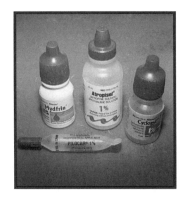

The screw-off caps of ophthalmologic drops are color-coded. Drops with red caps will dilate the pupil, those with green caps will constrict the pupil. Antibiotics and other preparations have a clear, white, or another color-coded cap. See color plate in center well.

WHEN INGESTED, JIMSON WEED CAUSES CLASSIC SYSTEMIC ANITCHOLINERGIC EFFECTS, INCLUDING FIXED, DILATED PUPILS

He had mild respiratory depression. After the left nostril was prepared with phenylephrine nose spray used to the shrink the mucosa, nasotracheal intubation was performed. It was originally not recognized that a small amount of the nose spray was inadvertently sprayed into the patient's left eye. Following successful intubation, gastric lavage was performed and the patient was stable. Re-examination revealed the left pupil to be fixed and dilated while the right pupil was normal and reactive. The level of benzodiazepine-induced coma had increased, and the patient was flaccid and unresponsive to deep pain. Because of the signs and symptoms, a diagnosis of cerebral herniation was made, and treatment was instituted to combat increased intracranial pressure. The patient was transferred on an emergency basis to a neurosurgical referral center by helicopter.

When the patient arrived at the referring institution, his level of consciousness had improved and a CT scan was normal. Laboratory evaluation confirmed a benzodiazepine and alcohol overdose. The patient awoke, but still had a unilateral fixed and dilated pupil. The pupil returned to normal in three to four hours. The contamination of the eye with the Neo-Synepherine nose spray was not recognized until a rather expensive and extensive investigation had occurred.

PSEUDO-CEREBRAL HERNIATION DUE TO PHENYLEPHRINE NASAL SPRAY

Roberts JR *N Engl J Med* 1989;320(26):1757

This is short report of yet another unusual pharmacological cause of a fixed and dilated pupil. This is actually a patient that I saw and reported, although it was a rather embarrassing situation. An unconscious 28-year-old man was brought to the ED suspected of having a benzodiazepine and alcohol overdose. The vital signs were normal, there were no signs of trauma, and initially the examination was nonfocal. The pupils were equal and reactive.

COMMENT: In my defense, other colleagues have related similar experiences. In this case, the physician was the culprit, but phenylephrine nose spray (Neo-Synepherine) is readily available over-the-counter and could easily be instilled by the patient. I have seen children who have had chemical mydriasis when they inoculated their eyes with this medication. I have also encountered a fixed and dilated pupil when TAC (tetracaine, epinephrine, and cocaine) solution inadvertently crept into the eye when it was used to anesthetize a supraorbital laceration. In that scenario, a child with obvious but minor head trauma was resting comfortably at nap time waiting for the physician. The scene caused a few minutes of anxiety in the ED staff when the fixed and dilated pupil was first discovered in the sleeping child with obvious head trauma.

Importantly, the pilocarpine eye drop test would likely be of little value in differentiating this particular cause of a fixed and dilated pupil. When the pupil is dilated because of an anticholinergic or atropine-like chemical, pilocarpine is competitively blocked from producing pupillary constriction. If the pupil is dilated because of an adrenergic mydriasis, such as would be seen with cocaine or Neo-Synepherine, the pilocarpine will produce a small pupil.

OPHTHALMOLOGY TRIVIA: CONJUNCTIVITIS AND CORNEAL EROSIONS

Conjunctivitis is frequently self-limited while corneal abrasions resulting from an epithelium torn loose from Bowman's layer may continue to recur

Fixed and dilated pupils may be seen following application of a scopolamine patch for motion sickness if some of the medication is inadvertently placed in the eye. A similar scenario is possible when the omnipresent jimson weed plant (seed, leaf, or stem) introduces enough atropine/scopolamine alkaloids into the eye to produce chemical mydriasis. Neo-Synepherine nose spray or TAC (tetracaine, epinephrine, and cocaine) local anesthetic solutions that gain access into the eye can also produce a chemical mydriasis.

Although a fixed and dilated pupil may suggest an intracerebral aneurysm, tumor, or CNS bleed, the specific diagnosis of local pupillary sphincter blockade by an anticholinergic medication is easily made in the emergency department if the affected pupil fails to constrict following the intraocular installation of 1% pilocarpine eye drops. This test may not work for local adrenergic causes of a dilated pupil (cocaine/phenylephrine), but it is specific for atropine-like blockade. Failure of a dilated pupil to respond to pilocarpine virtually rules out serious neurological causes.

This chapter consists of a potpourri of unrelated articles that make great cocktail party conversation and provide impressive trivia to dazzle the residents at your next conference.

INFLUENCE OF DRUG VEHICLE ON OCULAR CONTACT TIME OF SULFACETAMIDE SODIUM

Hanna J, et al *Ann Ophthalmol* 1985;17:560

The authors of this study attempted to evaluate the concentration of antibiotic solution that remained in the eye following installation of various concentrations of sulfacetamide sodium ointments and drops. Sulfacetamide is a commonly prescribed ocular antibiotic that is found in at least 24 ophthalmologic preparations. The drug is available as a solution and an ointment, and it's occasionally mixed with a steroid or vasoconstrictor. Numerous stabilizers, buffers, preservatives, and viscosity agents are used by various manufacturers. The authors were particularly concerned about the influence of drops versus ointment on the contact time of the antibiotics.

A standard amount of sulfacetamide sodium drops or ointment was applied to the conjunctiva of volunteers. A tear sample was taken before and for up to six hours after drug administration to assess drug concentration. Cultures of *Escherichia Coli* and *Staphylococcus aureus* were also tested in vitro against various concentrations of the antibiotic to determine what minimal inhibitory concentration (MIC) of sulfacetamide was required to inhibit the growth of these organisms. The concentration of the drops tested was 15% and 30%, and three ointment preparations were 10% sulfacetamide in various vehicles.

All of the sulfacetamide preparations promptly caused pain, irritation, and tearing when placed into the eye. The 30% drops produced intense tearing and ocular burning and even caused an unpleasant sensation in the throat when the preparation was swallowed. Overall, the ointments were less irritating than drops, but patients complained of an oily smell and unpleasant taste following ointment application. At first the ointment was greasy, but after a few blinks all preparations dissolved, and the solution was evenly spread throughout the eye.

As soon as 30 minutes following intraocular instillation of the 15% drops, a concentration of sulfacetamide in tears was below the level required to kill the test organisms. When the 30% solution was used, the concentration in tears remained high enough to be deemed effective against the bacteria for only two and a half hours. All three concentrations of ointment remained in therapeutic concentrations in the tears for approximately five and a half hours. The authors conclude that in order to obtain a MIC of topical sulfacetamide in the eye, drops would have to be applied every 30 minutes for the 15% solution and every two hours for the 30% concentration. Ointment, as a 10% preparation, could be applied four times a day to produce almost constant therapeutic drug levels in tears.

COMMENT: Eye drops are prescribed universally for signs and symptoms of conjunctivitis, and sulfacetamide-containing preparations are commonly used. There is no question that the 30% solution burns and is so irritating that most patients will not use this concentration more than once. If these drops are used in the ED immediately after a local anesthetic has been used, you probably won't appreciate how irritating the concentrated drops are. Therefore, if you are going to prescribe the drops, the 10-15% concentrations are most reasonable. These authors studied a 15% solution, but the 10% concentration is more widely available as Sodium Sulamyd and Opsulfa.

Numerous other authors have demonstrated that antibiotic drops maintain a concentration above the MIC for many bacteria for only a few minutes, yet drops seem to be universally effective when applied over much greater time intervals. I personally suggest using the drops every two hours for the first few days of acute conjunctivitis and prescribe, as my routine preparation of drops, 10% sulfacetamide. Drops are generally easier to apply than ointment if patients are treating themselves. Ointment can be messy and is more cumbersome because usually it has to be applied by someone else. Drops are also much easier to

OPHTHALMIC PREPARATIONS CONTAINING SULFACETAMIDE SODIUM

IsoptoCetamide	15% solution
Cetamide	10% ointment
IsoptoCetapred	10% solution, plus 0.25% prednisolone
Cetapred	10% ointment, plus 0.25% prednisolone
Bleph-10	10% solution
Blephamide	10% solution, plus prednisolone 0.2%, phenylephrine 0.12%
Blephamide SOP	10% solution, plus prednisolone 0.2%
Sulamyd 10	10% solution
Sulamyd 30	30% solution
Sulamyd ointment	10% ointment
Metimyd	10% solution, plus prednisolone 0.5%
Metimyd ointment	10% ointment, plus prednisolone 0.5%
Optimyd	10% ointment, plus prednisolone 0.5%
Vasosulf	15% solution, plus phenylephrine 0.12%
Vasocidin	10% solution, plus prednisolone 0.25%, phenylephrine 0.12%
Vasocidine ointment	10% ointment, plus prednisolone 0.5% phenylephrine 0.12%
Sulf-10 droppers	10% solution, in pure water
Sulphrin	10% solution, plus prednisolone 0.5% phenylephrine 0.12%
AK-cide	10% solution, plus prednisolone 0.5%

Source: Ann Ophthalmol *1985;17:560-4.*

get into a child's eye. If one really wants to be scientific, however, ointment should be prescribed instead of drops because of superior contact times.

Whenever the situation permits, I prescribe ointment instead of drops. The ointment melts quickly and is readily dispersed throughout the eye, but it must be placed directly on the inside lower lid (conjunctiva) or it will not get into the eye. A quick reflex blink or squint can keep all of the ointment from entering the eye so this is one disadvantage compared to drops. Once the topical anesthetic has worn off, ointment application may be more difficult. In addition, one must be careful not to injure the eye by touching it with the metal applicator tip of the ointment tube. Ointment seems to be the preferred antibiotic to place under an eye patch, but even with this approach, the drug does not remain in therapeutic concentrations until the next ED visit. Patches should be removed for the reapplication of ointment at least four times a day if one is truly concerned about infection. Ophthalmic neomycin does not burn initially, but it's best avoided because of a high incidence of hypersensitivity reactions. Polysporin ointment is a reasonable choice; it contains broad spectrum polymyxin and bacitracin, active against *Pseudomonas, H. influenza* and most Gram poitive organisms.

Although this study and others raise interesting questions, the findings are largely theoretical. Using antibiotic eye drops only four times a day is clearly not scientific because the eye is without an effective concentration of antibiotic for extended periods of time, but this regimen seems to cure the vast majority of patients with run-of-the-mill conjunctivitis. It's nice to look at MICs and antibiotic concentrations, but it's a big leap from the laboratory to clinical practice. One is readily reminded of urine cultures that show resistance to organisms in the laboratory, but the patient is repeatedly cured when supposedly ineffective antibiotics are given for only a few doses.

> NO CONVINCING DATA DEMONSTRATE THAT ANTIBIOTIC TREATMENT AFFECTS OUTCOME OR SHORTENS THE DURATION OF CONJUNCTIVITIS

EPIDEMIOLOGY AND DIAGNOSIS OF ACUTE CONJUNCTIVITIS AT AN INNER-CITY HOSPITAL

Fitch C, et al *Ophthalmology* 1989;96:1215

The authors of this prospective study begin their report by noting that the treatment of conjunctivitis is usually empiric, the disease is frequently self-limited, and in the majority of cases there is little need for extensive laboratory testing to determine an etiologic agent. There are occasional instances, however, where circumstances require a specific identification of the offending organism. The best example is neonatal conjunctivitis where *Chlamydia* and gonococcal conjunctivitis are more common. Chronic conjunctivitis unresponsive to standard medications also requires further laboratory investigation.

The authors attempted to find the specific cause of acute conjunctivitis in children and adults who presented to an inner-city hospital emergency center. To be eligible, patients had to be older than two months and have at least one eye that was red, inflamed, or irritated. The duration of symptoms had to be less than two weeks. Patients with obvious chemical, allergic, or foreign body conjunctivitis were excluded. Extensive culturing and staining were performed to evaluate a variety of bacterial and viral etiologies. Urethral samples were also obtained to assess the presence of *Chlamydia* organisms. Forty-five patients completed the study.

An etiology was proven in 34 of 45 cases (76%) and the remaining 11 patients (24%) could not be diagnosed with the study criteria. The following etiologies were found: viral, 36 percent; bacterial, 40 percent; and no definite cause, 24 percent. But the authors note that final assignment of an etiology, even when extensive lab tests were obtained, was difficult. All except one of the viral cases were due to adenovirus. One case of herpes simplex virus was discovered. Some cases yielded positive cultures for both bacterial and viral organisms. No cases of chlamydial conjunctivitis were found.

Bacterial cultures were positive in 43 of 45 cases, and more than half had more than one bacterial species isolated. The most common organism isolated was *Staphylococcus epidermidis. S aureus, Streptococcus pneumoniae, S viridans* and *Corynebacterium* were also isolated.

Gram and Giemsa stains of the tears were of minimal diagnostic help and were poor correlates to the final culture results. Importantly, there was no significant difference in the incidence, character, or degree of redness, itching, burning, type of discharge, photophobia, pain, crusting, blurred vision, or any other physical finding among the viral, bacterial, and nondiagnosed groups. In short, no clinical sign or symptom adequately distinguished viral from bacterial conjunctivitis. It was unclear whether the isolated organism actually caused the clinical findings

COMMENT: I like studies like this. It clearly limits the amount of time and effort required on the part of the emergency physician. It's a very small study, however, but surprisingly one of the few I could find on this relatively common pathology. In short, the data suggest that even with extensive laboratory evaluation, only three-quarters of cases of common conjunctivitis, thought to be of infectious origin, can be diagnosed with certainty. Even when expensive and time-consuming culture and staining tests are done, it's difficult to assign a specific etiology. Because you can't tell etiology by clinical appearance, one wonders how the authors accurately excluded allergic or other non-infectious causes of a red eye.

The lack of correlation between laboratory diagnosis and clinical diagnosis would support the strategy of most emergency physicians: treat all cases of conjunctivitis with antibiotics drops or ointments and reserve culturing, Gram's staining, and other diagnostic techniques for resistant cases or other special circumstances. One particular circumstance that should automatically prompt culturing would be a red eye in neonates, and it is imperative to include *Chlamydia* and gonorrhea cultures in these cases. The smear used to diagnose cervical *Chlamydia* is not accurate for an exudate from the eye because the gynecologic test requires cells. Actual viral culture medium should be used if one is searching for a virus. Patients who don't respond to antibiotics may also undergo diagnostic evaluation.

Even though less than half the cases of conjunctivitis are bacterial, it seems to be a waste of time, money, and effort to do anything other than prescribe antibiotics if your clinical diagnosis is conjunctivitis. It's also impossible to talk parents out of some prescription for pink eye so the solution to the red eye (unlike the diagnosis) is clear.

As a general rule, when I prescribe antibiotics for unilateral conjunctivitis, I also have the patient put the medication in the opposite eye every other time. I have seen no data to support this practice, and it doesn't make great theoretical sense if one considers the short half-life of topical antibiotics, but it seems like a good idea because conjunctivitis often spreads to the other side. The length of time that antibiotics should be used is also not well addressed in the literature. It makes sense to me to continue antibiotics for at least 24 hours after all signs and symptoms have disappeared.

I am amazed by the paucity of scientific investigation that has been done on this very common problem. Patients with red eyes that are irritated and have a watery or crusty discharge are automatically assumed to have an infectious etiology. This paper suggests that the clinical call is correct most of the time but not always. I am also amazed by the long-winded and seemingly erudite discussions in the literature that attempt to differentiate allergic, viral, and bacterial conjunctivitis based on certain signs and symptoms. Classically viral con-

RECURRENT CORNEAL EROSIONS

Patient:	31-year-old man
Date of presentation:	April 1979
Complaint:	Foreign body sensation in a red and painful eye
History:	Eye struck three days previously with fingernail
Diagnosis:	Slit lamp exam revealed minor corneal abrasion
Treatment:	Topical antibiotic
Outcome:	Healed uneventfully
Date of presentation:	June 1979
Complaint:	Foreign body sensation in a red and painful eye
History:	No history of trauma
Diagnosis:	De-epithelialization at site of previous injury
Treatment:	Patch
Outcome:	Healed uneventfully

Note: Patient returned with same complaint three additional times. Diagnosis made was epithelial breakdown at site of initial trauma. All healed with 24 hours.

Source: Ann Ophthalmol 1982,1113-4.

junctivitis presents with a clear, watery discharge, low-grade inflammation, a follicular appearance, and preauricular adenopathy. Bacterial conjunctivitis is supposedly associated with a mucopurulent discharge and more acute inflammation, including chemosis. Based on the literature, this distinction is probably bogus. Perhaps the compulsive ophthalmologist who deals with the red eye on a daily basis and spends hours behind a slit lamp can make a reasonable distinction of the various etiologies, but this article would suggest that an accurate etiologic diagnosis is probably impossible on clinical grounds alone.

These data would support a rather straightforward and simple approach to conjunctivitis in the ED unless there are extenuating circumstances. Many patients may be overtreated if all are reflexively treated with antibiotics, but therapy is generally benign. I have not seen convincing data demonstrating that antibiotic treatment affects ultimate outcome or shortens the duration of symptoms or illness, but it's probably difficult to do anything wrong in the treatment of simple conjunctivitis. The task of the emergency physician is to zero in on those cases where the neophyte might lump such things as glaucoma, herpetic infections, or corneal involvement into the same category as benign or self-limited conjunctivitis. (For a great discussion of the red eye, see *EM Clin NA* 1988;6(1):43.)

RECURRENT CORNEAL EROSIONS
Newsom S, et al *Ann Ophthal* 1982;14(12):1113

This short article highlights a problem that can be quite perplexing unless one is aware of the entity. It describes a syndrome of recurrent corneal erosions, an uncommon but well documented condition that may present to the ED. The authors describe the case of a 31-year-old man who was seen for a complaint of a foreign body sensation in a red and painful eye. His eye had been struck three days previously with a fingernail, and slit lamp examination initially revealed a seemingly minor corneal abrasion. The patient was treated with a topical antibiotic, and he healed uneventfully. Two months later, he presented with similar symptoms but without a history of new trauma.

Examination revealed an area of de-epithelialization at the site of the previous injury. The patient was treated conservatively and appeared to heal, yet returned on multiple

occasions with similar findings and a similar history that lacked new trauma. Each time, the erosions healed within 24 hours with conservative therapy.

This case report describes recurrent episodes of corneal erosion from spontaneous breakdown of the corneal epithelium. Most patients have a history of a previous uncomplicated minor corneal abrasion that seemed to heal well. Classically the patient will awaken in the morning with photophobia, tearing, and pain, classic signs of a corneal abrasion but without a history of trauma. Examination reveals an epithelial defect that is easily seen with corneal staining, but the pathology is more complicated than a simple abrasion. In essence, the epithelium has torn loose from Bowman's layer because the result of faulty healing of the original injury, resulting in loss of epithelial adhesion to the corneal basement membrane. The result is poor epithelial adhesion. Overnight the eye becomes dry, the lid "sticks" to the fragile epithe-

> FOR CONJUNCTIVITIS, PRESCRIBING DROPS WITH 10-15% ANTIBIOTIC SOLUTION IS MOST REASONABLE

CAUSE OF CONJUNCTIVITIS IN AN INNER CITY HOSPITAL

Viral etiology	36%
Bacterial etiology	40%
No cause found	24%

Source: Ophthalmol *1989;6:1215.*

lium, and the erosion is produced when the eye is abruptly opened.

The initial injury is usually from a fingernail, paper, a hair brush, or a tree branch, but there are no characteristics that could predict a future problem. In essence there is a faulty epithelium adhesion that holds up for a short period of time — months to years — only to break down spontaneously.

The main objectives in treating this recurrent erosion are first to recognize the problem, and then to institute therapy to reform a new basement membrane complex. Such therapies include hypertonic sodium chloride ointment, debriding, and a variety of topical preparations. The long-term use of soft contact lens also has been suggested.

COMMENT: This entity has been well described in an extensive review by Kenyon (*Int Ophthalmol Clin* 1979; 19:169). Recurrent corneal erosion is more of a curiosity than serious pathology for the emergency physician, and special therapy is best directed by a consultant. If you are unaware of this phenomenon, you may question the patient's history or otherwise be puzzled by the presentation. Symptoms that first start upon waking and progress during the day are classic. Most of the time, one assumes that the patient injured his eye during sleep, and the strange history is dismissed without any further attention.

There is little that the emergency physician can do to anticipate or prevent this syndrome. The initial injury appears to be rather benign and is treated in the standard fashion. Even recurrent erosions seem to heal quickly so they can be unappreciated for a long time. If the patient sees a different physician each time, it is likely that this diagnosis will be quite delayed or may never be made in the ED.

ACUTE NARROW-ANGLE GLAUCOMA: UNDERSTANDING THE BASICS

Primary open-angle glaucoma is the most common type of glaucoma, and it is a leading cause of blindness in this country

Acute narrow-angle glaucoma is an uncommon but well-known serious eye problem that may present to the emergency department. The pathologic process is also known as acute-angle closure glaucoma. It is a true emergency and an entity that is clearly distinct from the type of glaucoma known to the general public and the type usually encountered in the ophthalmologist's office. The majority of patients with this rarer type of glaucoma are almost always unaware of their congenital problem until some type of medical intervention inadvertently precipitates an ophthalmologic crisis. Occasionally the culprit is the nonophthalmologist physician who unwarily instills topical mydriatic agents into the eye for a relatively benign problem or to facilitate fundoscopy. The administration of systemic drugs with mydriatic side effects is also occasionally culpable. It is essential that emergency physicians be cognizant of the diagnosis and therapy of acute narrow angle glaucoma because failure to recognize it and failure to institute proper and timely emergency therapy can lead to blindness. This month's discussion will focus on the physiology of acute narrow angle glaucoma and how to identify patients at risk.

PREVENTION OF IATROGENIC ACUTE NARROW ANGLE GLAUCOMA

Bresler MJ, Hoffman RS
Ann Emerg Med 1981;10(10):535

Although this article is 15 years old, it's an excellent review of the etiology of acute narrow angle glaucoma (ANAG). The discussion also includes a description of a rather simple bedside technique that can be used in the ED to identify patients at risk for developing ANAG. This test should be done prior to inducing mydriasis in most patients. Mydriatic agents, such as phenylephrine (Neo-Synephrine) and atropine-like eye drops (Cyclogyl, Mydriacyl), are often used in the ED to facilitate fundoscopic examination or to treat various types of minor ocular pathology such as acute iritis.

The authors note that the term glaucoma refers to a group of diseases that have a common pathophysiology: increased intraocular pressure. Emergency physicians will rarely diagnose primary glaucoma, and medical intervention is rarely emergent, but failure to quickly recognize and expeditiously treat acute-angle closure glaucoma can lead to permanent loss of vision. The underlying pathophysiology of increased intraocular pressure in all types of glaucoma is an impeded outflow of aqueous humor from the anterior chamber. Normally, aqueous humor that is formed by the ciliary body in the posterior chamber flows throughout the anterior and posterior chamber. The fluid's path to the anterior chamber from its origin in the posterior chamber is through the pupil. In the anterior chamber, the liquid ultimately exits the eye and enters the venous system through a network of collecting channels (Schlemm's canal). The opening to this drainage system is at the junction of the root of the iris and the peripheral cornea. When the outflow of aqueous humor is blocked or hampered, glaucoma results (Figure 1).

Primary open-angle glaucoma is slow and insidious and is the most common type of glaucoma. It is a leading cause of blindness in this country. This type of glaucoma is chronic, slowly progressive, bilateral, and painless. Patients with primary open-angle glaucoma can safely undergo pupillary dilation. Primary glaucoma is idiopathic in origin.

Patients with an abnormal anatomic predisposition, specifically a narrow-angle at the outflow apparatus, do not have classic glaucoma, but can experience acute glaucoma. Narrow-angle glaucoma is not subtle; it's an acute and very painful phenomenon. In the absence of pupillary dilation, patients with an anatomically narrow anterior angle are only at theoretical risk for glaucoma, and they are asymptomatic. They have normal vision and essentially normal-appearing eyes except that the anterior chamber is noted to be shallow if it is evaluated. The drainage angle is functional but narrow. This angle is further narrowed when pupillary dilation causes the base of the iris to unfold in the anterior chamber angle and block the outflow tract, resulting in acute obstruction to the drainage of aqueous humor. Aqueous humor production continues unchecked, resulting in a sudden rise in intraocular pressure. The end result is blurred vision, severe pain, and often other systemic findings such as nausea and vomiting. Abdominal pain, diaphoresis, and bradycardia have also been reported.

Importantly, pharmacologic dilation of the pupil is a glaucoma-precipitating event only in patients with a shallow anterior chamber, and it is only this group of patients in whom mydriasis produces the problem. The purpose of this article is to assist the clinician in evaluating the depth of the anterior chamber by a simple bedside transillumination test. Theoretically, this test will identify patients at risk for acute glaucoma and will therefore alert the clinician that mydriasis may be harmful. Measurement of baseline intraocular pressure would be of no value in detecting patients at risk for acute narrow-angle glaucoma because prior to an attack they do not have increased intraocular pressure.

The test that is described requires only a penlight, and it's easily performed on even unconscious or uncooperative

CHARACTERISTICS OF GLAUCOMA

Type
Open angle glaucoma (primary)

Incidence
• Most common type of glaucoma
• Leading cause of blindness
• Bilateral process

Risk Factor
• Old age
• Positive family history
• Nearsighted

Pathophysiolocy
• Idiopathic rise in intraocular pressure, unrelated to decreased outflow of aqueous humor
• Optic nerve is slowly compressed with resultant atrophy

Course
• Slow, chronic insidious, progressive increase in intraocular
• Takes years to develop

Symptoms
• Painless, initially no visual symptoms, may see halo around lights
• Usually diagnosed by patient on routine eye exam by pressure/characteristic

Visual Loss
• Begins at periphery, progresses
• Slow and often not recognized by patient
• Visual acuity is normal until late in disease

Findings
• Eye appears normal
• Anterior chamber
• Cornea is clear
• Intraocular pressure increased, fundoscopic findings range 20 30 mmHg
• Pupil reacts normally/no redness

Source: James R. Roberts

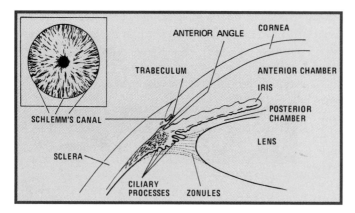

FIGURE 1. *Ocular anatomy with inset showing circumferential placement of Schlemm's canal.*

patients. Each eye is tested separately. The light source is held lateral to the eye being tested, with the light beam directed horizontally across the iris. In normal individuals, the entire iris is illuminated by the light, signifying a normal anterior chamber. If the anterior chamber is shallow, the light will only illuminate that half of the iris (the temporal area) that is adjacent to the light (Figure 2). Part or all of the opposite half (the nasal area) remains dark because the iris, in its shallow chamber, lies anterior to its normal position and obstructs the passage of light beyond the pupil. The beam of the light source must be properly placed, exactly perpendicular to the visual axis. Errors in interpretation may occur if the light beam is incorrectly aimed.

COMMENT: There are two basic types of glaucoma: open-angle and narrow-angle glaucoma. These two entities actually have relatively little in common except that the final common pathway leading to vision loss is increased intraocular pressure. In essence, however, they are completely different diseases. Primary open-angle glaucoma is the most common type of glaucoma, and it is a leading cause of blindness in this country. It is a slow, chronic, insidious, progressive increase in intraocular pressure, and a bilateral process. This type of glaucoma is painless, and it has no systemic symptoms. The external eye looks normal to both the patient and the physician, and it is usually diagnosed by abnormal fundoscopic findings or abnormal intraocular pressures discovered on a routine eye examination. The intraocular pressure in open-angle glaucoma is elevated but generally not to the extent as is seen with acute glaucoma. This is the type of glaucoma that occurs with old age, but there is a family history of glaucoma in many

patients and it is more common in those who are nearsighted. The rise in intraocular pressure is idiopathic in nature but related to a decreased outflow of aqueous humor. The pathophysiology is chronic and progressive pressure on the optic nerve results in optic nerve atrophy and vision loss. Importantly, visual acuity is generally normal until the late stages of the disease, so merely testing visual acuity will not pick up most early cases. To make things even more insidious, primary open-angle glaucoma initially causes peripheral vision loss only and slowly progresses centrally. Patients can adapt to this slow peripheral vision loss until a surprisingly large visual field loss is finally documented. Occasionally patients will complain of a halo around lights, but it is truly a silent disease.

Closed-angle glaucoma is much less common, and it is actually not even bona fide glaucoma until some precipitating event suddenly increases intraocular pressure.

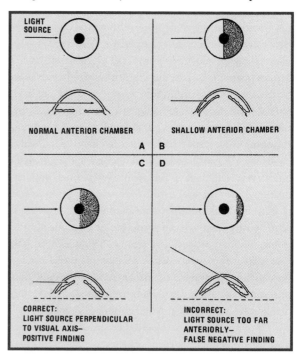

FIGURE 2. *Anterior chamber depth and transillumination test. (A) Normal anterior chamber with negative transillumination test. (B) Shallow anterior chamber with positive transillumincation test. (C) Shallow anterior chamber with correctly placed light source yielding true positive test result. (D) Shallow anterior chamber with incorrectly placed light source yielding false negative test result.*

Patients with closed-angle glaucoma essentially have normal eyes, including normal vision and normal intraocular pressure until the pathology makes itself known in an acute manner. These patients have a congenital deformity where the anterior chamber is shallow. It is more common in far-sighted individuals, and it occurs more commonly in the elderly as the lens enlarges. Acute angle-closure glaucoma is generally a problem in the 40-50 year old age group, younger in age by a few decades when compared to open-angle glaucoma, but the risk increases with age as the lens enlarges. There is a hereditary component. Importantly, if one were to evaluate the fundus and measure the intraocular pressure in the absence of symptoms, they would be normal.

When the pupil is dilated in susceptible individuals, the iris contracts, bunches up around the drainage network, and acutely blocks the egress of aqueous humor. Most patients have no idea that they are at risk, but they quickly realize something is wrong when an acute attack is precipitated. Some patients may give you a history of headaches that are initiated by darkness, the classic description being headache or eye pain when the pupil dilates after going into a movie theater. Such questions, however, are often forgotten during the ED history. Curiously, the eye pain often subsides when the patient goes to sleep because the pupil will constrict, the angle opens, and the intraocular pressure decreases.

When the pupil is widely dilated, most commonly with eye drops, the intraocular pressure rises rapidly (usually over a number of hours) and severe symptoms are quick to follow. Acute glaucoma is almost always a unilateral process even if a systemic process is culprit. Patients usually describe severe headaches, vomiting, and blurred vision, although curiously they can also complain of abdominal pain. Bradycardia and diaphoresis have been described (vagally mediated?) and the severity of the non-eye symptoms can thwart the correct diagnosis. This diagnosis is easy to miss! The headache and systemic symptoms are often so severe and so impressive that the symptom of blurred vision is underappreciated by both clinician and patient. In its early stages, the eye itself can look deceptively benign. The most common misdiagnoses are intracranial hemorrhage, vascular headache, brain tumor, sinusitis or a variety of nonophthalmological entities. While the patient with open-angle glaucoma has a normal-appearing eye, patients with full-blown acute glaucoma will have a cloudy cornea, a diffusely reddened eye (the most intense redness is around the limbus), and the pupil

CHARACTERISTICS OF GLAUCOMA

Type
Closed angle glaucoma (also angle closure

Incidence
• Uncommon
• Usually unilateral

Risk Factor
• Shallow anterior chamber (congenital)
• Farsighted
• Old age: 40-60 (lens enlarges)
• Hereditary

Pathophysiolocy
• Sudden block of drainage of aqueous humor when angle closes
• Precipitated by mydriasis, usually iatrogenic

Course
• Patient is asymptomatic, normal vision and normal intraocular pressure until attack is precipitated
• Takes few hours to days after myadriasis to precipitate

Symptoms
• History may include headaches precipitated by darkness
• Sudden onset of severe headache, eye pain, vomiting, abdominal pain, bradycardia, diaphoresis
• Severity of attack and systemic symptoms prompt misdiagnosis

Visual Loss
• Vision is blurred, looking through frosted
• Halos around lights
• Visual activity decreased markedly and suddenly

Findings
• Eye appears abnormal
• Cloudy cornea
• Pupil often dilated and poorly reactive
• Redness mainly around limbus
• Ocular pressures exceed 30mmHg
• Eye may be tender or feel hard

Source: James R. Roberts

is usually slightly dilated and poorly reactive. In the early stages, these eye findings are not prominent and could be easily missed unless one is thinking about this disease.

The ocular pressure is usually very high, generally greater than 40 mm Hg when measured by tonometry. It has been stated that eye will be tender or feel hard (like a

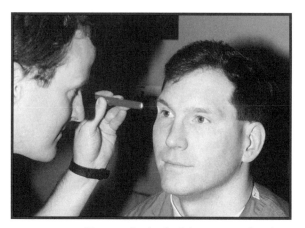

FIGURE 3. *To assess the depth of the anterior chamber and hence the potential for pupillary dilation to precipitate acute glaucoma, a penlight is held laterally and a light beam is directed medially. To avoid false testing, the light beam should be exactly perpendicular at the line of sight when the patient looks forward (parallel to the coronal plane of the face). The light beam should pass through the medial and lateral canthus simultaneously and the amount of iris that is illuminated is observed. See color plate in center well.*

marble), but these are inaccurate ways to diagnose acute angle-closure glaucoma. The cornea becomes cloudy or hazy because it is edematous. The condition often gives the sensation that the patient is looking through frosted glass rather than blurred vision or double vision. The intense

redness, due to conjunctival edema, is noted around the limbus and is quite characteristic. Perilimbal injection is also called a ciliary flush, and this pattern of conjunctival redness should alert the clinician that there is something wrong with the cornea. Viral or bacterial conjunctivitis will produce peripheral redness, sparing the limbus.

The test described in this report is relatively simple and straightforward, and it should be mastered and routinely practiced by any clinician who places mydriatic agents into the eye. Importantly, this test only delineates patients at risk and does not diagnose acute angle-closure glaucoma. It is important to direct the beam of the light exactly perpendicular to the line of sight. If the flashlight is held parallel to the floor, lateral to the eye being tested, and aimed first at the ipsilateral ear and then brought anterior and aimed at the base of the nose or medical canthus, most errors will be eliminated. The light source should be directed from lateral canthus to medical canthus and never be anterior to the frontal plane of the face (Figure 3). It's important to note, however, that this test is not foolproof and is operator dependent.

Although one should always ask the patient about a history of glaucoma, most patients with a narrow anterior chamber will not be aware of their dangerous predisposition. Patients with the more common open-angle glaucoma are more likely to know their diagnosis, but these patients can have their eyes safely dilated. It is a common misconception that no patient with glaucoma can undergo mydriasis; in fact, the only patients at risk are those with shallow anterior chambers. Occasionally patients will be tangentially told about their predisposition by an ophthalmologist, usually with a warning that doctors should not dilate their eyes. Some patients will offer subtle symptoms, such as complaining about visual problems (halos) or pain when they are in a dark room (as the pupil dilates), but most will not have a clue about their potential problem.

THERAPY FOR ACUTE ANGLE-CLOSURE GLAUCOMA

The local effects of nebulized medications used for the treatment of asthma/COPD can precipitate acute glaucoma

Although acute angle-closure glaucoma and primary open-angle glaucoma both have increased intraocular pressure as their etiology, the diseases are distinctly different in onset, clinical presentation, and prognosis. Emergency physicians do not become involved in either the diagnosis or treatment of open-angle glaucoma, and most of us probably see patients every day with this entity but fail to recognize it.

Acute angle-closure glaucoma, on the other hand, is an ophthalmologic emergency that can be caused by a physician dilating the pupil of an individual with a shallow anterior chamber, resulting in an abrupt rise in intraocular pressure. This type of glaucoma is not a subtle problem; it's very symptomatic, and quickly brings patients to the ED. The unfortunate and often confusing issue is that acute glaucoma is so symptomatic and the eye findings and eye complaints are often deceptively mild at first that both patient and physician tend to look for nonophthalmological pathology. In the elderly with severe headache, vomiting, and blurred vision, higher on the differential diagnosis list are intracranial hemorrhage, brain tumor, CNS infection, and vascular headache.

A simple bedside test can identify patients at risk for acute glaucoma by demonstrating a narrow anterior chamber, the specific anatomical predisposition for acute angle-closure glaucoma. In concluding the discussion of acute glaucoma, I'll look at a relatively newly described precipitant: the local effects of nebulized medications used for the treatment of asthma or chronic obstructive pulmonary disease (COPD). Finally, the treatment of acute angle-closure glaucoma is discussed with a particular reference to those procedures that should be immediately instituted in the ED.

> ### ACUTE ANGLE-CLOSURE GLAUCOMA AS A COMPLICATION OF COMBINED BETA-AGONIST AND IPRATROPIUM BROMIDE THERAPY IN THE EMERGENCY DEPARTMENT
>
> Hall S *Ann Emerg Med* 1994;23(4):884

This interesting report may be a harbinger of future problems, and the concept should be recognized by emergency physicians. The author describes a single case of bilateral acute angle-closure glaucoma (AACG) following outpatient asthma therapy in the ED. In this report a 66-year-old woman presented to the ED complaining of a severe headache and loss of vision in both eyes of eight hours' duration. She also reported nausea and a sandpaper-like sensation in both eyes. She had been treated in the ED 36 hours previously for an exacerbation of asthma, and her therapy consisted of four doses of nebulized albuterol (Proventil, Ventolin) and four puffs of ipratropium bromide (Atrovent) from a metered dose inhaler. The therapy was successful, and she was free of wheezing, discharged, and started on a prednisone taper. She had no eye complaints at discharge. There was a past history of acute angle-closure glaucoma, and she had received an iridotomy. She was on no ophthalmologic medication, but she was taking multiple maintenance asthma medicines upon presentation and after discharge.

EPs PROBABLY SEE OPEN ANGLE GLAUCOMA EVERY DAY BUT FAIL TO RECOGNIZE IT

On examination, she was alert but quite hypertensive (254/122 mmHg). There was no fever, and the neck was supple. Positive findings included photophobia, significantly decreased vision in both eyes that allowed her only to count fingers or detect motion. One pupil was fixed in mid-position, and the cornea was clouded. Tonometry demonstrated significantly elevated intraocular pressures and ophthalmologic consultation confirmed acute angle-closure glaucoma despite the previous iridotomy. She received standard therapy for acute glaucoma (mannitol, beta blockers, eye drops, and pilocarpine drops) and underwent emergent bilateral iridotomy. She subsequently did well.

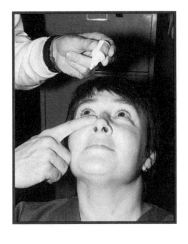

The authors note that many elderly patients have undiagnosed narrow-angle glaucoma, and they are asymptomatic until the pupils are dilated. Usually the problem is precipitated by eye drops that dilate the pupil, but previous authors have documented that beta-adrenergic agents and ipratropium bromide can precipitate acute glaucoma in susceptible individuals. Acute angle-closure glaucoma (AACG) has been reported with each agent alone, but the combined therapy with the beta agonist and an anticholinergic agent is more common and the drugs are thought to be synergistic.

Previously available only via a metered dose inhaler, ipratropium bromide is now available as a solution for use in a nebulizer. It is predominantly an anticholinergic (atropine-like) bronchodilator that is used for emphysema and asthma. Ten previous cases of AACG following nebulized ipratropium were documented by the author, and most of them occurred when combined with albuterol. Curiously, all previous case reports have been described in hospitalized patients undergoing maintenance therapy, and this is the first report where such an event occurred following short-term treatment and discharge from the ED. Importantly, this patient was totally asymptomatic from a glaucoma standpoint upon discharge and did not experience symptoms immediately.

Although most patients are unaware of their predisposition for AACG, the author suggests that before administering these types of asthma medications to patients at risk, one should ask questions about a history of glaucoma or symptoms suggestive of previously undiagnosed acute attacks. A penlight may be used to estimate the anterior chamber depth (described in

Prior to the instillation of eye drops, the medial punctum is occluded with gentle finger pressure and held closed for a few minutes. This will limit the systemic absorption of medication by decreasing the amount of drug drained by the nasolacrimal duct. Some eye drops, such as beta blockers (Timolol) can cause significant systemic effects, especially after the repeated administration required to treat acute glaucoma. Some authors suggest tightly shutting the eyes as an alternative to finger pressure. See color plate in center well.

the previous chapter), but this is not always reliable and is operator dependent. In AACG, patients are asymptomatic until the pupil is dilated, the outflow of aqueous humor is blocked, and intraocular pressure quickly rises, so measuring intraocular pressure prior to therapy is not helpful. In addition, the fundoscopic examination will be normal in the absence of symptoms.

It is generally believed that the pupillary dilation occurs secondary to local rather than systemic effects of the medications. Minimizing the amount of mist that is available to the eye may be beneficial. Pretreating patients at risk with prophylactic pilocarpine or choosing medications that do not cause pupil dilation are other options. However, it is often impossible to choose alternative agents when faced with a patient with significant bronchospasm. Using protective eye wear or administering the drugs via a hand-held system instead of a face mask may also decrease ocular exposure to medication.

COMMENT: With the recent availability of ipratropium solutions, this anticholinergic (atropine-like) medication is often mixed with a beta agonist to treat bronchospasm. A significant amount of nebulized medication may inadvertently enter the eye as the patient takes a break from the treatment, allowing the nebulized drug to flow onto the face. I have commonly observed the tired asthmatic holding the steaming nebulizer next to the face, bathing the eyes with the medicated mist. Ipratropium is a drug that is commonly used for older patients with COPD exacerbations, and this is the population at highest risk for acute glaucoma.

Acute glaucoma can be a difficult diagnosis in the ED. Any elderly patient who presents with headache, decreased vision, and vomiting would probably be first investigated for a CNS infection, subdural hematoma, subarachnoid hemorrhage, or some other serious intracranial pathology. This patient's significant blood pressure elevation could have easily prompted the diagnosis of a hypertensive crisis. Although acute glaucoma will eventually cause a red eye with a cloudy cornea and a significant decrease in vision, in its early stages ocular findings may be quite subtle and easily overshadowed by vomiting and headache. AACG should be in a differential diagnosis of any elderly patient with severe headache, and it should be particularly high on the list when the patient complains of any eye symptoms.

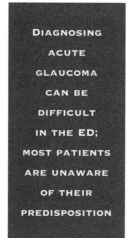

DIAGNOSING ACUTE GLAUCOMA CAN BE DIFFICULT IN THE ED; MOST PATIENTS ARE UNAWARE OF THEIR PREDISPOSITION

The author's suggestion to limit ocular exposure to mists that cause pupil dilation are probably reasonable, as is the use of a penlight to detect a shallow anterior chamber prior to drug administration. But AACG is clearly an unusual event, and it's probably not standard of care to evaluate all elderly patients with asthma or COPD with penlight examination prior to instituting bronchodilator therapy. It is key to make the correlation of these agents with the symptoms of acute angle-closure glaucoma should patients present with suspicious symptoms. It is surprising that this patient presented so late (34 hours) after ED therapy, but the drug regimen at home was not detailed. The bilateral process suggests some systemic effect of the drugs in producing mydriasis. There is no reason why this episode couldn't have occurred from the repeated home use of the bronchodilators, so the previous ED visit may not be totally responsible and is certainly not a prerequisite for this scenario.

MANAGEMENT OF ACUTE ELEVATED INTRAOCULAR PRESSURE: PART II, TREATMENT

Kooner KS, Zimmerman TJ
Ann Ophthalmol 1988;20(3):87

This is one of few journal articles I could find in the recent literature that describes the management of acutely elevated intraocular pressure in acute angle-closure glaucoma. (See also *Ann Ophthalmol* 1984;16(12):1101.) Many emergency medicine textbooks contain the same information, and I have reviewed the overall therapy in the accompanying table.

The authors note that the management of angle-closure glaucoma should be aggressive regardless of the degree of elevation of intraocular pressure. The treatment consists of four basic interventions, all instituted simultaneously. Importantly, medical therapy is only a temporizing measure until definitive surgery, in the form of a peripheral iridectomy, is performed.

The authors note that pain, nausea, and vomiting may require antiemetics, narcotics, or sedatives, before or during glaucoma therapy. Topical beta blockers are used to decrease aqueous humor production and to facilitate corneal penetration of pilocarpine. Apparently beta blockers change the corneal epithelial lining to some degree and allow pilocarpine to penetrate more readily. Although pilocarpine should be instituted simultaneously, it may not effectively enter the anterior chamber until intraocular pressures are lowered. In addition, the ischemia and resultant paralysis of the pupillary sphincter from the increased intraocular pressure may block the miotic effect of pilocarpine (*Arch Ophthalmol* 1972;87(1):21). In rare instances, pilocarpine will actually worsen an attack by increasing the relative pupillary block (a complex mechanism that I don't understand and one that cannot be readily anticipated). Carbonic anhydrase inhibitors can be given by any route in order to decrease aqueous humor production. The standard drug for this indication is acetazolamide. Mannitol or glycerin are osmotic diuretics that rapidly decrease intraocular pressure.

COMMENT: The treatment of acute glaucoma is relatively easy; it's the diagnosis that's difficult. One caveat that should be emphasized is that beta blocker and pilocarpine eye drops can produce systemic side effects when used repeatedly for the treatment of acute glaucoma. Pilocarpine can cause cholinergic effects, and beta blockers are well known to cause bradycardia and bron-

EMERGENCY DEPARTMENT TREATMENT OF ACUTE ANGLE-CLOSURE GLAUCOMA
All treatments are instituted simultaneously

Agent	Regimen	Rationale	Comment
Pilocarpine eye drops (2%-4%)	One drop every 15 minutes for two hours, then every 4 hours as needed to produce miosis,* allowing aqueous humor to exit	Miosis pulls the peripheral iris from the trabecular meshwork and opens the drainage angle and canal,	• May not be effective until other agents lower intraocular pressure • Frequent use may cause systemic cholinergic symptoms
Timolol eye drops (0.5%) (Timoptic) or Betaxol eye drops 0.5% (Betopic) Cardioselective beta blocker that may be safer in pulmonary disease	1 drop initially; repeat in 10 minutes, then hourly* 1 drop initially; repeat in 10 minutes, then every 12 hours*	Lowers intraocular pressure and decreases aqueous humor production	• Intraocular pressure drops within 30-60 minutes • May facilitate penetration of pilocarpine; may cause significant systemic effects (bronchospasm and bradycardia)
Acetazolamide (Diamox)	500 mg STAT (oral, IM, IV), followed by 250 mg every 6 hours	A carbonic anhydrase inhibitor that decreases production of aqueous humor	• Can cause paresthesias of fingers, hyperchloremic metabolic acidosis. Use with caution in sulfa allergic patients
Mannitol 20%	1-2 grams/kg IV over half hour	Osmotic agent that lowers intraocular pressure and decreases aqueous humor production	• An alternative is oral glycerol (50%): 1-1.5 gm/kg or 1.5-3 ml/kg
Antiemetics, narcotics, sedatives	As needed	Symptomatic relief	• Pain, vomiting can be severe
Telephone	Call ophthalmologist	Laser surgery (iridectomy) usually required	

Occlude punctum to decrease systemic absorption.

Source: James R. Roberts, MD

chospasm in susceptible individuals. Up to 80 percent of the dose of drug administered by eye drops can enter the general circulation via absorption from the nasal fossa. Heart block, significant bradycardia, congeestive heart failure, exacerbation of asthma, and intermittent claudication have all been reported after the use of beta blocker eye drops.

It is generally advised that the medial punctum be occluded with a finger for three to four minutes following the installation of these drops in an effort to avoid uptake by the tear drainage system, and eventual absorption into the systemic circulation from the nasal mucosa. This relatively simple but important adjunct is frequently omitted, and one can quickly notice systemic side effects when these medications are repeatedly used in an effort to control intraocular pressure. As an alternative to finger pressure, some authors suggest that the patient tightly shut the eyes after drop administration.

SECTION IV

SWALLOWED FOREIGN BODIES

FISH BONES IN THE THROAT

Fish bones in the oropharynx, larynx, or esophagus are a serious problem that cannot be ignored

*P*atients frequently present to the ED complaining of a sharp pain in the throat or trouble swallowing after eating fish. Usually each is convinced that there is a bone stuck in his throat. This can be a frustrating problem for the physician in terms of diagnosis and for the patient in terms of anxiety or symptomatic relief. A foreign body of the oropharynx, larynx, or esophagus is clearly a serious problem that cannot be ignored, and the literature is filled with case reports of disastrous consequences, such as aortic or GI perforation or septic complications from either a known or totally unexpected foreign body.

This is a discussion of the clinical approach to patients that may have a fish bone lodged in their throat. Some cases can be handled entirely by the emergency physician, although ENT referral is commonly required. Even though this is a frequently encountered scenario, the literature addresses it only sporadically. In fact, when I reviewed two recent ENT books, the topic was not even discussed.

FISH BONES IN THE THROAT

Knight LC, Lesser TH *Arch Emerg Med* 1989; 6:13

This is an informative study of adult patients who presented to the ED with persistent sharp pain in the throat after eating fish. The authors emphasize that retained fish bones can result in serious septic complications and note a previous report where two patients died from such a retained foreign body (*BMJ* 1984;289:424). The purpose of the report was to determine the site and frequency of impacted fish bones, to define the role of x-ray, and to determine the need for endoscopy.

Their protocol dictated that patients who had total dysphagia be referred for immediate endoscopy, but 71 patients with nonserious symptomatology were identified and included in the trial. All patients had direct examination of the mouth and oropharynx and mirror examination of the pharynx and larynx. The neck was examined for tenderness, masses, or emphysema, and all patients had a soft tissue lateral neck x-ray. If a bone was seen on the radiograph, the patient was referred directly for ENT evaluation. If the clinical examination and x-ray were negative, the patient was discharged and told to return for ENT follow-up in 48 hours, if their symptoms persisted. Two days later they were again examined. It's unclear from this report whether they were all endoscoped at this revisit. All were endoscoped if the pain persisted for two weeks.

Interestingly, only 15 of 71 patients (21%) had a fish bone identified at any time. Fourteen (93%) of these bones were identified on the initial ED examination, and, surprisingly, 13 of them were readily seen by direct or mirror examination. The bone was impacted in the base of the tongue in eight patients, in the tonsil in three, and in the posterior pharyngeal wall in two. All were easily removed under direct vision.

Only five of 15 bones (33%) were visible on plain x-ray. In 56 of the original 71 patients, a bone was not identified, and patients were told to return in 48 hours if their symptoms persisted. The symptoms usually resolved, but 15 patients (27%) had persistent complaints at 48 hours. None had a bone subsequently identified and all but four were asymptomatic in two weeks. Follow-up failed to discover an etiology in these four individuals. Two of the four patients had symptoms at three months after a negative endoscopy.

In this study, the majority of patients presenting with symptoms of an impacted fish bone had no demonstrated pathology, and their symptoms spontaneously resolved in 48 hours. The authors postulate that their symptoms were due to a minor abrasion or other local trauma, but they did not totally discount the fact that a fish bone could

Some fish bones can be easily removed in the ED, and most patients can localize the general area where a fish bone has lodged. This patient consistently pointed to the left submandubular area, and a fish bone was found impaled in the left tonsil, almost exactly where the patient indicated. See color plate in center well.

have been the culprit, yet passed spontaneously within the first 48 hours.

The most common area for the bone to lodge was the base of the tongue or the tonsil. The authors caution that saliva strands can either obscure or impersonate a fish bone, and they advise caution when attempting to extricate the suspected bone. The authors believe that the plain x-ray is of limited value in a presence of a normal physical

examination. One may see indirect evidence of a fish bone (soft tissue swelling or subcutaneous air), but these radiographic signs may take 12 hours to develop fully.

It's concluded that a fish bone can be found in only one of five patients that present with symptomatology. But if the bone is present, it's usually easily visible in the oropharynx. If the bone is not identified on examination, a lateral neck x-ray is suggested, but one should not rely on a negative radiograph to rule out a retained bone. If the x-ray and physical exam are normal, the authors believe it's reasonable to discharge these patients to return at 48 hours if symptoms persist. They specifically believe that referral for immediate endoscopy is unwarranted if only minor symptoms are present.

A PROSPECTIVE STUDY ON FISH BONE INGESTION: EXPERIENCE OF 358 PATIENTS
Ngan JH, et al *Ann Surg* 1990;11(4):459

This study for the University of Hong Kong is a prospective evaluation of 358 patients who complained of the following symptoms after eating fish: foreign body sensation, pain on swallowing, rest pain, blood-tinged saliva, or feeling of obstruction. All patients had an initial oral examination, and if a bone was not identified, they were evaluated with a plain lateral neck radiograph and fiberoptic endoscopy. All patients were followed until the symptoms completely subsided.

Fish bones were found in 117 of 358 patients (33%). The initial oral exam permitted visualization and removal of the offending bone in 21 cases (6%). Flexible fiberoptic endoscopy was performed in the remaining 281 cases. With this procedure, 94 bones were identified, 82 were retrieved, and 12 bones were dislodged and swallowed. Two bones were initially missed by endoscopy.

One was removed when persistent symptoms prompted a repeat endoscopy, and a bone was found lodged in the posterior tongue. In the second case, a bone was noted on the radiograph and required repeat endoscopy under general anesthesia for removal. Interestingly, three patients who had ingested fish heads had a large triangular fish bone lodged in the hypopharynx. These were easily seen on x-ray, and all were recovered with rigid endoscopy, but one patient suffered a mucosal tear and two required lengthy procedures to retrieve the bone.

Of the 35 patients who refused initial endoscopy, one developed a retropharyngeal abscess within two weeks. The other 34 patients were asymptomatic at four-week follow-up.

In this study, the predictive value of symptoms was quite poor. Although the majority of patients with a fish bone had a sensation for a sharp pricking pain on swallowing (predictive value 76%), the usefulness of any of the other symptoms in actually predicting the presence of a fish bone was questionable, with an overall predictive value of less than 50 percent. Likewise, the value of a plain radiograph was marginal — it had only a 32 percent sensitivity. However, when a bone was seen on x-ray, it was 91 percent specific, with an overall predictive value of 66 percent. Soft tissues and calcified laryngeal structures were misinterpreted as fish bones in 18 of 54 positive radiographs. Therefore, only 31 percent of bones were identified by x-ray.

When a fish bone was present, the patients could localize the area of lodgement by pointing to the general location in the mouth, neck, or chest. On endoscopy, bones were found close to the anatomic vicinity indicated by the patient.

The authors conclude that most swallowed fish bones become lodged in the oral cavity or oral pharynx, and that a good percentage (27%) can be removed directly without formal rigid endoscopy. A complete oral examination is mandatory, and when combined with flexible endoscopy, the vast majority of fish bones can be identified and removed without morbidity. Once fish bones are in the hypopharynx, they can be associated with the need for lengthy procedures, treatment failures, and mucosal tears during removal. The authors believe that flexible endoscopy is required in all patients complaining of an impacted fish bone if it cannot be visualized on direct oral examination.

COMMENT: Although only about a third of patients who think they have a bone in the throat actually have such pathology, all patients who complain of a foreign body of the throat should be taken seriously. Nonchalantly attributing even vague symptoms to anxiety or a benign mucosal scratch can be disastrous. Even relatively smooth or rounded objects that remain impacted in the esophagus have the potential for serious problems, and a fish bone can perforate the esophagus in only a few days.

As noted by the authors of the first study, as early as 1936 the famous physician Chevalier Jackson appreciated the potential for serious complications when the following mistakes are made: the physician fails to consider the possibility of a foreign body, does not elicit a proper history, is skeptical of the patient's claim, treats the condition with apathy, incorrectly awaits spontaneous passage, or attempts to attribute signs and symptoms to other medical conditions. Although the authors of these two studies have somewhat different opinions as to the work-up of a sus-

PATIENTS PRESENTING WITH COMPLAINT OF INGESTED FISH BONE

	Number of Patients	Number of Bones Removed
Total	71	15
Fish bones seen at initial presentation	15	15
Patients still symptomatic at 48 hours	15	0
Patients still symptomatic at 2 weeks	4	0

Source: J Accid Emerg Med *1989;6:13-16.*

SITES AT WHICH FISH BONES WERE FOUND

Site	Number visible	Number on x-ray
Base of tongue	8	3
Tonsil	3	0
Posterior pharyngeal wall	2	1
Aryepiglottic fold	1	0
Upper esophagus	1	1*

*Indirectly inferred.

Source: J Accid Emerg Med *1989;6:13-16.*

pected fish bone, both describe similar clinical scenarios.

Most patients who present with a sensation of a bone caught in their throat will not have a bone identified after a complete evaluation. The incidence of actually finding a bone in these two reports is 21 percent and 33 percent. Therefore, about 75 percent of the patients who come to the emergency department will not have a bone identified.

It is impossible to say how many of these patients actually have a bone that is not documented on the initial visit but spontaneously passes over the next few days. The current thinking is that in the absence of a retained fish bone, the sensations described are due to minor trauma of the

PREDICTION OF FISH BONE PRESENCE BY SYMPTOMS AND PLAIN RADIOGRAPH

Predictive Symptom	Sensitivity	Specificity	Value
Foreign body sensation	0.94	0.06	0.31
Pain on swallowing	0.83	0.21	0.24
Rest pain	0.71	0.30	0.44
Blood-stained saliva	0.13	0.73	0.20
Sense of obstruction	0.25	0.71	0.42
Sharp pricking sensation*	0.90	0.74	0.76
Plain radiograph**	0.32	0.91	0.66

* 65 patients evaluated
** 310 patients evaluated

Source: Ann Surg 1990;11(4):459-62.

GI tract when the bone is swallowed. Even though the symptoms are attributed to a mucosal tear or minor laceration, it is extremely uncommon to identify such pathology clinically. Because the GI tract regenerates so quickly, it is not uncommon for a superficial injury to heal within 48 hours, so this commonly held belief may be correct. Don't expect to see bleeding or a mucosal defect. If you do see bleeding, think seriously about an acute perforation.

Some physicians place diagnostic value on the response to swallowing viscous lidocaine or symptomatic relief following the use of other anesthetic solutions. If the pain

goes away, it confirms the suspicion of minor trauma and rules out a fish bone. I have not seen this contention verified in the literature, however, I would caution that one should never assume that a significant foreign body is absent just because the pain disappears when someone swallows a local anesthetic. Anesthetics can provide initial relief or facilitate examination, but they have no diagnostic role and their repeated use is unwarranted and potentially dangerous. A 2% viscous lidocaine solution contains 20 mg/mL absorbable lidocaine. Because the average adult swallow is 15 mL, each bolus of this anesthetic contains 300 mg lidocaine. It's well absorbed orally and can quickly lead to toxicity should the patient be given a bottle to take home.

The ideal ED approach is first to examine carefully the patient's oral cavity. This is best done with the patient sitting in a chair, the use of a bright head lamp, a tongue blade, and spraying the pharynx with an anesthetic. I prefer to use 10% lidocaine spray. Because many fish bones are seen in the oral pharynx with just a flashlight and tongue blade, it's certainly justified to avoid the knee jerk response of ordering an x-ray before you examine the patient. I have personally removed fish bones stuck in a tonsil, the tongue, or soft palate, and the report by Knight and Lesser indicates that the majority of impacted bones can be seen on initial examination.

These authors are also correct in stating that strands of saliva can mimic a fish bone and therefore one must be extremely careful about blindly grasping at the posterior pharynx with a hemostat in an effort to pick out an imaginary bone. Interestingly, patients are able to identify the general location of pathology in the cervical area so ask them to point to the bone and look in these areas more carefully. A number of authors have demonstrated that patients can accurately tell if a foreign body is on the right or left side and can identify the general level of impaction.

The literature is divided over the need for immediate endoscopy. Fiberoptic nasopharyngoscopy now allows all patients to be examined in the ED on their initial visit. This is a technique that is becoming more available and is easily mastered by the emergency physician: I urge its routine use. It's a lot easier to perform than a mirror exam. The fiberoptic scope is used mainly for diagnosis. If a bone is seen deep in the throat, it's best to leave it there and call for the endoscopist to remove it in the OR. Some physicians will examine the supine patient's oropharynx and larynx with the standard curved blade of the laryngoscope that's used for intubation. This allows a good view of the proximal structures, but not all awake patients can tolerate this examination. It's a reasonable option in the middle of the night if the fiberscope is unavailable.

If the initial work-up is normal, I will advise the patient to eat a piece of bread in hopes that it will pick up an occasional unseen bone. I have not seen this studied, but patients do it all the time at home and it's a common recommendation. I see no harm in doing it.

It's best to work out a prospective arrangement with your ENT consultant, but there is general agreement that if the direct visualization and fiberoptic examination and plain radiographs are negative, the minimally symptomatic patient can be safely discharged. All should have a 24- to 48-hour revisit. Clearly the majority of patients with an initial negative examination will be asymptomatic in two to three days. Although there is always that nagging question of a retained fish bone that becomes asymptomatic only to announce its presence with a septic event or an aortic rupture later, there is general agreement that asymptomatic patients need not be endoscoped. Certainly if the patient is spitting blood, cannot swallow, or has respiratory involvement, aggressive endoscopy is indicated. Note that occasionally a repeat endoscopy or lateral neck x-ray may be required should symptoms persist.

RADIOLOGY OF FISH BONE FOREIGN BODIES IN THE NECK

Karr AJ *J Laryngol Oralog* 1987; 101:407

This is a brief article that describes two patients who had pain in the throat after eating trout or halibut. Both had negative soft tissue x-rays of the neck yet laryngoscopy revealed a fish bone in each case. Based on these cases, the authors experimentally x-rayed the bones of 17 common species of fish in a cadaver model to determine radiopacity. Cod, haddock, halibut, and monk fish had consistent radiopaque bones, but mackerel, herring, salmon, and trout demonstrated no radiopacity. It did not matter if the bone was fresh or had been cooked. This author presents a table showing the relative radiopacity of bones of various species.

COMMENT: This article is frequently quoted, but I believe it has significant limitations. Specifically, all of the halibut bones were considered radiopaque when examined in the cadaver yet one of the patients given as an example had ingested halibut and had a negative x-ray. Physicians

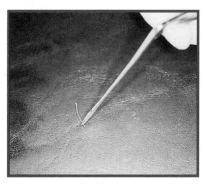

Bones lodged in the throat are difficult to see and can resemble strands of saliva. Be careful when exploring with your hemostat. See color plate in center well.

tend to overestimate the ability of plain radiographs to detect small fish bones in the throat. A plain film is of very limited value, and clearly a negative x-ray does not rule one out. Although Goldman states that about 75 percent of bones will be visible on x-ray (*Ann Otol Rhinol Laryngol* 1951;60:957), probably the best accuracy one can hope for is about 30-40 percent with the type of fish eaten today.

One is often frustrated trying to figure out if that little speck of calcium is a calcified ligament, a fish bone, or some other artifact on the x-ray. It helps to have a book or normal radiology variants handy. In the Ngan et al paper, 18 of 54 (33%) radiographs were false positives. Large bones may be obvious on the film, but particularly in elderly patients where laryngeal structures tend to calcify, a lateral neck x-ray has limited value. One may be lucky enough to see soft tissue swelling or entrapped air — indirect evidence of a retained foreign body — however, this may not occur for the first 12 hours. Therefore, I don't hesitate to repeat the film if one was negative two days earlier and symptoms persist.

When looking for a fish bone, there seems to be no particular added benefit of xeroradiography (*Radiology* 1979;133:218). CT, MRI, or ultrasound might be useful in unusual cases, but they are an expensive alternative to endoscopy. A number of fancy radiology tests have been devised that seem to offer no great benefit, although some physicians continue to use them. The barium swallow may outline a fish bone, but coating the throat with thick layer of barium will make endoscopy very difficult.

Others have suggested swallowing a piece of cotton

soaked in barium to limit this coating effect with the hope that the ball itself or a few radiopaque strands of cotton will hang up on a foreign body. Importantly, if a barium swallow is to be done with a cotton ball, it should be done under fluoroscopy so any changes of motility of the cotton ball can be evaluated. Yet others have suggested a barium swallow followed by a glass of water to wash out residual barium hoping that a few flecks will remain on the foreign body. There is a lot of folklore surrounding the barium study and the cotton ball technique, and I have never seen them evaluated prospectively. I personally think their value is a myth or extremely limited. Given the availability of endoscopy, I don't use them.

SUMMARY: A number of reasonable options exist, but I suggest the following approach to patients with a history of eating fish who develop subsequent pain upon swallowing. First of all, even though less than half have an impacted fish bone, believe the patient when he tells you there is something caught in the throat!

Secondly, examine the patient under proper lighting, local anesthesia, and positioning with the expectation that you may well see the offending foreign body with only a flashlight and tongue blade.

Third, don't rely on the relief of pain with a local anesthetic to signify that the symptoms are due to minor mucosa trauma. If the initial examination is negative, order a plain lateral neck x-ray and ask for soft tissue technique, but don't rule out the fish bone if the x-ray is negative or if a barium swallow is negative. Don't hesitate to

LOCATION AND OUTCOME OF FISH BONES

Location	Total	Removed	Dislodged
Oropharynx	73	67	5
Laryngopharynx	18	17	1
Hypopharynx	18	12	5
Oral cavity	6	6	0
Esophagus	2	1	1
Total	117	103	12

Source: Ann Surg *1990;11(4):459-62.*

reorder the neck film if symptoms persist because indirect evidence of the fish bone may take a while to evolve.

Master the technique of fiberoptic nasopharyngoscopy (or mirror laryngoscopy) and perform it routinely on the initial visit. If these steps are negative, discharge is reasonable if symptoms are minor and follow-up is available in 48 hours. In the meantime, let the patient eat. An option is to defer endoscopy for 48 hours if patients have minimal symptomatology. Aggressively evaluate patients whose symptoms persist for more than 48 hours, even if it means a repeat endoscopy.

PEDIATRIC COIN INGESTION

Even children with no symptoms can have an esophageal foreign body, and problems can persist if it is not removed

Children are forever putting anything and everything into their mouths, and it's not unrealistic to expect that sooner or later all practicing emergency physicians will come across a child who may have swallowed a coin. Usually the history is straightforward and the clinical course benign, but it's clear that the diagnosis may be quite subtle, the retained foreign body (FB) may be asymptomatic or mimic other pathologic conditions, and occasionally the outcome can be disastrous.

The clinical approach to this problem seems to vary among otolaryngologists, pediatricians, and emergency physicians so I would like to review the basic concepts and put the issue of treatment into perspective, using logic that integrates all of the relevant disciplines.

COIN INGESTION: DOES EVERY CHILD NEED A RADIOGRAPH?

Hodge D, et al *Ann Emerg Med* 1985;14(5):443

This study was designed to determine whether all children who have swallowed a coin require a radiograph and whether symptomatology is predictive of a retained esophageal FB. During a one-year period, pediatricians at Children's Hospital of Philadelphia were able to identify 80 children who presented to the ED within 24 hours of possible coin ingestion.

All children received a chest x-ray that included the cervical esophagus, and abdominal films were also obtained in some children. The authors termed cases as positive when the coin was located above the diaphragm, and negative if the coin was below the diaphragm or was not seen (presumably never ingested). The mean age of the children was four years. Most (48%) ingested pennies, but nickels, dimes, and quarters were also swallowed.

About one-fifth of the children had choking and coughing at the time of ingestion. Immediate vomiting, dyspnea, chest pain, and drooling also occurred. Choking and coughing disappeared quickly, but the other initial symptoms frequently persisted. On the average, one-half hour elapsed from presentation to when the first radiograph was obtained, and even after this short interval, the majority of coins were subdiaphragmatic (55%). No coin was detected in 14 percent, but 18 percent were lodged in the cervical esophagus and 13 percent were in the mid-lower esophagus. No patient with a negative radiograph had signs or symptoms and all patients who were symptomatic in the ED had a positive film.

All coins either passed or were removed. Almost half (40%) of the coins spotted in the esophagus passed spontaneously into the stomach within a five-hour observation period and eventually 70 percent of those swallowed passed to this benign location. The Foley catheter technique removed the coin or forced it into the stomach in all 10 patients (13%) who underwent this procedure. Four children (5%) underwent esophagoscopy. No complications were noted in any case, and there was no long-term morbidity.

Seventeen percent of the 66 children without any clinical signs or symptoms had an esophageal coin. Because the mean age of these children was three years, the authors contend that the absence of symptoms was not attributed to the inability of patients to verbalize their complaints. The most important sign correlating with a positive radiograph was the ability of the child to localize the coin.

The authors conclude that all children presenting to the ED with coin ingestion should receive a chest radiograph that includes the neck, esophagus, and gastric air bubble. If a child complains of symptoms in the ED, it is highly likely that a coin is present. Because an occasional child may be totally asymptomatic with a coin in the esophagus, the authors believe that the lack of signs and symptoms does not rule out the FB nor does it negate possible delayed complications. The authors believe that it unwise to give telephone advice on this subject.

COMMENT: Once a coin has reached the stomach, it is of little clinical consequence. The maximum transit time for such foreign bodies in children is five days (*Prog Pediatr Radiol* 1969;2:286). About one-third of the children in this study (31%) who arrived in the ED with a positive history had the coin still lodged in the esophagus. Half of these children were asymptomatic with a FB in an area at high risk for significant complications. All the children who had signs and symptoms (able to localize the coin, choking, drooling, vomiting, or chest pain) had a coin in the esophagus. It's interesting to note that even children can tell you if the coin is present; if they point to the neck or chest, the FB will invariably be present and lodged in the general vicinity indicated. Because a retained

esophageal FB is such a high-risk condition, it makes utmost sense to me to x-ray all children if coin ingestion is suspected, even if they are completely asymptomatic.

I have discussed this issue with colleagues in pediatrics, and some advocate a position that has been termed dangerous by the authors of this study. Specifically, they feel that if a child is asymptomatic, a radiograph is not needed. I was surprised to discover that a routine radiograph is not advocated for asymptomatic children by all authors and not deemed necessary by many clinicians.

Caravati et al take such a contrary stance (*Am J Dis Child* 1989;143:549). In their prospective study of 162 children, a surprising 59 percent of patients advised to have

RADIOGRAPHIC FINDINGS VS. SYMPTOMS IN THE EMERGENCY DEPARTMENT

	Radiograph (%)*	Radiograph (%)**	Total
Symptoms	14 (100)	0	14
No symptoms	11 (17)	55 (83)	66
Total	25 (31)	55 (69)	80

*Coin supradiaphragmatic.
**Coin subdiaphragmatic or not seen.

Source: Ann Emerg Med *1985;14:443-446.*

an x-ray by a poison center had the suggestion countermanded by the patient's private physician, even though 19 percent were symptomatic at the time of ingestion. No difference in morbidity was demonstrated between asymptomatic children who were and were not x-rayed. The conclusion of this frequently quoted study was that asymptomatic children who can tolerate fluids need not be routinely x-rayed if follow-up is available. This may be the case, however, these children were only followed for five days.

Schunk et al reported that 77 percent of pediatricians in Salt Lake City responding to a telephone survey would not routinely x-ray asymptomatic children (*Am J Dis Child* 1989;143:546). However, when Schunk prospectively studied 57 children with possible coin ingestion, the absence of signs and symptoms did not reliably exclude the presence of an esophageal coin. Specifically, 30 percent of their patients with foreign bodies in the esophagus were totally asymptomatic. The bottom line is this: An x-ray is a non-invasive, minimally expensive test, many retained coins are totally asymptomatic, and a silent esophageal FB is a time bomb waiting to explode. I just can't buy the approach that forgoes a routine x-ray.

There are two other issues of importance with regard to radiographs. The film should include the area from the nasopharynx (not only neck) to the rectum. Often this can be done with a single large radiograph plate, particularly in a small child. There have been reports of orally ingested coins that have ended up in the nasopharynx which were missed when only the chest or cervical esophagus were included on the film. In one report, a nasopharyngeal coin was initially missed by x-ray and not diagnosed until seven weeks after ingestion (*Postgrad Med* 1988;64:201). A coin in the stomach or intestines is of little clinical consequence, but it's always helpful to know if the coin was actually ingested; it just ties up the loose ends. Occasionally one is surprised by other radiopaque foreign bodies ingested at a previous time.

A smooth coin could theoretically cause problems, such as intestinal obstruction, although that would be extremely unusual. Still, I prefer to tell the parents to check the stool and return to the family doctor for follow-up x-rays if they don't find the coin within seven days. Usually it passes, but the parents just get tired of mashing up the stool with a fork in an asymptomatic child and forget my advice. Frequently the family doctor opts not to pursue it.

The next issue is to define the proper radiograph to obtain. Coins usually never lodge in the trachea, but the literature always makes the point that one need order only an AP radiograph to check for the coin's orientation. Invariably the round front or back of the coin is visible, signifying that the coin has not turned in an AP direction (on edge) to pass through the vocal cords and is, in fact, in the esophagus. A coin in the trachea is clinically extremely obvious and even a dime would have a hard time passing through the vocal cords of a child. I've seen plenty of coins in the esophagus, but have never heard of one in the lungs. However, there are numerous reports of multiple coins lying stacked on top of each other in the esophagus, presenting an impression of a single coin if only an AP film is obtained. This is of no great consequence if all the coins end up in the stomach five hours later, but should one of the multiple coins be vomited or removed with a Foley catheter or endoscope, the physician may think all is well while other coins are left to erode slowly into the aorta!

The purist would argue that following removal, one should take a repeat single AP film to document that multiple coins were not ingested. If a lateral film demonstrating a single coin were obtained initially, and a single coin is recovered, there is no need to repeat the radiograph for confirmation. I have personally seen three coins stacked on top of each other in the esophagus of a small child yet only one was suggested when a single AP x-ray was obtained. I may be overly paranoid, but I always order both an AP and lateral film to evaluate coin ingestions. One could, however, reasonably argue that only the lateral film is required, and I have occasionally adopted this approach. Finally, one must differentiate a coin from a button battery. The battery can resemble a coin, but is usually identified by a double ring sign. Because batteries rapidly cause esophageal injury, one does not have the luxury of waiting 24 hours for it to pass as one does with a coin.

DELAYED DIAGNOSIS OF COIN INGESTION IN CHILDREN

Savitt DL, Wason S *Am J Emerg Med* 1988;6(4):378

This very informative paper presents the case histories of five children with respiratory or GI complaints without a history of coin ingestion. Ultimately all had an impacted esophageal coin proven to be the cause of their symptomatology. The first case is an 8-month-old boy who was playing with a quarter and had a choking episode. The report from the mother was that she successfully retrieved a coin from the mouth and thought the problem was solved. However, the patient had multiple subsequent episodes of choking and coughing when fed solid foods. The family physician had been contacted initially and several times during the following months when feeding continued to be problematic. The parents were reassured that this was normal in an 8-month-old started on solid foods. When another physician was consulted, two pennies were found in the esophagus. Both were removed through an endoscope, and the child immediately ceased having feeding difficulties.

A 1-year-old boy presented to the ED with a three-week history of irritability, poor feeding, coughing, wheezing, and occasional fever. He had been evaluated by physicians an amazing four times during the prior three weeks and had been discharged with various diagnoses, including otitis media and gastroenteritis. When the child demonstrated bilateral wheezing that failed to clear with an injection of epinephrine, an x-ray was taken that revealed an esophageal coin at the level of the aortic arch where it was impinging on the trachea. All symptoms immediately resolved following removal of the coin.

In another case, a 13-month-old girl carried the history of bronchiolitis and had been treated with theophylline and antibiotics. When she failed to improve, a chest x-ray was taken that demonstrated a coin in the esophagus. In another case, a 9-month-old boy presented with a week's

ROENTGENOGRAPHIC LOCATION OF COIN COMPARED WITH PRESENCE OF SYMPTOMS AT INGESTION

	Symptoms	No Symptoms
Esophagus	11	2
Not in esophagus	15	38
Total	26	40

Source: AJDC 1989;143:549-551.

history of congestion. He had also been diagnosed as having bronchiolitis and was started on theophylline. Because of persistent tachypnea and fever, a chest x-ray was ordered that demonstrated a coin in the upper esophagus with marked tracheal compression.

Finally, a 4½-year-old boy came to the ED with a bizarre history of neck pain and intermittent arching of his neck. The first diagnosis was a pharyngeal inflammatory process, but an x-ray revealed a coin in the upper esophagus.

These authors advocate that an initial x-ray should be ordered in all cases of possible coin ingestions. All five patients in this series were misdiagnosed with respiratory or gastrointestinal problems that were actually due to an unsuspected coin. Importantly, two additional coins were found in the first case after the mother had successfully removed one, substantiating the fact that multiple coin ingestions are frequent. In young children, an esophageal FB can cause partial obstruction and mimic GI pathology or compress the trachea and produce a clinical scenario that closely resembles asthma or bronchiolitis. Coins that do hang up in the GI tract frequently do so in the upper

esophagus where they can easily compress the airway.

The authors point out that rare tragic complications of a retained esophageal FB are well referenced and include esophageal perforation, tracheoesophageal fistula, mediastinitis, and aorto-esophageal fistula, a uniformly fatal condition. It is not uncommon for an esophageal FB to be retained silently for many months, only to become symptomatic when the history of the possible ingestion is long forgotten.

The authors also reiterate that the absence of symptoms does not guarantee that a coin was not swallowed or has passed to a benign location. They suggest that new onset wheezing in a pre-school child, localized neck pain without other obvious explanation, symptoms of feeding difficulties, or wheezing not responsive to bronchodilators should all prompt radiographic evaluation for a possible esophageal FB.

COMMENT: This is a great paper that should be read by all those physicians who think an asymptomatic child with a possible coin ingestion can be followed without the aid of a radiograph. It is amazing how long a FB can remain silent in the esophagus, and the authors of this paper cite literature references where significant pathology developed many months after an unrecognized coin ingestion. Glass et al report nine children with respiratory difficulties secondary to esophageal foreign bodies, and in eight cases, the missed diagnoses and mistreatment amazingly persisted for up to one year (*Laryngoscope* 1966;76(4):605). In addition to supporting routine x-rays, the message here is that when children present to the ED with long histories of seemingly hard to treat respiratory or gastrointestinal difficulties, think esophageal FB. This also applies to psychiatric patients and those with mental retardation.

The timeliness of the diagnosis is a clinically important issue for another reason. Foreign bodies of the esophagus are more difficult to remove when prolonged impaction leads to anatomic injury such as edema, swelling, and necrosis. This can occur quite rapidly (in a matter of 2-3 days), and for this reason the Foley catheter manipulation is not recommended for coins that have been entrapped for more than 48 hours.

This thought-provoking paper demonstrates how easy it is for a child to ingest a coin surreptitiously and to have it not suspected initially by either parent or physician. It must have been very embarrassing for the physicians who saw these patients initially to find out that their diagnoses were incorrect and the symptoms were actually due to an esophageal FB.

The clinical approach to a known esophageal coin has not been prospectively studied in detail. This is fertile ground for emergency medicine research. There are two scenarios where the course of action is clear. In the first instance, the patient is coughing, in respiratory distress, or drooling, and is unable to swallow liquids. This condition almost always is due to an upper esophageal coin, and it necessitates urgent removal, either with a Foley catheter or endoscope. Once swallowed, a coin is usually out of the reach of your fingers or the laryngoscope, but I have removed coins from the oral pharynx of two infants with my hands. Parents seem adept at this, often using a Heimlich maneuver, or hitting the back of a child held upside down. Once the coin is below the pharynx, it doesn't cause acute airway obstruction so such maneuvers should not be attempted. In the other scenario, the FB is in the stomach or intestines, and these patients can be sent home for elective follow-up. I prefer to have parents check the stool for the coin, and if it is not found within a week, a repeat radiograph is suggested. Some would argue that this is excessive, and it may be in most cases.

Children with asymptomatic esophageal foreign bodies

OBJECTS COMMONLY INGESTED BY CHILDREN

Coins	Buttons	Marbles
Bones	Toys	Beverage can tops
Balloon	Pins	Nuts, seeds
Jacks	Hair clips	Screws, nails

Source: Am J Emerg Med 1988;6:378-381.

present the most difficult treatment scenario. There is relatively good evidence that suggests one can safely wait 12, and probably 24, hours before progressing to invasive treatment. Surprisingly, in many studies a coin is removed as soon as the diagnosis is made, without waiting to see if it will pass spontaneously. My approach is to allow the asymptomatic child to eat and drink (usually peanut butter crackers from the vending machine and a soft drink), and then x-ray the patient again in a few hours, sooner if they tell you the FB sensation has gone away. I have recently been putting nitroglycerin paste on the skin to promote

esophageal relaxation, but I don't know if this is helpful. Intravenous glucagon has not been studied carefully for treatment of pediatric coin ingestions, and I don't routinely use it. The drug might be helpful but only for coins at the GE junction. If the coin does not pass within 3-4 hours of ED observation, I will then contact my pediatric/ENT consultant and allow him to make the decision. Most of the time, they opt for admission to the hospital with re-evaluation 12-24 hours later and subsequent endoscopy if the coin has not passed. (Hopefully, they will x-ray the patient just before they put the child under general anesthesia). A case can be made for the Foley catheter technique to be used immediately for coins of the upper esophagus, but I initially try to have the child drink (not eat), even with foreign bodies in this area. If she can't drink or continues to vomit, I call for help. Most coins in the mid to lower esophagus will pass in a few hours, especially after eating or drinking, so I will be more patient with these children.

I have not been discharging patients to even reliable parents because I greatly respect esophageal foreign bodies, and it's too easy for the parents to wait 3-4 days while the asymptomatic coin becomes further embedded in esophageal mucosa.

Once you consult ENT, you are probably guaranteeing endoscopy in lieu of more conservative measures that seem to be favored by pediatricians. Radiologists and emergency physicians have experience with the Foley catheter technique, but this procedure is tricky and should only be used with coins that have been impacted less than 12 hours and are in the upper esophagus. Unlike an impacted bolus of meat in an adult, underlying esophageal pathology is not usually suspected when a coin gets hung up.

SUMMARY: In my opinion, the following statements summarize the problem.
• If the history suggests coin ingestion, obtain an x-ray that evaluates the entire body. Remember that multiple stacked coins appear as one coin in PA films. Unless you are certain that a single coin is present, document removal with a post-procedure film.
• Symptomatology is not predictive of a potentially dangerous FB.
• If a patient states a coin is in the throat, it's almost always there and in the general area indicated.
• Immediately remove coins that are causing significant symptoms, but be patient with lower esophageal coins that are asymptomatic or mildly so. Frequently allowing the child to eat or drink pushes the coin into the stomach.

Don't allow esophageal foreign bodies to remain in the esophagus. It's not clear exactly how long is considered "safe," but most can be watched for 12-24 hours.

• When there is acute airway compromise, the coin may be proximal enough for a Heimlich maneuver, your fingers, a laryngoscope, or a pat on the back while held upside down.

• Consider upper esophageal foreign bodies in children with atypical or prolonged respiratory or gastrointestinal complaints.

• Children with esophageal coins do not need a work-up for underlying pathology.

ESOPHAGEAL FOOD IMPACTION

The condition frequently calls for endoscopic removal and mandates follow-up of the esophagus and swallowing mechanism

The most common cause of esophageal impaction is a bolus of meat. The diagnosis of food impaction is relatively straightforward, but the treatment is less clear. A number of therapeutic measures have been suggested to relieve the obstruction, including pharmacologic means and endoscopy. Although meat impaction can often be relieved in the ED, the situation frequently calls for endoscopic removal and always mandates a follow-up evaluation of the esophagus and swallowing mechanism.

INTRAVENOUS GLUCAGON IN THE MANAGEMENT OF ESOPHAGEAL FOOD OBSTRUCTION

Glauser J, et al *JACEP* 1979;8(6/0:228

This article is the first report in the emergency medicine literature that focuses specifically on the use of intravenous glucagon to relieve an obstructing bolus of food. The authors present the case histories of two individuals who had food lodged in the esophagus and presented to the ED four to five hours postimpaction. A barium swallow study demonstrated complete esophageal obstruction by a bolus of meat. Both patients had relief of symptoms within a few minutes following the intravenous administration of 1 mg of glucagon.

In 1979 the use of glucagon was a relatively new modality, and the authors claim that at the time the article was written there were only 11 recorded cases documenting the use of glucagon for this purpose. Of those 11 cases, five patients obtained relief and there were six failures that eventually required endoscopic removal. Prior to the use of glucagon, the treatment of esophageal food impaction consisted of only two specific modalities: enzymatic digestion of the food bolus and endoscopic removal. The risk associated with the enzymatic approach was recognized quite early and likely prompted the investigation of other less dangerous treatment protocols.

The exact treatment regimen suggested by the authors includes an initial contrast study to confirm obstruction and to localize the level of pathology. This is followed by a 1 mg bolus of intravenous glucagon, given after a test dose to check for hypersensitivity. If there is no relief within 20 minutes, an additional 2 mg bolus of glucagon is then administered. If the bolus of food passes with glucagon, a follow-up esophagram is ordered. If the food is still impacted, the authors advise esophagoscopy to remove it. Based on available data, the authors predict that approximately half of the cases will respond favorably to glucagon.

ESOPHAGEAL FOOD IMPACTION: TREATMENT WITH GLUCAGON
Trenkner S, et al *Radiology* 1983;149:401

This prospective study of 19 patients was undertaken to determine the efficacy of intravenous glucagon in relieving esophageal food impaction and to evaluate the specific underlying esophageal pathology that could predispose to this condition. Four patients who presented with impacted food in the upper or middle esophagus were excluded from this study because glucagon is thought to only have an effect on the lower esophagus. As with the previous study, the authors used a barium swallow initially to identify the presence of a foreign body and to determine its location.

In the protocol, IV glucagon was given in a dose of 0.5 to 2 mg, followed by ad lib water. If the foreign body passed, a barium esophagram was ordered to determine the etiology of the impaction. If the bolus had not passed in one to two hours, endoscopy was undertaken.

Glucagon therapy resulted in clearing the food impaction in seven of 19 patients (37%). Two patients had their obstruction relieved when they vomited after receiving glucagon. Importantly, all but one patient had an abnormal esophagus when subsequently evaluated by endoscopy or barium swallow. The most common pathology was distal esophageal narrowing due to strictures or rings. Other esophageal pathology included hiatal hernia or esophagitis. No cases of cancer were detected.

The authors conclude that although glucagon is successful in less than half of cases of esophageal food obstruction, its use is indicated because it is safe and may be effective. They note that because esophageal food impaction usually occurs in conjunction with some underlying abnormality of the esophagus, it is mandatory to evaluate such patients for coexisting pathology.

COMMENT: The use of glucagon for this purpose was first reported in 1977 (*Radiology* 1977;125:25), and almost all emergency physicians are familiar with its use for the treatment of food impaction. It's my impression, however, that many physicians overestimate the efficacy of glucagon therapy. Glucagon is worth a try, but it will be effective in less than half the cases and is ineffective in impactions due to tight, fixed constriction. There are no large prospective, double-blind series of patients treated with glucagon, and the literature supports this drug only through anecdotal case reports. The Trenkner et al article is probably one of the most scientific in the literature, but it does not include a control group.

Meat impaction occurs most frequently in the distal esophagus, probably because that is where constrictive pathology is likely to occur. The problem can occur in any age group, but it is more common in elderly patients, probably for a number of reasons. Most importantly, advancing age is associated with esophageal pathology such as strictures and rings. In addition the elderly are more likely to have dentures and may not chew food properly. This results in swallowing a large bolus. Another predisposing factor is drinking alcohol with one's meal, making the patient less aware of his eating habits. (That's why your mother told you to eat slowly and chew your food well.) Once the food is impacted, it does not take long for the patient to show up in the ED, often drooling, in pain, and unable to keep down liquids. Many are unwilling to take a test swallow in the ED because they know they will vomit in a few minutes.

Glucagon is thought to be effective through its relaxation of the lower esophageal sphincter. The drug has been used for many years for its inhibitory effect on the alimentary tract, and it is utilized in radiographic studies where hypotonicity of the GI tract is desired. Glucagon does not produce changes in esophageal peristalsis. Importantly, because the drug has no physiologic effect in the upper or middle esophagus, it would not be expected to be of any value in the treatment of impactions in these areas. Although glucagon is almost always mentioned in the treatment of food impaction, there is no reason why it could not be given for lower esophageal coins or other smooth foreign bodies. When it's successful, glucagon usually works in a few minutes. The physiologic effects last for only about 15-20 minutes.

There are a few contraindications to glucagon use. True hypersensitivity is uncommon, although it is not unusual for patients to vomit, particularly following rapid intravenous administration. Giving a test dose for hypersensitivity is a good idea, but it's not always done. Hyperglycemia may occur with glucagon use, but it is of little clinical significance and blood sugars need not be monitored. Pheochromocytoma and insulinoma are generally considered contraindications. The hyperglycemia that results may cause an insulinoma to secrete insulin and produce hypoglycemia. Glucagon may cause a pheochromocytoma to release catecholamines. If either hypoglycemia or a catecholamine excess occurs, you just might look like a star by diagnosing these very rare tumors. Most authors suggest a 1-2 mg dose, and there does not appear to be a benefit from using higher doses. A l mg dose of glucagon costs our hospital pharmacy $14.

In addition to glucagon, adjunctive medical treatment to relax the esophagus includes diazepam (Valium), nitroglycerin, atropine, and calcium channel blockers, such as nifedipine. I have been unable to find any hard data on the use of these additional medications, and their efficacy, while theoretically attractive, is questionable. I have personally used glucagon for the treatment of food impactions, but have had only about a 20-30 percent success rate. I also routinely use sublingual nitroglycerin prior to glucagon and intravenous narcotics for pain control.

AGES OF PATIENTS WITH ESOPHAGEAL FOREIGN BODIES

Age Range, in Years	No. (%) Patients
0-10	30 (19)
10-20	13 (8)
20-30	12 (8)
30-40	14 (9)
40-50	20 (12)
50-60	24 (15)
60-70	23 (14)
70-80	17 (11)
80-90	6 (4)

Source: Arch Otolaryngeal, 1981;107:249-251.

Although this seems to make theoretical sense, I'm not sure if they are of any additional value. Importantly, one should allow the patient to drink water after glucagon has been given to get an extra boost from esophageal peristalsis. If the food passes, the patient will quickly tell you of your success; the relief is not subtle.

The use of radiographic procedures to document an esophageal food impaction prior to therapy requires some comment. Patients know when food is stuck, and they can accurately identify the level of impaction in the esophagus, so I don't buy the concept that one needs to do a routine pretreatment contrast study. Plain films are of no value, except if a large bone has also been ingested. The results of a contrast study rarely alter the course of action. ENT consults have varying opinions on this, but the majority of those I have consulted do not require a contrast study prior to medical therapy or endoscopy.

The more aggressive consultants rush to the ED with their endoscopes as soon as they hear about the case, eschewing any further investigation or therapy. Except in unusual circumstances, such as psychotic or mentally retarded patients, the diagnosis of the food bolus is usually straightforward. If one opts for a contrast study, one has the option to use either Gastrografin or barium. Gastrografin is generally preferred over barium: it is a clear, iodinated liquid that does not cloud the endoscope as does barium. Secondly, if there is a perforation, either with endoscopy or from retching, Gastrografin in the mediastinum is not as harmful as barium. However, aspirated Gastrografin can produce pneumonitis or pulmonary edema. If aspiration is a possibility, it's much better to have barium in the trachea than Gastrografin. If you need a contrast study, these problems can be largely avoided by using the new low osmolality iodinated contrast agents (such as Amipaque, Omnipaque or Hexabrix) that produce less reaction in both the lung and mediastinum (*Radiology* 1988;169(1):141).

The high incidence of esophageal pathology associated with food impaction mandates a routine follow-up evaluation of the esophagus. Esophageal cancer is an extremely uncommon cause of food impaction, although it should always be considered. Most patients have some sort of benign pathology, in the form of a ring or stricture. Following the successful removal of a bolus of food in the ED by glucagon, it's reasonable to send the patient for an outpatient study rather than to do it immediately or have them admitted to the hospital.

Although endoscopy is clearly the definitive treatment, I almost always give glucagon/nitroglycerin a try prior to calling my ENT consultant. The reason for this is that many of them would rather use a scope than try a questionably effective medication, and I have found that calling a consultant virtually guarantees that a patient will get endoscopy. Endoscopy, with its therapeutic ability and diagnostic capabilities (including biopsy) has virtually replaced the contrast study. A food bolus in the esophagus can be tolerated for a number of hours, although it should be considered an urgent situation. While endoscopy can safely wait until morning, patients should not be discharged from the ED prior to removal.

ESOPHAGEAL PERFORATION FOLLOWING MEAT IMPACTION AND PAPAIN INGESTION
Holsinger TW, et al *JAMA* 1968; 204 (8):188

This is a single case report of a disastrous complication of attempted enzymatic digestion of an esophageal meat impaction with papain. The authors describe a 39-year-old woman with an eight-hour history of acute esophageal obstruction that occurred while eating pork. Papain treatment apparently cleared the obstruction in six hours, but 12 hours after papain was initiated the patient developed a perforated esophagus, with frank necrosis of the esophagus being noted. The patient died on the tenth hospital day after a chest tube eroded into the descending thoracic aorta.

This is not the first report of death secondary to papain use, and as early as 1959 the potential fatal consequence of this commonly suggested routine was noted (*Ann Otol Rhinol Laryngol* 1959;68:890). In animal studies, prolonged exposure to papain consistently results in some injury to the normal esophageal wall, and produces severe pulmonary injury if aspirated. It is believed that the proteolytic enzyme may have an even more detrimental effect on an ischemic esophagus and result in digestion of that section of the esophagus that is damaged by a bone or pressure necrosis. If papain remains in contact with the esophagus for a number of hours, subsequent perforation by endoscopy may be more likely.

COMMENT: Prior to the 1960s, papain had been used for years to relieve meat impaction. Most older clinicians have used it many times without problem, and one older series describes it being safe and quite successful: in one study, 16 of 17 patients had their impactions relieved without complications (*Ann Otol Rhinol Laryngol* 1945;54:238). Papain is a proteolytic enzyme commonly found in meat tenderizer, and the substance does slowly dissolve meats. Papain has received terrible publicity from a few case reports, and everyone now seems to condemn its use. I was, however, quite surprised to find a description of papain use in three major textbooks of emergency medicine. One

noted potential problems, but none had a strong objection to its use. Although the risk of esophageal perforation due to enzymatic treatment is probably equal to that of rigid esophagoscopy, most emergency physicians would not even consider using this enzyme. Given the availability of glucagon and the safer flexible endoscope, I agree that papain is probably a dinosaur that should be relegated to medical history. The fear is that the enzyme will dissolve even a normal esophagus if it is left in contact with the mucosa for prolonged periods. It usually requires a number of hours to be effective while the enzyme pools in the proximal esophagus. In the old days the rate of perforation was about equal with papain and rigid endoscopy (about 3%), but endoscopy has become a much less risky procedure. Because the mortality rate from esophageal perforation is close to 50 percent, it is prudent to avoid papain in the ED because it has been linked to this disastrous complications.

Another serious complication from the use of meat tenderizer for esophageal food impaction has been noted by Hall et al (*Chest* 1988;94(3):640). These authors report a case of hemorrhagic pulmonary edema due to the pul-

MEDICAL THERAPY FOR ESOPHAGEAL IMPACTION

Agent	No. (%) Attempt	No. (%) Successes
Diazepam	27	8 (29)
Glucagon	14	6 (43)
Meperidine hydrochloride	10	0
Atropine sulfate	7	1 (14)
Atropine meperidine	2	1 (50)
Atropine diazepam	2	1 (50)
Papain	1	1 (100)

Source: Arch Otolaryngeal *1981;107-249-251.*

monary aspiration of a solution of Adolph's meat tenderizer. The patient apparently inhaled some of the papain concoction and developed severe respiratory distress. In a follow-up animal experiment, the authors instilled meat tenderizer into the lungs of experimental animals and noticed hemorrhagic pulmonary edema to occur within five minutes.

ACUTE ESOPHAGEAL FOOD IMPACTION TREATED BY GAS-FORMING AGENTS

Rice B, et al *Radiology* 1983;146:299

This is a description of a technique that utilizes carbon dioxide production to force a bolus of food from the distal esophagus into the stomach. The authors describe the cases of eight patients who were successfully treated by the oral administration of a combination of tartaric acid and sodium bicarbonate. The specific cocktail consists of 15 mL of tartaric acid (18.7 g/100 mL) followed by 15 mL of sodium bicarbonate (10 g/100 mL). When these components are combined in the esophagus, carbon dioxide is produced, distending the esophagus and propelling the impacted meat into the stomach. This procedure was successful in all eight cases, and there were no complications. The authors note the potential for vomiting and aspiration, or even esophageal perforation due to increased intraluminal pressure with this regimen, but they have not had these complications nor has it been reported in the literature. The authors note that all patients were treated within six hours of impaction and stress that obstruction lasting longer than 24 hours may be a relative contraindication due to esophageal injury from pressure necrosis.

Interestingly, as noted in other reports on esophageal meat impaction, underlying esophageal disease was present in all cases, again emphasizing the need for follow-up evaluation.

COMMENT: I have not had personal experience with the gas-forming regimen, although it appears to be worth a try in selected cases. Certainly it should only be done in cases of recent ingestion, but those are the individuals who usually present to the ED. Mohammed et al (*Clin Radiol* 1986;37(6):589) report some success (57%) with impacted esophageal FBs with a similar technique that allowed patients to drink 100 mL of a carbonated beverage. Kaszar-Seibert et al went one logical step further and combined glucagon with a gas-forming agent (*AJR Am J Roentgenol* 1990;154: 533). In this report 14 adults were administered 1 mg of IV glucagon, then while sitting upright, they drank a 30 mL solution of E-Z gas (sodium bicarbonate, citric acid, simethicone), followed by 240 mL of water. Almost immediate relief was obtained in 75 percent of cases. Interestingly, our pharmacy does not carry either E-Z gas or tartaric acid, but (unknown to the pharmacy) E-Z gas is stocked by our radiology department.

As a final comment, one should probably never succumb to the temptation of trying to push a meat impaction

USE OF GLUCAGON TO TREAT ESOPHAGEAL IMPACTION

Patient Age	Sex	Foreign Body	Dose, mg	Successful?	Esophageal Pathology
76	M	Meat	0.5 x 2	No	HH, S
82	M	Food	NA	No	HH, E, S
61	M	Pork bone	1.0 x 2	No	Diverticulum
70	M	Meat	0.5 x 3	No	HH, E, R
78	F	Food	1.0	Yes	HH, E, R
80	F	Meat	2.0	No	None known
48	F	Meat	1.0 x 2	Yes-V	HH, E
65	M	Meat	1.0 x 2	No	HH, E
68	M	Food	1.0	No	HH, E, S
63	M	Meat	1.0 x 2	No	S
60	M	Meat	1.0	No	HH, S
54	M	Meat	1.0 x 2	Yes	HH, E, S
73	M	Meat	1.0	No	HH, E, R
71	M	Meat	2.0	No	E, S
58	M	Meat	2.0	Yes	HH, E, R
40	F	Meat	1.0 x 2	No	HH, E, R
67	F	Meat	2.0	Yes	HH, E, S
21	M	Meat	1.0	Yes-V	HH, S
72	F	Meat	1.0	Yes	HH

HH - Hiatal hernia
S - Stricture
E - Esophagitis
R - Mucosal ring
V - Vomited

Source: Radiology *1983;146:299.*

into the stomach with the use of nasogastric or oral gastric tube. This is a blind procedure that can result in esophageal perforation. Although I have heard of colleagues who have used it successfully, I strongly recommend against its use.

There is one report of successful extraction of meat with the use of an oral gastric tube as a suction device (*Dig Dis Sci* 1980;25(2):100), but I believe the only instrument that should go down the esophagus is an endoscope.

SECTION V

FINGERTIP PATHOLOGY

EVALUATION AND TREATMENT OF SUBUNGUAL HEMATOMA

Subungual hematoma can prompt the hardiest soul to seek treatment, which usually means simply relieving the pressure and hence the pain

Emergency physicians frequently deal with patients who have suffered trauma to the digits. This chapter begins a series of discussions on the clinical approach to fingertip problems by reviewing the treatment of subungual hematoma (SUH).

An SUH is a painful problem that can bring the most hardy and stoic construction worker to the ED for immediate treatment. Even narcotics may fail to relieve the pain produced by an expanding subungual hematoma as it compresses the sensitive nail bed, and some method to release the pressure is usually required. There are few controlled studies in the literature that critically evaluate various therapeutic modalities, treatment recommendations vary greatly, and unsubstantiated clinical dogma about this entity is rampant.

Although it's not a major digit-threatening injury or rarely even an ultimate cosmetic concern, a subungual hematoma is usually treated by an emergency physician, who should be expert in the care of this injury. The key to a successful outcome of any fingertip injury is to know when to be conservative and when to be aggressive. Many emergency medicine textbooks devote little time to the evaluation and treatment of SUH, and housestaff usually learn from on-the-job experience. Some continue to repeat the mistakes of an equally misinformed mentor because even otherwise seasoned physicians are not cognizant on the issues involved in the treatment of fingertip injuries. Mismanagement can lead to prolonged morbidity or even occasionally permanent deformity.

TREATMENT OF SUBUNGUAL HEMATOMAS WITH NAIL TREPHINATION: A PROSPECTIVE STUDY

Seaberg DC, et al *Am J Emerg Med* 1991;9(3):209

This nicely done study was designed to determine if simple nail trephination alone would adequately treat uncomplicated SUH without producing or fostering associated cosmetic or infectious complications. This is the only study I could find that prospectively attempts to answer this rather common question. Over a period of two years, 48 patients who presented to the ED with SUH were entered into the study. Patients were excluded if they had disruption of the nail itself, if the nail was loose or the border was violated, or if previous nail deformities existed. Therefore, the study population included only patients with a closed hematoma, an intact nail, and without laceration of the external skin or disruption of the nail proper. An underlying distal phalanx fracture did not exclude patients from the protocol.

Ages of the subjects ranged from 3 to 60 years. All patients underwent radiographic analysis and were treated with electrocautery trephination and expression of the subungual blood. Antibiotics were apparently not prescribed. Postoperative treatment included splinting of fractures in extension for one week. Patients were followed for at least six months after the injury for evaluation of deformities, dysfunction, or signs of infection.

The size of the hematoma was rated relative to the nail surface area. The SUH involved more than 50 percent of the nail surface in more than half of the patients; 30 percent had an associated fracture. Although most patients with underlying fractures had a greater than 50 percent hematoma, there was no close correlation between the size of the hematoma and the presence of a fracture. There were no complications directly related to the trephination, and there were no cases of soft tissue infection, osteomyelitis, or permanent significant nail deformity. A few patients were noted initially to have

> PROVIDE SIMPLE NAIL TREPHINATION IN ALL WITH SUH, ORDERING X-RAYS ONLY AS NEEDED

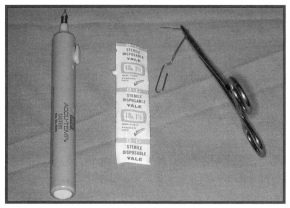

A number of devices are available to trephine the nail. The heated paper clip is an inexpensive and disposable apparatus. See color plate in center well.

ridges in the nail at the site of trauma; however, at three months these ridges had grown out and the nails appeared normal. It took an average of four months for a new nail to grow following trephination. Importantly, these excellent results were achieved regardless of the size of the SUH

or the presence of an underlying tuft fracture.

The authors question the need for routine radiographs in all cases. They conclude that patients with uncomplicated SUH will obtain excellent results with simple nail trephination without removal of the nail or suturing of the nail bed. This conclusion is contrary to other authors, who suggest routine removal of a nail in order to repair all nail bed lacerations. The authors emphasize that their study examined only cases where the nail and nail margins were completely intact, and their conclusions may not be applicable to extensive crush injuries or complex nail disruptions. They also believe that the electrocautery device provides the most ideal method for rapid and painless trephination. If a fracture is present, routine protective extension splints are also suggested. There appears to be no role for routine antibiotic coverage, even if the phalanx is fractured.

COMMENT: It is certainly undesirable for any patient to end up with a permanently deformed nail. It's clear, however, that some physicians are truly in a clinical fog when it comes to evaluating and treating common injuries. When I discussed this problem with my colleagues, I was amazed that their clinical approaches varied so widely. Even erudite pontification was accompanied by a lot of shoulder shrugging.

The majority of fingertip injuries can be handled in the ED, but it's paramount to pay close attention to detail. It is most important to put the natural evolution of the injury into proper prospective when deciding on therapy; too much treatment can be as harmful as too little. This study provides convincing evidence that conservative treatment for uncomplicated SUH is ideal.

Most EPs approach SUH with this philosophy and simply trephine the nail and discharge the patient, but it's easy to get sidetracked with aggressive nail removal and fancy nail bed repairs after a cursory reading of the hand surgery literature. Few emergency medicine texts devote a detailed discussion to this common problem, and because hand surgeons rarely see these minor injuries except when there are complications; therefore, the entire medical literature is sketchy. One of the most lucid and detailed discussions of fingernail injuries can be found in a 25-year-old article by Ashbell (*J Trauma* 1967;7:177) and a 10-year-old article by Rosenthal (*Orthop Clin North Am* 1983;14(4):675). These are a bit dated in their approach to some fingertip injuries, but the discussions about nail and nail bed injuries should be required reading for all EPs.

Impressively, and despite much clinical paranoia and unreferenced warnings in the literature about SUH, there were no signs of permanent nail deformities in any patient in this study. Only 48 patients were studied, but because my waiting room is not filled with fingers permanently deformed by this everyday injury, I am convinced that the authors' conclusions are valid. The lack of infectious complications — particularly in those patients with underlying fractures — is also comforting. Although some physicians routinely prescribe antibiotics following trephination when there is a tuft fracture, based on the theory that such injuries are actually compound fractures once drainage is performed, there is absolutely no data to support this protocol.

I was surprised that so many of my colleagues steadfastly held to this tenet. I believe one is on firm ground by

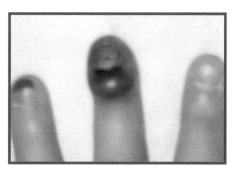

SUBUNGUAL HEMATOMA

Size of hematoma relative to nail surface	Presence of fractures	
	No	Yes
<25%	10	1
25-50%	7	3
>50%	16	10

Source: Am J Emerg Med *1991;9:209-210.*

withholding antibiotics posttrephination of an uncomplicated SUH even with an underlying fracture. I have never personally seen or heard of osteomyelitis in such cases, and it's certainly theoretically possible. In a related but not identical scenario, there are numerous studies suggesting no antibiotic coverage for other types of fingertip injuries, even those with partial amputations, exposed bone, or open tuft fractures (*Ann Emerg Med* 1983;12:358). I would be slightly tempted to use three to five days of post-

trephination antibiotics in the presence of an underlying fracture in immunocompromised patients (perhaps diabetics) or those with peripheral vascular disease, but certainly routine antibiotics are overkill. Tetanus toxoid is theoretically a good idea, but I could find no cases of tetanus from nail trephination.

This subungual hematoma was initially inadequately drained with one small hole, and the blood accumulated again when the exit became clogged. The result is a large collection of clotted blood with extension under the nail fold, necessitating drainage of the subcutaneous collection and removal of the nail.

In a related study, Simon and Wolgin (*Am J Emerg Med* 1987;5:302) evaluated 47 adult patients with SUH to determine the association between the hematoma, associated fractures, and the presence of occult lacerations of the nail bed. The fingernail was removed to check for the presence of a "repairable laceration" in patients with an SUH greater than one-fourth of the nail bed. They discovered that 60 percent of patients with an SUH greater than half of the nail had a "laceration requiring repair." The incidence of repairable laceration rose to 95 percent when there was an associated fracture. Patients were not followed for cosmetic results, and the authors did not define "repairable."

These authors, however, suggest that fingernails should be routinely removed, the nail bed explored, and lacerations sutured if the SUH is greater than half of the nail surface or if there is a phalanx fracture. In my opinion, this aggressive stance is not substantiated by the data and seems to be blatant over-treatment for a minor injury that will heal nicely with a more conservative approach. Once removed, it may take four to five months (1 mm per week) for a new nail to grow back. This is a long time to go without one's fingernail!

The nail bed certainly must be lacerated if an SUH is present, and the hematoma is the consequence of physical disruption to a highly vascularized tissue. The contention that all nail bed lacerations must be meticulously approximated to avoid future nail cosmetic abnormalities is, however, open to debate. I believe this recommendation is clearly disproven by the Seaberg et al study. The intact nail is an ideal splint that provides integrity to the matrix and ensures close approximation of any laceration. One need only try to remove a nail to be convinced that the nail is normally firmly attached to the nail bed. Such stabilization is probably as good as can be accomplished with suturing the nail bed. If the nail remains attached at its margins, it's best to leave it be, even though the inner portion may be partly separated from the nail by the interposed hematoma.

Significant crush injuries, those that involve lacerations of the nail itself or the nail margin, or injuries that avulse the nail, are completely different cases that should be approached in a different manner. In cases where a nail bed laceration extends to the skin or the nail is split, disrupted, or avulsed, it is generally agreed that the nail should be completely removed and the nail bed inspected and carefully repaired.

It is difficult to talk patients out of a routine x-ray for minor crush injuries of the fingernail. I would order x-rays if specifically requested by the patient, if there were gross deformity or if it were important to predict accurately how long the pain would persist. Usually a fracture can be ruled out if there is no tender-

> **ADEQUATE HOLES SHOULD BE MADE TO ENSURE DRAINAGE, BUT ANTIBIOTIC COVERAGE IS UNNECESSARY**

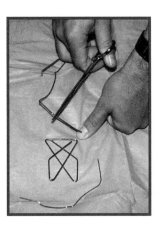

A large paper clip (or clamp), heated until red hot by a butane lighter and held with a hemostat, can be used for nail trephination. A digital block is advised, and it may require two or three attempts before the nail is penetrated.

ness when longitudinally compressing the fingertip or carefully palpating the distal fat volar pad. Displaced phalanx fractures should always be reduced, but with an SUH and an otherwise normal appearing fingertip, I generally try to avoid x-rays. The presence or absence of an underlying crack in the distal phalanx is of no importance to initial therapy. Laborers, typists, or musicians may require an x-ray because fractures may mandate light duty or time off from work because of pain. A documented fracture may mean the difference between a few days and a few

weeks of disability compensation.

Although no one disagrees that an SUH requires trephination, there is a wide variety of personal preferences for the trephination device and many variations on the actual procedure. Some patients can tough out the trephination, but I find it more desirable and easier to obtain proper drainage with local anesthesia. I routinely perform a digital block with long-acting bupivacaine prior to nail trephination. I'll agree that the procedure can be done relatively painlessly if one gently uses the electrocautery, being careful not to exert downward pressure on the nail bed. If the cautery device is used, a large hole (3-4 mm) or multiple drainage holes should be placed. A single small hole may clot and the hematoma can reform. The cautery is theoretically a single-use device, making this an expensive procedure. Many hospitals re-use them, but not with the blessings of the infection control committee.

I usually opt for the large paper clip (cheap and disposable) and butane lighter approach. Some physicians avoid this technique because it requires some painful pressure and because carbon particles may be deposited (unsightly yet benign). Be sure to hold the heated paper clip with a hemostat. Two or three tries are usually needed before the nail is punctured. Again, multiple holes should be made. Blood usually spurts out under pressure and then slowly drains over the next few days. Gentle pressure will initially squeeze out most of the remaining blood (it rarely clots), and the patient can soak the finger in cool salt water for a few days. It's a good idea to advise patients that the original nail may fall off if there was significant blunt trauma, but this is unusual or obvious at the time of injury. Subungual blood usually does not clot even after a few days, but one argument made to drain even small blood collections is that slow bleeding can continue and delaying evacuation may promote clotting.

Many SUHs are produced from injuries that cause excessive flexion to the distal phalanx. Therefore, one should always check for avulsion of the extensor tendon (mallet finger). In the excitement of draining the hematoma, this injury may be missed and produce a noticeable cosmetic deformity if treatment is not initially correct. Some authors advise prepping the nail with alcohol before cautery. I don't usually do this, but if it's done, be certain that the alcohol is dry because it will catch on fire with the cautery (and produce a nearly invisible flame).

Lastly, some unusual entities can masquerade as a sub-ungual hematoma so don't assume that all dark patches under a nail are blood collections. Such things as malignant melanomas, Kaposi's sarcoma, pigmented nevi, glomus tumors, and splinter hemorrhages from endocarditis could cause some embarrassment if they were inadvertently assumed to be a simple SUH.

In summary, it seems logical to provide simple nail trephination in all patients with SUH, with ordering routine x-rays dictated by the individual situation. Adequate holes should be made in the nail to ensure continual drainage. Routine antibiotic coverage is unnecessary, even if there is a tuft fracture. If the nail is loose, split, or the laceration extends past the nail margin, the nail should be removed, the laceration of the nail bed repaired, and the nail reapplied as a dressing. Obviously all displaced fractures should be reduced and splinted as appropriate.

FINGERNAIL AVULSION AND INJURY TO THE NAIL BED

The emergency physician can and should repair most fingertip injuries by following a few basic principles

Fingertip injuries are complex, as is the clinical approach to patients with traumatically avulsed nails, crush injuries, or significant nail bed lacerations. As with subungual hematomas, discussions in medical textbooks tend to be inadequate about the more complex fingertip injuries that can result in cosmetic or functional deformities. Armed with a few basic principles and the time to use them, however, the emergency physician can and should repair the majority of fingertip injuries that do not require extensive revision or fancy grafts or flaps. The fingertip is rather forgiving and recovers quickly, and usually one can obtain adequate cosmetic results when a few basic rules are followed.

THE DEFORMED FINGERNAIL, A FREQUENT RESULT OF FAILURE TO REPAIR NAIL BED INJURIES

Ashbell TS, et al *J Trauma* 1967;7(2):177

This article is rather dated, but it remains a classic description of nail bed injuries. Some of the information concerning grafts and flaps for the treatment of fingertip injuries is dated and not currently advocated, but the discussion on nail bed injuries is timeless.

The authors note that medical textbooks frequently neglect the subject of the absent, deformed, or split fingernails as a result of injury. The proper primary treatment of the nail and nail bed will prevent most fingertip deformities and minimize cosmetic or functional problems. This review article is based on the authors' experiences with more than 3,000 nail bed and nail root injuries and is accompanied by numerous instructive illustrations and diagrams.

The author notes that it is important to understand the anatomy of the nail bed and nail root and the intricacies of nail growth in order to treat injuries adequately. (Figure 1.) Nails are ectodermal appendages covering the dorsal aspects of the digits. These structures provide both protection and integrity to the fingertip and allow precise and delicate touch, skilled hand functions, and the ability to pick up tiny objects. These functions are disrupted when the anatomy is disrupted. The distal border of the nail is free, but the proximal border is tucked into a fold and is covered with a skin flap called the eponychium or cuticle.

The nail is attached at its lateral, distal, and proximal borders. The nail bed (also called the matrix), upon which

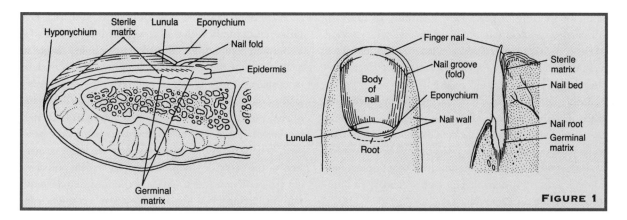

FIGURE 1

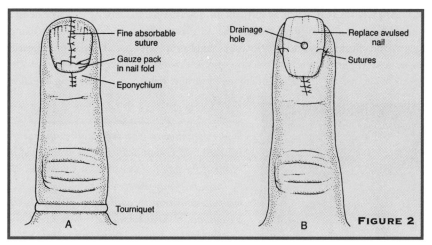

FIGURE 2

the fingernail lies, anchors the dermis to the periosteum of the distal phalanx. Growth takes place in the nail root, also called the germinal matrix or lunule. The lunule is the pale crescent-shaped structure easily recognized under the proximal portion of the nail. Importantly, the nail is not firmly attached at the lunule and only weakly attached to the root. Because the nail is formed in the germinal layers of the root, loss or deformity of the nail root results in permanent loss or permanent deformity of the nail. As the nail grows distally, the more superficial cells become cornified. Distal to the lunule, the nail is firmly attached to the nail bed (also termed the sterile matrix). Complete regrowth of an avulsed nail usually requires four to five months (1 mm per week).

There are a few well-supported treatment principles that must be adhered to when approaching fingertip injuries. A basic tenet includes thorough cleaning with minimal debridement of the nail bed and nail root. It is paramount to reposition and repair disrupted nail beds and nail roots accurately. Improper alignment will be followed by deformed nails, and close approximation of the nail bed is an absolute necessity. It is also important to preserve the skin folds surrounding the nail margins. Adhesions between the eponychium, nail bed, and root are prevented by maintaining this space with either the replaced nail or gauze packing. (Figure 2.) Wide scars or misalignment in the skin fold can

FIGURE 1. *Anatomy of the fingernail. The fingernail rests on the nail bed, also termed the matrix. This distal nail covers the sterile matrix; the proximal nail arises from and covers the germinal matrix. The tissue adherent to the proximal dorsal nail is the eponychium (also termed the cuticle), and the potential space between the nail and the eponychium is the nail fold.*

FIGURE 2. *A laceration involving the nail bed, germinal matrix, and skin fold must be carefully approximated. First, the nail is completely removed. Fine absorbable sutures are placed under a bloodless field provided by a finger tourniquet. The avulsed nail or a gauze pack is gently placed between the matrix and eponychium for two to three weeks to prevent scar formation (A). If the original nail is replaced (the best option), it may be sutured or taped in place (B). A large hole in the nail will allow for drainage. The old nail is pushed out by a new one. If the nail matrix is replaced quickly and atraumatically, the nail may act as a free graft and grow normally.*

result in splitting or permanent deformity of the nail. Although some deformities may be repaired with excision of the scar tissue and revision at a later date, often this is a permanent deformity. Finally, fractures of the distal phalanx should be anatomically reduced.

Other injuries that are noted include ingrown nails when the lateral folds are not maintained, widened nails that result from unrepaired lacerations or nonreduced fractures, narrow nails that result when the nail bed is allowed to grow inward because lacerations were not approximated, and protruding nonadherent nails secondary to unreduced dorsally displaced fractures.

COMMENT: This article is difficult to describe and should be read in order to appreciate the numerous diagrams and illustrations. Although complicated crush injuries resulting in significant tissue loss and/or deformity are best treated by a consultant, many common hand

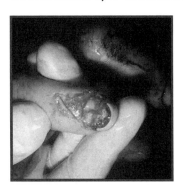

Under digital block with bupivacaine, the essential bloodless field is obtained by a tourniquet, and the extent of the nail bed laceration is determined. The nail may be gently removed by spreading small scissors placed between the nail and nail bed, allowing the nail bed to be anatomically repaired with 6-0 absorbable sutures. See color plate in center well.

An easy way to obtain a clean operative field is to put a sterile glove on the patient and cut out the involved finger. This does away with annoying paper drapes. Note a Penrose drain used as a tourniquet. A tight-fitting glove allows one to roll back the latex to the base of the finger for use as a tourniquet. See color plate in center well.

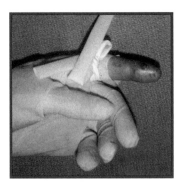

injuries seen in the ED can be handled by the well informed E.P. I would like, therefore, to summarize some basic principles that should be mastered by all those who attempt to repair fingertip injuries. As with most injuries, the initial repair largely determines the final outcome. Plastic surgeons can fix some things, but not even the most skilled consultant can undo all damage done by an uninformed primary physician.

A common injury is shown in figures 3, 4, and 5. A minor crush injury with avulsion of the base of the nail is a common complication of getting one's finger caught in a door. Because the nail is not as firmly attached at the base or lunule as it is to the distal nail bed, the flexion injury avulsed only the base and the proximal nail now lies on top of the eponychium. Occasionally the entire nail bed may be avulsed, but more often than not the bed is only lacerated. When attempting repair, one first checks for an avulsion of the extensor tendon. In the excitement and anxiety of a crush injury, this may be overlooked, and the resultant mallet finger may actually be more of a cosmetic concern than the nail injury. Always test the finger for the ability to fully extend the distal tip. With these injuries, an x-ray is usually mandatory because fractures should be reduced. Minor fractures are easily reduced, but some may require surgical fixation.

Following digital block with bupivacaine, the nail can be removed to facilitate surgical repair of the nail bed. The least traumatic way to remove the nail is to place the closed blades of small iris scissors between the nail and nail bed and gently advance and separate the blades. A scalpel can be used, but this tends to lacerate the bed. A tourniquet is an essential part of any procedure, and it is unthinkable to proceed without one. I also like to prep the avulsed finger, put a sterile glove on the patient, and cut out the involved finger slot to obtain a sterile field. (Figure 6.) This does away with annoying paper drapes that invariably fall off, and it certainly impresses a surgeon who may be wandering through the ED. If you choose a tight-fitting glove, you can just cut off the tip and roll the material proximally to base of the finger; this squeezes out venous blood for less oozing and also makes a nice tourniquet.

Once the nail is removed, it is washed, not debrided or trimmed, and kept for possible use as a dressing. The proximal portion of the nail is soft and pliable. It is best to leave this area intact rather than to trim it; just make sure this area lies flat when replaced in the nail fold. It should be noted that the loss of the nail itself is actually a minor problem. If the nail root is repaired properly, a new nail will grow and be indistinguishable from the original one.

The nail bed is now ready for repair. The aim of the surgery is to provide a flat, smooth surface on which the new nail will grow and to approximate the nail root where a new nail will originate. Uneven nail beds will lead to permanent grooves and ridges in the regrown nail. As noted, failure to repair the root of the nail can cause a wide scar to form and lead to a permanently split nail. The actual nail bed repair should be accomplished with absorbable sutures, usually 6-0 size. Amazingly, I still see residents perform intricate repairs of nail beds with nylon sutures that must be removed. Importantly, do not extensively debride the nail bed. The tissue in the nail bed is extremely hardy and resilient, and, unlike skin, tenuous flaps frequently survive when approximated. Less than perfect closure or coverage often gives a better cosmetic result than extensive debridement. Grafting may be required in some cases. Small detached pieces of bone may be carefully removed prior to closing the nail bed. Displaced fractures can usually be easily reduced.

After the nail bed repair is performed, it is most important to preserve the eponychial space and skin folds surrounding the nail, either by replacing the avulsed nail or with a gauze packing. This prevents adhesions between the eponychium and nail bed/root. It's easiest to replace the patient's own nail because packing this small space with gauze is technically more difficult. The entire original nail is gently repositioned with forceps after the nail fold is cleared of blood clots. Make sure the soft edges of the proximal nail lie

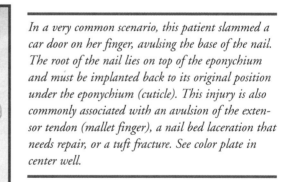

flat in the fold. I personally place a few drain holes in the replaced nail and then suture it in place, but it may be held tightly with steristrips. Nylon sutures (4-0) will penetrate the lateral skin and nail and hold it firmly in place during dressing change and hand washing. Don't put sutures through the nail root.

Antibiotics are optional. This is a concept that is difficult for many physicians to accept, especially if the pha-

lanx is fractured. I usually don't prescribe them unless the patient is immunocompromised. It's not unreasonable, however, to use three or four days (but not 10 days) of a first-generation cephalosporin, but prophylaxis has been studied and there are no data demonstrating a benefit. For the first few days, a plaster volar splint rounded at the end to protect the fingertip is helpful. Elevation is stressed. I opt for a wound check in three days with a dressing change. I remove the sutures or the gauze packing in two weeks. At this point, the raw nail bed is much less sensitive and occasionally the replaced nail has begun to grow. If the nail does not take as a graft, a new nail will slowly push off the replaced nail. Tell the patient that the final results will not be evident for 4-5 months.

DRESSING OF THE NAIL BED FOLLOWING NAIL AVULSION

Dove AF, et al *Hand Surgery (Br)* 1988;13(4):408

Following nail avulsion, the raw nail bed is often dressed with a variety of supposedly nonadherent materials. Patients may experience considerable pain at the time of dressing change because despite manufacturer's claims, these dressings invariably stick to the nail bed. Removal causes bleeding, so that even a replacement dressing becomes adherent as well. A variety of impregnated materi-

In a very common scenario, this patient slammed a car door on her finger, avulsing the base of the nail. The root of the nail lies on top of the eponychium and must be implanted back to its original position under the eponychium (cuticle). This injury is also commonly associated with an avulsion of the extensor tendon (mallet finger), a nail bed laceration that needs repair, or a tuft fracture. See color plate in center well.

als and sponge-type dressings have been advocated to facilitate the growth of new epithelium, allow passage of oxygen and fluid from the wound site, and to make dressing changes easier and less painful for the patient. The authors of this paper compared a polyurethane sponge, paraffin-gauze, and the replacement of the avulsed fingernail as dressings for injured nail beds.

The 156 cases described in this paper included patients

with injuries severe enough to require removal of the fingernail for repair of an injury. Patients with diabetes or peripheral vascular disease were excluded. Dressings were applied according to manufacturers' recommendations. The avulsed nail was anatomically positioned and held in place with a dressing (without suturing). Dressings were changed at 7, 14, and 21 days. During the dressing change, the patients recorded their pain scores and nurses noted the adherence properties of the dressing, signs of infection, and extent of healing.

Those whose nail bed dressings consisted of the replaced nail had significantly less pain at the first redress-

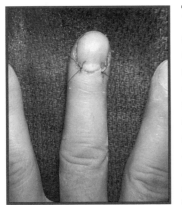

Without trimming or debriding, the base of the avulsed nail is carefully replaced in the nail fold (between the eponychium and teh nail bed). This step is critical to avoid synechia formation and a resulting split nail. Although it was not done in this case, it would be desirable to put a few holes in the replaced nail to allow drainage of the nail bed. The replaced nail may be sutured in place, but avoid putting sutures in the nail root. In two weeks the sutures are removed. The nail may grow normally or be pushed out by the new nail. See color plate in center well.

ing compared to other modalities. Although the difference in pain was not statistically different among the groups at the second and third dressing change, there was a tendency toward the replaced nail group to continue to have less pain. Likewise, the adherence of the dressing was significantly greater in the sponge and gauze group compared to the replaced nail group. There was no difference in the rate of healing or incidence of infection.

The authors were not able to show any advantage of the synthetic dressings over native nail replacement. Nails were not sutured in place as recommended by some authors, but they were simply tucked under the nail fold and held in place with a gauze dressing. Even when only half the nail was left, it was a suitable dressing and appeared to be enough to reduce the pain and adherence of the overlying

dressing. Most of the replaced nails (37 out of 49) remained in place with this simple technique, and some replaced nails took as a free graft and grew normally following replacement. The authors advocate nail replacement as the dressing of choice in patients with fingertip injuries with nail avulsion.

COMMENT: This study basically demonstrates that there is no such thing as a nonadherent nail bed dressing. I have had similar clinical experience so I routinely replace the patient's lost nail, even when only part of the original structure is available. I do, however, continue to see patients in follow-up that have gauze placed over the nail bed only to have them bleed when changed or require digital block for removal.

One could make the point that it is not routinely necessary to remove dressings that are stuck to the repaired nail beds. Some colleagues merely place a piece of Vaseline gauze over the sutured nail bed and allow it to separate spontaneously in two to three weeks. Only the overlying, bulky absorbable dressing is periodically changed, eliminating the pain and bleeding that invariably accompanies attempts to replace an entire dressing. This approach works well and is not particularly problematic, although I still believe that the replaced nail is the easiest way to protect the healing nail bed, pack the nail fold, and to provide a natural splint for the healing injury. Even if it is only partially present, the native nail can be replaced to provide a physiological dressing. Minimally traumatized avulsed nails can actually grow normally if carefully replaced in their proper anatomic position.

Photographs and drawings courtesy of Clinical Procedures in Emergency Medicine, *2nd ed., Roberts JR, Hedges JR, editors, Philadelphia, PA: W.B. Saunders Co., 1991.*

THE CLINICAL APPROACH TO PARONYCHIA

Physicians tend to recommend an overly aggressive approach to paronychia, which is usually a simple problem with a simple solution

Paronychia is a rather common and often painful and annoying digital infection that frequently brings patients to the ED in search of relief. Most infections are minor and can be easily treated with rather conservative methods, but occasionally surgical intervention or other aggressive or prolonged therapies are required.

The neglected or mismanaged case can end disastrously. There are surprisingly little objective data in the medical literature dealing with the treatment of this common problem, probably reflecting the fact that most patients do well. I could not find a single prospective study that evaluated treatment protocols or outcome, and even review articles and textbooks are often superficial or incomplete. I have been impressed, however, that some of my colleagues, and even oft-quoted textbooks, tend to recommend an overly aggressive approach to what is usually a simple problem with a simple solution. When dealing with a paronychia, as with any infection involving the hand, it is paramount for the clinician to know when to be aggressive and when to be conservative.

PARONYCHIA

Randell P *Aust Fam Physician* 1985;14(5):377

Although brief and quite superficial, this is one of the few articles that I could find that discusses the treatment of the common paronychia. A paronychia is an acute or chronic inflammation or infection of the periungual tissue. An acute paronychia generally begins as a red, hot, swollen, and tender area on the skin surrounding the proximal fingernail. It can quickly become quite painful. Clinically it first appears as a cellulitis, and if left untreated it can progress to an abscess. Once pus has localized, drainage can be accomplished relatively easily and the patient experiences rapid relief of symptoms. Many cases seem to develop spontaneously, but some patients can recall an episode of trauma, such as a puncture wound. Children can develop a paronychia from sucking their fingers. The infection usually involves the fingers (especially the thumb and index finger), but the toes may also be affected.

A chronic paronychia can develop, particularly in individuals whose hands have repeated exposure to moisture and repeated minor trauma. The chronic form involves slow, progressive swelling of the lateral or posterial border of the nail folds and scarring associated with discoloration or physical changes of the nail. Unlike the acute bacterial paronychia, which generally involves a single finger, the chronic infection can affect a number of fingers simultaneously.

A chronic paronychia is often caused by a fungal infection, which should always raise the possibility of immunosuppression. A paronychia can be mistaken for psoriasis or Reiter's disease. Tumors such as squamous cell carcinoma or malignant melanoma, cysts, the primary chancre of syphilis, warts, or foreign body reactions can occasionally mimic a paronychia.

Careful local treatment is generally curative. Patients with chronic paronychia should be investigated for yeast infections. Once cured, attention to local nail care can help prevent a recurrence. Failure to cure a paronychia rapidly should prompt specialized culture techniques, proper referral, or occasionally a biopsy.

COMMENT: This is a very superficial article that attests to the fact that this subject is neglected in the medical literature. Reading the current medical literature will leave the student with many unanswered questions, unproven therapeutic recommendations, and can even instill incorrect approaches. I could not find a single prospective study that compared various treatment modalities, nor could I find a recent detailed review article. Most of the articles in the literature are written by hand surgeons who see complicated or advanced cases and base their treatment recommendations on their skewed experience. In many instances, the rather benign paronychia is included with a discussion of much more serious and complicated hand infections, such as felon, human bite, deep space infections, or purulent tenosynovitis. One need only quickly peruse the literature to conclude that many textbooks are overly aggressive in their recommendations for the therapy of a paronychia.

Theoretically, for a paronychia to develop there has to have been a break in the skin — usually from a hangnail, puncture, or trauma — with local inoculation of bacteria. The infections are polymicrobial and involve a number of aerobic and anaerobic organisms. Bacteria that normally inhabit the skin or mouth are usually found if the infection is cultured. Many patients with paronychias bite their nails, suffer repeated minor trauma, or have chronic skin conditions or occupational predispositions.

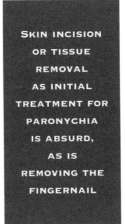

SKIN INCISION OR TISSUE REMOVAL AS INITIAL TREATMENT FOR PARONYCHIA IS ABSURD, AS IS REMOVING THE FINGERNAIL

It's helpful to consider the common bacterial paronychia in two contexts. The first scenario would be the subacute infection where patients present with minor pain, swelling, redness, and tenderness in the periungual area, without obvious fluctuance, drainage, lymphangitis, or adenopathy. The history is usually not specific for an etiology, and the process insidiously develops for no apparent reason. At this point, the process is basically a cellulitis, but sometimes pus has drained spontaneously or the brave patient performs self-treatment, and the infection is already on the road to recovery. Patients in this category will likely respond to conservative treatment.

Although there are no data, most physicians defer drainage attempts unless there is obvious pus and recommend three to four days of a broad spectrum antibiotic in addition to hot soaks. I have found it difficult to convince some patients to soak their fingers with enough regularity to ward off pus formation. Nevertheless, when pus is absent, conservative home care is the most reasonable course. In fact, there is no surgery to recommend unless pus is present; one is dealing with a simple cellulitis. I advise patients to soak their affected finger in a coffee cup filled with very hot tap water (not boiled water or sterile saline) for 10 minutes, four times a day. It sounds simple enough, but it's difficult to do religiously. If you give patients some Betadine or similarly bright colored additive it may increase compliance because it focuses attention on a bona fide "medical procedure;" that is, soaking in an antiseptic. Because the skin is closed, the antiseptic should offer no great medical benefit over the local heat, but it can increase compliance because it focuses attention on the hot soaks.

Each time the finger is soaked — and it should be for 10 minutes by the clock — the patient can take an oral antibiotic. Long-acting antibiotics are usually more patient friendly, but if one couples the antibiotic with the soaking, the soaking may be more likely to be done. There are no data identifying the proper antimicrobial, but a short course (maximum four to five days) with penicillin would be a reasonable approach (see following discussion), and it may be curative in this early stage of cellulitis.

Many physicians, however, question the need for antibiotics at all at this stage, but I tend to prescribe them unless the process is obviously minor. After soaking the finger, an antibiotic ointment and gauze dressing or Band-

Aid are applied. Follow-up is not scheduled and not required unless the condition worsens. X-rays, cultures, and laboratory tests are unnecessary, but tetanus prophylaxis is suggested.

The second scenario involves a more complicated or advanced condition where conservative measures fail or the patient presents with frank pus. In these cases surgical treatment is indicated (Figures 1, 2, 3). I hesitate to use the word surgery because this means skin incision to most physicians. In this case, however, initial drainage can be accomplished without an actual skin incision. I was amazed to find that many textbooks recommend incising the skin rather than the more reasonable approach of draining this localized pus collection by simply lifting up the eponychium.

It is important to realize that a paronychia is not an actual subcutaneous abscess, like a boil or infected sebaceous cyst, but a skin cellulitis over a collection of pus that has formed in the potential space under the cuticle. Incising the dorsal skin of the eponychium only compounds the injury and is clearly not the way to drain pus under the cuticle. Skin incisions should be avoided as the initial treatment. I cannot understand why most textbooks written for primary care physicians have diagrams involving skin incision or tissue removal as the initial treatment; it's downright absurd! Incising the skin in the fingertip of a diabetic can relegate them to four to six weeks of slow healing. Contrast this to the few day's healing time associated with more conservative procedures that eschew actual skin incision. Likewise, removing the fingernail, as suggested by many authors, is gross over-treatment for the first visit. Pus from a paronychia rarely makes its way underneath the fingernail. The presence of a true subungual abscess is an indication for a nail removal or wide trephination, but this rarely occurs with a paronychia.

Some patients can tough out a gentle physician's lifting up of the cuticle, but I prefer to perform all drainage procedures under a digital block with long-acting bupivacaine. The only disadvantage of the long-acting anesthetic is that the finger should not be individually soaked in hot water until sensation returns, to avoid thermal injury. (One can get around this by soaking an adjacent unanes-

thetized finger at the same time). Following digital block, the eponychium (cuticle) is separated from the underlying nail. This is done atraumatically by advancing a scalpel blade, scissor blade, or 18 gauge needle into the nail fold. The instrument is always kept parallel to the nail so the skin is not actually incised. One merely gently lifts the eponychium until there is spontaneous flow of pus that has collected in the nail fold. Once the eponychium is loose, a blunt instrument, such as a hemostat (not a scalpel)

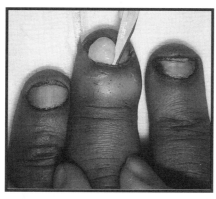

A paronychia is a collection of pus under the cuticle, not a cutaneous abscess per se. Instead of incising the skin, simply lift up the cuticle with a blade or scissors, spread the eponychial space with a blunt instrument, and pack the space open for 24-36 hours to promote drainage. Removing the nail or incising the overlying skin should be avoided whenever possible, which is most of the time. See color plate in center well.

finishes the job by being swept from side to side to the base of the infection to break up loculations. Irrigation of the cavity is probably not necessary.

A loose gauze pack is then placed in the eponychial fold to ensure continued drainage. I advise patients to begin soaking (with the pack in place) as soon as they get home. I have discovered that many of my colleagues bandage this infected area and tell the patient not to touch it for two days. In my opinion, this is a big mistake that only enhances skin maceration and bacterial growth.

Patients should be rechecked within 24 to 36 hours. The initial pack is removed and the wound inspected. Packing can usually be removed without anesthesia after soaking in peroxide to soften the gauze. If the infection is well on its way to recovery, additional packing is not needed. If there is still considerable drainage, the nail fold may be irrigated, reopened, and packed a second time. This requires another digital block. Patients can remove the second pack themselves (after soaking at home) in another 24 hours, and follow-up is determined by clinical response or degree of patient anxiety. If the periungual skin has been under significant pressure, an outer layer of skin may blister or peel (Figure 4) within 24-48 hours of drainage. This is not serious, but the dead skin should be debrided.

Following removal of the packing, there is usually a small cavity that remains open. This is the potential eponychial space where the pus has accumulated. It will quickly be obliterated when the infection is cured. When this space still exists, it can be easily filled with an antibiotic ointment and covered with a large Band-Aid or dressing. Soaking should continue for another two or three days after the pack has been removed. Once the paronychia has healed, the patient is advised to keep the periungual area

dry and to use skin softeners to avoid cracking. I also advise against biting the fingernails or removing hangnails with the teeth.

X-rays, laboratory tests, and cultures are not generally necessary, even if pus is obtained. It's probably impossible to convince some physicians that abscess cultures are not necessary, but there are voluminous data to support this suggestion. Further testing, cultures, and fungal scrapings may be warranted in the immunocompromised patient or in those who have poor response to therapy or suffer recurrences.

There is no evidence that oral antibiotics are necessary for the treatment of uncomplicated, easily drained paronychias in patients with normal immune systems. If there is significant cellulitis, antibiotics can be supported. Although I usually prescribe three or four days of penicillin for antibiotic coverage to complement local care, 10 days of the newest third-generation cephalosporin or some similarly exotic, recently introduced antibiotic is clearly unwarranted. Penicillin or ampicillin/clavulanate appear to be reasonable choices based on culture data (see following discussion), but in my experience patients given any antibiotics seem to do well, even with penicillin. The antibiotic debate is unresolved, but the key is to use reasonable clinical judgment and not be dogmatic. If $25 of an antibiotic will prevent a revisit, the cost is certainly justified. Prescribing inexpensive penicillin or erythromycin is a theoretical acceptable compromise.

Patients should be relatively asymptomatic in four or five days. Those who have recurrent problems or do not respond adequately — especially if pus was drained — should be considered to have complicated infections, a possible foreign body, or an unusual organism, and should

ORGANISMS ISOLATED FROM 28 PATIENTS WITH PARONYCHIA

Aerobic, Facultative, and Candida Isolates (N)		Anaerobic Isolates (N)	
Gram-Positive Cocci			
χ-Hemolytic streptococci	3	Peptostreptococcus species	5
Υ-Hemolytic streptococci	5	P. magnus	8
Group A β-hemolytic streptococci	2 2	P. asaccharolyticus	1
		P. prevotii	3
Group D streptococci	8	P. anaerobius	1
Staphylococcus aureus S. epidermidis	2	Streptococcus intermedius	1
Gram-Negative Cocci			
Neisseria species	1		
Gram-Positive Bacilli		Eubacterium lentum	1
Gram-Negative Bacilli			
Klebsiella pneumoniae	2	Fusobacterium nucleatum	4
Eikenella corrodens	3	Bacteroides species	3
Acinetobacter species	1	B. fragilis	2
Candida albicans	4	B. melaninogenicus	4
		B. intermedius	3
		B. oralis	1
		B. bivius	1
		B. oris-buccae	1
Total	33		39

Source: Ann Emerg Med 1990;19:994-996.

be referred to a consultant. It's probably a mistake to follow patients for a number of weeks trying to cure a smoldering infection with each member of an ED group trying his favorite regimen. The recognized complications of a neglected paronychia are osteomyelitis or extension to the flexor tendon (tenosynovitis) or fat pad area (felon). Occasionally patients must be admitted for intravenous antibiotics or require more extensive surgery, but such cases should be the exception.

Importantly, patients who fail to respond should be considered to have a herpes infection, termed the herpetic whitlow, or a fungal cause. These variations are usually clinically evident after a few days of nonresponse. Herpetic infections will be discussed in detail in the next chapter, but suffice it to say that patients with herpetic infections of the mouth or genital area, concomitant with their paronychia, or a paronychia associated with vesicles on the periungual skin, should be considered as having this viral infection. Although of no great clinical consequence, herpetic infections are slower to resolve and should not be treated with overly aggressive incisions or antibiotics. To emphasize, patients with skin infections that do not respond as expected should be investigated for unusual organisms, osteomyelitis, possible cancer, occult foreign bodies, or immunocompromise in the host (especially AIDS).

AEROBIC AND ANAEROBIC MICROBIOLOGY OF PARONYCHIA

Brook I *Ann Emerg Med* 1990;19(9):994

This report analyzes the microbiology of 28 patients who underwent surgical drainage for a paronychia of the finger. Patients ranged in age from 19 to 48 years, and there were 20 women and eight men. Aerobic and anaerobic cultures were obtained from the infected area by either swabbing the wound or by directly aspirating fluid. Careful culturing techniques were done to ensure optimal anaerobic growth. A variety of culture media was used to ensure maximum recovery of fastidious organisms. An average of 2.6 isolates per specimen were identified, with a total of 72 organisms being recovered from the 28 specimens. A pure culture of a single anaerobic organism was present in five (18%) patients, and a pure culture of a single aerobe in eight (29%). Mixed aerobic and anaerobic cultures were the norm, and were found in 54 percent. The specific organisms identified are shown in the table. There was no consistent pattern or combination of organ-

isms. In four cases, *Candida albicans* was cultured, and *Eikenella corrodens* was isolated in three patients.

Based on culture results, the authors conclude that paronychias are usually infected with a number of mixed aerobic and anaerobic organisms. The presence of aerobic bacteria is thought to be due to direct inoculation of the fingers with mouth flora, as can occur in biting the fingernails or sucking the fingertips. The organisms recovered were those that commonly colonize either the oral cavity or the skin. Interestingly, a few cases of *E. corrodens* were discovered. This organism accounts for some cases of human bite infections and is also normal flora of the mouth.

The author attempted to discuss the proper selection of antibiotics for these mixed infections, but could not recommend an ideal empiric choice. Most pathogens isolated should theoretically respond to clindamycin or amoxicillin/clavulanate. The presence of anaerobic bacteria, some gram-negatives, and *E. corrodens* make first-generation cephalosporins a less than perfect choice. It is recommended that cultures be done if antibiotic therapy is contemplated.

COMMENT: Most textbooks state that staphylococci are the most common pathogen found in paronychias. However, *Staphylococcus aureus* or *Staphylococcus epidermides* was isolated in this study in only two of 72 cultures. Clearly such infections are polymicrobial, including aerobes, anaerobes, and both Gram-positive and Gram-negative cocci and bacilli. In a related study of the bacteriology of paronychia in children by the same author (*Am J Surg* 1981;141(6):703), similar results were reported. Specimens from the paronychia of 33 children demonstrated a 20 percent incidence of pure anaerobic cultures, 27 percent pure aerobic cultures, and 46 percent mixed aerobic and anaerobic flora. In that report, there were 3.6 isolates per specimen. Numerous organisms were identified, including *C. albicans.*

Certainly no single antibiotic will provide complete coverage for the array of bacterial and fungal pathogens cultured from paronychias. Because the vast majority of paronychias are easily cured with simple drainage procedures and local treatment, systemic antibiotics probably play little clinical role. In fact, antibiotics are unlikely to be curative if one considers the polymicrobial nature of the infections. Just because someone receives 10 days of treatment with an expensive antibiotic and the paronychia goes away does not prove that the antibiotics were helpful.

Because there are no prospective studies evaluating the

true role of antibiotic treatment of paronychia and because no antibiotic will cover 72 pathogens, I would interpret the data in this study to argue strongly against the routine use of antibiotics. Likewise, I see no reason to culture paronychial pus routinely; how does one interpret a report of three organisms, all with a different antibiotic sensitivity? These infections are essentially abscesses, and there are good data demonstrating that antibiotics are of no additive value for the treatment of cutaneous abscesses that are adequately drained. In immunocompromised patients, particularly diabetics, those with peripheral vascular disease, or those with AIDS, cancer, or recurrent paronychia, however, a culture and antibiotics are warranted. It's also possible that antibiotics will short-circuit an early paronychia that is still only a cellulitis and not yet a drainable abscess, so antibiotics may play a yet undefined role in the early phase of the infection.

I disagree with the authors of this study; I would not routinely culture a paronychia just because I was prescribing antibiotics. Unless one does aerobic, anaerobic, fungal, and viral cultures, the full benefit of this laboratory investigation will not be gleaned, so why be only half-scientific? It is impossible to prospectively or empirically choose the proper antibiotic in all cases, but it seems reasonable to choose penicillin, erythromycin, clindamycin, or ampicillin/clavulanate if one opts for treatment. Because anaerobes are so common, penicillin may not be a bad choice, but the data are just not available. There's always the concern that penicillin will not cover staphylococci, but anaerobes and streptococcal species are more common isolates.

Evidence linking *E. corrodens* to a paronychia is interesting and thought-provoking. *E. corrodens* is a gram-negative rod that is normal oral flora, and it has been reported to cause nasty infections from human bites. This organism has an unusual sensitivity. It's sensitive to penicillin and ampicillin, but resistant to oxacillin, methicillin, nafcillin, clindamycin, and often to cephalosporins. Is this another reason to choose penicillin? Suffice it to say that long courses of expensive antibiotics are not routinely required and should never be substituted for drainage follow-up or further investigation. This area is ripe for prospective multicenter research from some energetic emergency physicians.

Chronic paronychia most often represent an occupational problem or a fungal infection. Repeated exposure to trauma, water, or irritating chemicals can prolong healing of a paronychia. *C. albicans* is the most common fungal pathogen. *Candida* can be cultured or diagnosed from a potassium hydroxide slide test, and it may cause physical changes in the fingernail. Consider underlying diabetes or immunosuppression in patients with proven *Candida* paronychia. Mycostatic cream is curative, but infections are difficult to eradicate and therapy must be used for a number of weeks. Chronic fungal nail infections will not be cured by creams, and can take many months to go away with oral antifungal drugs. It's best to refer such patients to a dermatologist.

HERPETIC WHITLOW: AN UNUSUAL PARONYCHIA

Herpetic hand infections are uncommon and therefore are often misdiagnosed or treated inappropriately

A unique type of paronychia is caused by the herpes simplex virus. Herpetic hand infections are uncommon and are therefore often misdiagnosed or treated inappropriately. Herpes simplex infections can, however, produce a rather annoying and angry-looking paronychia infection called a herpetic whitlow. The importance of this entity is that it should be recognized for its self-limited clinical course. Surgical incision should not be performed, hospitalization is not required, expensive antibiotics are useless, and occasionally the process can signal immunocompromise in an otherwise well-appearing patient.

HERPETIC WHITLOW OF THE DIGITS
Haedicke GJ, et al *J Hand Surg (Br)* 1989;14(4):443

This is probably the largest series every reported on the epidemiology and treatment of herpetic whitlow. The authors describe their experience with 10 patients — all medical and paramedical personnel — who presented with a digital infection of the fingertip characterized by pain, swelling, erythema, and vesicle formation. Four patients had undergone surgical incision and drainage procedures and had been prescribed antibiotics for a presumed bacterial infection. None of the subjects had a history of previous herpetic infections. The clinical diagnosis was that of a herpetic paronychia, or herpetic whitlow. The authors treated herpetic whitlows with twice daily washing with soap and water and the application of mercurochrome and a dry sterile dressing. Two of the 10 patients were treated with oral acyclovir, but the effect was not discussed. All patients had complete healing, usually within two to four weeks. There was no permanent disability or disfigurement, and no recurrences in a two-year follow-up. None of the patients developed AIDS or were found to have other diseases that would cause them to be immunocompromised.

The authors emphasize that a herpetic whitlow often may be associated with systemic influenza-like symptoms. The process should be suspected in patients with concomitant conjunctivitis, dermatitis, or oral or genital vesicular lesions or in those known to be herpes carriers. The finger lesions consist of a group of vesicles or blisters, overlying a beefy red and swollen skin. This process commonly involves the periungual area, but any part of the finger may be affected. Occasionally satellite vesicles extending beyond the confines of the larger lesion may be noted.

The herpetic infections in this report were presumed to have been caused by direct inoculation of the fingertip with the herpes simplex virus. The condition is more frequent in dental and medical personnel who deal with patients with herpetic gingivostomatitis or genital herpes. The treatment of this viral infection is conservative. Importantly, one should eschew surgical intervention. Even though the infected area can be associated with lymphangitis or adenopathy and can manifest a systemic febrile response, the herpetic whitlow is self-limited. It is important to recognize these infections as viral in origin to avoid a deep incision that will delay healing or induce secondary bacterial infection. Misdiagnosis can also prompt expen-

sive testing or prolonged hospitalization. Oral acyclovir will probably shorten the clinical course and may be particularly beneficial in immunocompromised patients, but there are no data.

COMMENT: Early in the clinical course, it may be impossible to distinguish a herpetic whitlow from bacterial paronychia. Key to making a clinical diagnosis is finding an alternate site of a herpetic infection. More likely, however, the diagnosis would be suggested from the presence of vesicles on the periungual skin. Small raised irritated bumps can appear before actual vesicles, and this appearance is distinctly different from the homogeneous, smooth cellulitis-like swelling seen with a bacterial path-

10 PATIENTS TREATED FOR HERPETIC WHITLOW

Age of patient	Gender	Occupation	Signs/symptoms	Duration of signs before treatment, days	Previous treatment	Duration of disability
28	F	Nurse	Painful vesicles, erythema, swelling	10	I&D, oral antibiotics	4 weeks
24	F	RT	Painful vesicle	5	None	2.5 weeks
38	F	Nurse	Painful vesicles, erythema	7	I&D, oral antibiotics	3 weeks
23	F	Nurse	Necrotic vesicle with pain, erythema, mild tenosynovitis	10	I&D, oral antibiotics	3 weeks
24	F	RT	Painful vesicle	5	None	2-5 weeks
48	F	Nurse	Painful vesicle	14	I&D, oral antibiotics	1 month
32	F	Orthodontist	Painful finger, diffuse extremity pain, axillary adenopathy	5	None	3 weeks
34	F	Nurse	Painful vesicle	5	None	1 month
33	F	Pathologist	Painful vesicle	7	None	2 weeks
27	F	Nurse	Painful vesicle	10	None	4 weeks

RT, respiratory therapist

Source: J Hand Surg (British Volume) 1989;14B:4:443-445.

ogen. Viral infections should not be associated with pus formation, and markedly indurated skin without fluctuance may be another tip-off. This infection also is seen often in medical personnel. The patients in this review were nurses, respiratory therapists, an orthodontist, and a pathologist. Individuals with cold sores (fever blisters) who bite their fingernails are another high-risk group.

Like other herpes skin infections, the patient with a herpetic whitlow may relate itching, burning pain, tingling, or other sensations a few hours or days before there is an obvious infection. Herpetic skin infections can be extremely painful or annoying; just ask anyone with cold sores. Many of the diagnostic subtleties of herpetic infections may be missed if a quick or superficial history is taken. Secondary bacterial infection is possible, and may confuse the clinical picture as well as laboratory tests. In the uncomplicated case, cultures should be negative for bacteria and the CBC should not demonstrate a leukocytosis, but routinely ordering these tests is probably overkill. Characteristically, herpetic hand infections take two to three weeks to resolve, whereas bacterial infections resolve much more quickly. A common scenario may be the patient who has had a few visits to a physician, but his problem persists despite undergoing drainage and an adequate course of a broad-spectrum antibiotic.

One must always consider herpetic whitlow as a primary manifestation of AIDS. Theoretically, acyclovir or famcyclovir should shorten the clinical course, but prospective studies are lacking. A controlled study will probably never be done because this is such an unusual condition. I would definitely consider oral antiherpes therapy in all patients. Although the infection is self-limited, it's probably not unreasonable to offer a prescription for the antiviral medication in normal patients (if they can afford it) because the process is very annoying and can be prolonged. Acyclovir ointment under an occlusive dressing may help, but I have not been unimpressed with topical acyclovir for other herpes infection so I usually opt for systemic therapy. At least 200 mg given five times a day should be prescribed. Famcyclovir, 500 mg TID, is a good alternative. Be sure to caution medical/dental personnel about the potential for transmission of the virus to their patients. I would prescribe antiherpes therapy to hospital employees to shorten the course and advise that they don't

HERPES SIMPLEX INFECTIONS CAN PRODUCE A PARONYCHIA INFECTION THAT HAS A SELF-LIMITED CLINICAL COURSE

work around patients (especially in the nursery, cancer ward, or AIDS unit) until the infection is completely cleared. Viral shedding is thought to cease when the skin heals and vesicles are gone.

Viral cultures are generally unnecessary. A Tzanck test can be diagnostic (but only about 70 percent of the time), but I doubt if it's available in most hospitals on a stat basis. To perform a Tzanck test, obtain a scraping of tissue — not just fluid — from the base of a vesicle and air dry it on a slide. The specimen is fixed and stained to reveal the diagnostic multinucleated giant cells. The microbiology technicians in my hospital never heard of the Tzanck test. I later found out that it was done in the cytology laboratory at a cost of $50 for the smear preparation plus whatever the pathologist charges for interpretation.

Viral cultures are definitive but likewise expensive and unavailable for the acute diagnosis. Fluorescent antibody tests and serologic tests can be useful, but there are false positive and negative reactions and they are rarely used for this problem. Patients who have herpetic whitlow should be cautioned against possible self-contamination of their eyes and for the potential to spread the virus to other individuals. Those with recurrent herpetic infections at any site should always be considered for HIV testing. Most patients with a herpetic paronychia are not immunocompromised so the first episode does not require investigation. Although most herpetic whitlows will occur in the periungual area, the vesicular legions can occur in the toes and anywhere along the finger and still meet the definition of herpetic whitlow.

The term "whitlow" has a number of meanings, but it is usually associated only with herpes infections of the finger. Some authors also use whitlow to describe a classic felon or any painful process near the end of the finger (*J Hand Surg [Br]* 1989; 14(4):446).

HERPETIC WHITLOW: EPIDEMIOLOGY, CLINICAL CHARACTERISTICS, DIAGNOSIS, AND TREATMENT

Feder HM, Long SS *Am J Dis Child* 1983;137(9):861

This article describes the characteristics of herpetic whitlow in a children's hospital. The authors discuss the case histories of five children with the infection and two pediatric residents who cared for children in the hospital. The authors note that herpetic whitlow is uncommon in the general population, but it is thought to be distinctly unusual in infants and children. Prior to this report, herpetic whitlow was always reported in association with herpetic gingivostomatitis or severe trauma (stress reaction) in the pediatric age group. The first two cases involve 8-month and 6-month-old infants who had herpetic whitlow as the sole manifestation of a herpes simplex infection. Neither infant had an associated herpes infection elsewhere, trauma, or known exogenous exposure to the virus. The clinical pre-

DIAGNOSING HERPETIC WHITLOW

Test	Approximate Cost
Papanicolau test	$28
Tzanck test	$28
Viral cell culture	$45
Immunofluorescence	$55
Complement fixation or neutralization	$26
Antiserum or herpes titer	$17

Source: J Hand Surg (British Volume) 1989;14B:4:443-445.

sentation was similar in both cases. The infants were hospitalized because of pain, swelling, and redness of the finger, presumed to be a bacterial infection. Both were febrile, with a temperature as high as 102°F. Both children were admitted because they did not respond to outpatient antibiotics and were treated with intravenous antibiotics for presumed cellulitis or osteomyelitis in the hospital, but there was no rapid improvement. The disease was finally identified when vesicles developed. The Tzanck test was positive in only one child. Both children recovered completely.

A 10-month and a 20-month-old infant are presented to emphasize a herpetic soft tissue infection caused by a known exogenous or endogenous source. One child who sucked his thumb developed a herpetic whitlow, and it was noted that he had a few previously unrecognized herpetic vesicles and ulcers on the gingival mucosa. The finger and mouth lesions both cultured positive for herpes simplex

virus type 1 virus. Another child was treated for a presumed bacterial infection of the thumb until it was discovered that the mother had recurrent herpes labialis and bit her infant's fingernails. Presumably the infection was transmitted from the mother to the child in this manner. Both the mother's saliva and the infant's thumb had positive cultures for the same herpes strain.

The authors also report the case of 15-year-old girl who presented with fever, malaise, and a warm erythematous index finger associated with lymphadenopathy. She was found to have genital herpes lesions and cultures of her finger and labial lesions revealed herpes simplex virus type 2. In the final cases, the authors describe two pediatric residents who developed systemic symptoms in association with an erythematous swollen finger. One presumably contracted a herpetic whitlow after intubating a neonate who had an overwhelming herpes simplex viremia. The cultures from the infected resident and the baby were both positive for herpes simplex virus type 2. In the second case, a resident developed a herpetic whitlow following the accidental piercing of his thumb with a lancet that had been contaminated with the virus.

The authors note that the characteristics of a herpetic whitlow include delay of vesicle formation and a tingling or burning sensation that precedes frank swelling or erythema. Systemic signs and symptoms are also common, particularly in young children. Fever, lymphangitis, lymphadenopathy, and constitutional symptoms are well described with herpetic whitlow. Although the vesicles in these patients appeared to have pus, further investigation revealed a clear serosanguinous fluid that cultured positive for the herpes virus. Both herpes strains (types 1 and 2) can cause the disease, and recurrences are seen in about 20 percent of patients.

The route of transmission appears to be multifactorial and includes autoinfection from a primary herpes source (either gingivostomatitis or a genital infection) or exposure to an exogenous source. The potential for medical personnel to become infected is stressed. The authors note that herpes simplex virus has been recovered in the saliva of ostensibly normal adults so transmission is possible even without overt lesions.

COMMENT: In the absence of vesicles or a known active herpes infection source, it would be very difficult initially to make the diagnosis of herpetic whitlow in an infant or young child. Such cases would likely be treated as a bacterial cellulitis or osteomyelitis until the characteristic lesions surfaced. Because the infection resolves spontaneously, many cases undoubtedly are never diagnosed correctly. One tip-off may be the presence of significant fever and systemic complaints, distinctly unusual for a bacterial paronychia. Interestingly, this report comes from a children's hospital where such unusual infections should be routinely diagnosed early, yet these children were in the hospital for a number of days and received intravenous antibiotics for alternate diagnoses.

The transmission of herpes virus to medical personnel is one of significant importance. It appears that in one case, a resident contracted the infection from merely intubating an infected infant. Although some of us don't wear gloves during intubation, here's another reason why it's probably a good idea. As more information becomes available about the epidemiology of herpes infection, it is clear that many patients are carriers and actively excrete the virus in saliva, urine, and vaginal secretions in the absence of recognizable lesions or obvious clinical infection *Arch Intern Med* 1978; 138(9):1418 and *N Engl J Med* 1992;326:1533). Particularly in hospitals that care for patients with AIDS, the potential for physicians to be exposed to herpes viruses in patients without obvious lesions is significant.

HERPETIC WHITLOW, THE GREAT TOE

Feder HM Jr.
N Engl J Med [letter] 1992;326 (19):1295

This is short report of a rather unusual type of herpetic whitlow. The authors note that some parents have the strange habit of biting off their babies' toenails and fingernails. Folklore has it that cutting a child's nails before a year turns them into thieves. Many parents are also afraid of injuring the baby's finger tips if sharp scissors or clippers are used. The authors report a three-year-old girl who was first examined for a great toe infection characterized by a red, swollen, tender, and warm periungual area. Fever, lymphangitis, and adenopathy were present. The child was treated with antibiotics for a presumed bacterial soft tissue infection. Within the next few days, vesicles developed, and a Tzanck test was positive. Culture of the clear fluid from a blister was positive for herpes simplex virus type 1 and negative for bacteria. It was discovered that the mother had recurrent herpes simplex labialis (fever blisters) and had an outbreak two weeks previously. The mother also stated that she occasionally bit her child's toenails. The infection resolved over the next week with symptomatic therapy. The authors report this case to further emphasize the need to be aware of this viral infection and again stressed the caveat to avoid incision and expensive long-term antibiotic therapy.

COMMENT: This is a good example of a herpetic infection being caused by oral-digital transmission. A common source in adults is the individual with a fever blister who bites the fingernails. In children, the most common way is to suck the finger during an outbreak of herpetic gingivostomatitis. This case is a little unusual in that it occurred in the big toe and could easily be confused with an ingrown toenail, foreign body, or bacterial infection. I must admit that I don't ask the parents of infants with toe problems whether they bite the toenails, but perhaps it should be part of the routine history.

SECTION VI

PAIN CONTROL IN THE EMERGENCY DEPARTMENT

ANESTHETICS AND ANALGESICS: THE USE OF VISCOUS LIDOCAINE

Studies show that physicians commonly withhold narcotics or don't administer adequate dosages

Emergency physicians must have at least a working knowledge of every subspeciality in medicine, but because the field is so diverse, it is difficult to become an in-depth expert on any single topic. When it comes to acute pain relief, however, the EP should know more than anyone else on the medical staff. Because pain relief is such a large part of everyday emergency medicine, one must be cognizant of the issues involved in pain relief from many causes, with cases ranging from the infant and pregnant woman to post-operative, trauma, and urology patients. It's easy to give a narcotic, although most of us use them all too infrequently and often in ineffective doses. There are, however, many tricks of the trade or unusual or unique uses for anesthetics or analgesics in the ED.

Before I discuss specific modalities, I review an article that reiterates the conclusions from every other study that has been done on the use of analgesics by physicians and house staff. In essence, most physicians do an extremely poor job when it comes to managing or relieving acute pain.

ANALGESIC USE IN THE EMERGENCY DEPARTMENT

Selbst SM, Clark M *Ann Emerg Med* 1990;19(9):1010

This is a retrospective review of 112 pediatric and 156 adult patients (a few months to 97 years of age) who were treated in the ED for selected painful conditions. The specific painful conditions were sickle cell crises (20%), lower extremity fractures (31%), and second or third degree burns (49%). The authors note that other studies have concentrated on inpatients while this report looks particularly at acute pain in the ED. Other authors have repeatedly concluded that narcotics are commonly withheld altogether or patients suffer severe pain or distress because inadequate dosages are used. When it comes to children, physicians — including pediatricians — are even more stingy. Children who have the same diagnosis as adults are less likely to receive appropriate narcotics.

Of the 268 patients, 15 percent were admitted because of their pain or injury, although children were rarely admitted (0.6%) compared to older adults. Amazingly, only 40 percent of the patients with acutely painful conditions received any analgesics at all in the ED, and children were much less likely than adults to receive pain relief (28% vs. 60%, respectively, received analgesics). Burns in particular were undertreated in children; only 15 percent received pain medication. Only 37 percent of all patients with lower extremity fractures received analgesics. When narcotics were given, 12 percent of patients received less than the usual recommended initial dose.

Although emergency physicians were more liberal than pediatricians in ordering analgesics for children, both specialties were culpable. For those patients who were discharged from the hospital with painful conditions, only 45 percent received prescriptions for analgesics (35% of the children and 76% of the adults).

The authors conclude that most patients who present to the ED with acute painful conditions do not receive appropriate analgesics. It's admitted, however, that it is difficult to determine the actual amount of pain experienced in a retrospective study. The authors suggest that pain management is rarely addressed in medical training, and the topic receives little attention in textbooks.

Physicians have unfounded fears about causing respiratory depression or addiction in patients that often limit their use of narcotics. The alarming fact of this study is that children are much less likely than adults to receive analgesics for similarly painful conditions. It is speculated that children may not voice pain as much as adults for fear of a painful injection, and it's suggested that one make special efforts to observe subtle clues in children that may signify the need for pain relief.

COMMENT: Hypotension and respiratory depression are legitimate concerns when one prescribes narcotics, and certainly other issues take precedence during a resuscitation. There is, however, no excuse for withholding pain medications when safe analgesia is possible. The subject of the inappropriate use of analgesics is a textbook in itself, but suffice it to say that the majority of physicians tend to undertreat patients who are in pain, and patients treated in the ED are also shortchanged. There are many reasons for this shortcoming, but most of the time it is due to the physician's unrealistic concern about narcotic overdose, the potential for addiction, skepticism about the degree of pain, or the fear of masking or exacerbating medical conditions.

It is distressing to read the statistics in this study and, despite evidence that shows that neonates experience pain, there is still a misconception that younger patients tolerate pain better than adults. I could never understand why the same physician who religiously avoids venipuncture or an intramuscular dose of antibiotics for fear of hurting the pediatric patient gives plain acetaminophen for a painful earache or thermal burn or doesn't even address the issue of pain control in a child with a fracture unless the parents ask for it.

The subject of addiction is a fascinating one, but I find it difficult to believe that anyone becomes addicted to Demerol because it's given too freely in the ED for a kidney stone or fractured femur. In fact, there is evidence to suggest that the chance for addiction is greater when pain medication is withheld and the patient must suffer and then plead for an injection than if they are given narcotics on a routine basis. In my opinion, every time the patient has to ask for a pain shot because pain control is not at least addressed, it's an error on the doctor's part.

Finally, many residents have concerns about giving narcotics to patients that they believe fit the profile of a drug abuser, fearing they will get "beat" out of some Demerol or morphine. I have personally been wrong in my bias a number of times and have learned that a patient is not a drug abuser just because he has back pain and requests a brand name narcotic. I don't think twice about getting swindled out of a single injection of a narcotic in borderline cases. It probably happens quite frequently. Although I would hesitate to give a prescription for 50 Dilaudid to a patient who was a classic drug abuser (from out of town, physician can't be reached, allergic to everything else, carrying his own MRI showing a bulging disc three year ago), I would think no more than two seconds before I gave a single injection in the ED unless the patient was blatantly bogus.

THE EMERGENCY DEPARTMENT TREATMENT OF DYSPEPSIA WITH ANTACIDS AND ORAL LIDOCAINE

Welling LR, Watson WA
Ann Emerg Med 1990;19(7):789

This is one of only a few articles that addresses the common routine of administering a therapeutic GI cocktail to patients with dyspepsia of unknown origin. Although plain antacids are most commonly used for the symptomatic treatment of gastroesophageal reflux, gastritis, or peptic ulcer disease, occasionally local anesthetics are added to increase potency. The authors administered either 30 ml Mylanta II (34 patients) or 30 ml of the antacid plus 15 ml of 2% viscous lidocaine (300 mg; 39 patients) to individuals with dyspepsic complaints, such as burning epigastric pain, nausea, or belching. Prior to and after treatment, patients rated their pain on a linear analogue pain scale. The improvement on the pain score was significantly better in the group that received antacid plus lidocaine versus those who receive lidocaine alone (35% and 69%, respectively, experienced acceptable pain relief).

A specific diagnosis was often not made and 26 percent of the patients eventually received a diagnosis of a condition not usually associated with dyspepsia. Most patients were discharged with the label of nonspecific abdominal pain, peptic ulcer disease, or gastritis/esophagitis. Interestingly, there was no relationship between the discharge diagnosis and the response to treatment, indicating a significant placebo response. Most patients did not return for follow-up. Although there were no adverse events secondary to therapy, two patients had significant cardiovascular disease, including one with angina and another who returned in cardiac arrest from a mesenteric thrombosis. The authors note that most patients with nonspecific dyspepsia have no etiology identified on follow-up testing, and therefore symptomatic relief is often prescribed before the specific diagnosis is known.

The authors caution against the possible side effects of multiple doses of viscous lidocaine and note that they administered only a single 300 mg dose. The authors conclude that a single dose of antacid plus viscous lidocaine is an appropriate treatment modality for the relief of acute dyspepsia in the ED, even when the exact etiology of the pain is unknown. They caution that the response to therapy should not be considered diagnostic of gastrointestinal disease.

COMMENT: Hardly a day goes by that the EP does not administer some sort of GI cocktail for the treatment of an unknown but presumably benign gastrointestinal disorder. It goes without saying, however, that myocardial infarction and many other life-threatening conditions can present as indigestion and get amazingly better with antacids. It can be disastrous to underestimate the placebo effect of the hospital, a caring nurse or physician, a little nasal oxygen, and some strange-tasting medication; such a regimen can make even cancer pain much better. Therefore, it is essential to reiterate the authors' caution that the response to pain is diagnostic of nothing!

Other authors have attempted to utilize viscous lidocaine in the ED. Fifteen years ago, Schwartz suggested that viscous lidocaine could aid in the differential diagnosis of chest pain (*JACEP* 1976;5(12)). He administered 20 cc (400 mg) of viscous lidocaine to 60 patients with chest and/or epigastric pain in whom the diagnosis of GI or cardiac pain was suspected. A positive response was the dramatic or complete relief of symptoms within 10 to 15 minutes. Serum lidocaine levels were minimal in the few patients studied (maximum=0.55 μg/ml), well below the antiarrhythmic therapeutic level (2-5 μg/ml).

Six patients in this study ultimately had an myocardial infarction (MI) or angina, none of whom had a positive response to the lidocaine. No patient with a positive response had an MI. This author concludes that the response to lidocaine may aid in diagnosis (e.g., a positive response suggests GI pathology), but the incidence of those with true cardiac arrest who will respond to lidocaine is unknown. Antacids/lidocaine may provide welcome relief to the patient with severe GI discomfort, but I firmly believe that it's dangerous to consider the response to a GI cocktail as even semi-diagnostic.

The caution about the overuse or chronic administration of viscous lidocaine is well warranted. Note that each milliliter of 2% viscous lidocaine contains 20 mg of a

VISCOUS LIDOCAINE

- *Available as a 2% gel*

- *2% means 2 grams in 100 ml*
  or
  2000 mg in 100 ml
  or
  20 mg per ml

- *Average adult swallow = 15 ml = 300 mg lidocaine*

- *Average child swallow = 5 ml = 100 mg lidocaine*

Source: James R. Roberts, MD

potentially toxic drug, most of which is absorbed from the GI tract. The bottom line is that discharged patients should never receive a prescription for viscous lidocaine even though it may have been a therapeutic triumph in the ED.

The authors also note that many combinations of drugs make up the omnipresent GI cocktail, including antispasmodics (Donnatal), sucralfate (Carafate), Pepto Bismol, and simethicone. There is little objective data to label any concoction superior. I'm a firm believer in the enhanced therapeutic effect of adding lidocaine to antacids, but it is difficult to prove that any oral regimen is better than placebo (*J Clin Gastroenterol* 1986;8(suppl 1):72). Because recipes differ so greatly, it's important to specify the exact contents of the GI cocktail. I once saw a patient with an acute allergic reaction, and the chart did not state what components were used. This patient subsequently claimed an "allergy" to all ulcer medicines.

My GI cocktail consists of 60 ml of antacid, 10 (not 15) ml of viscous lidocaine, and 10 ml of Donnatal elixir, occasionally followed by two Carafate tablets dissolved in water. This is clearly shotgun therapy and is aimed at treating anything from esophageal spasm to gastritis to ulcers, and I have had some remarkable cures. I have, however, also cured at least two myocardial infarctions and made one aortic dissection feel much better so I have no misconceptions that this is in any way, shape, or form a diagnostic maneuver. This study appears to prove that the topical anesthetic provides some additional pain relief to antacids alone. It makes sense to include this in one's initial treatment arsenal, as long as the previously mentioned caveats are understood.

SEIZURES SECONDARY TO ORAL VISCOUS LIDOCAINE

Hess GP, Walson PD *Ann Emerg Med* 1988;17(7):725

This article reports adverse effects to the oral administration of viscous lidocaine in two children. In the first case, a 1-year-old girl with gingivostomatitis was prescribed viscous lidocaine, one teaspoon every four hours, for symptomatic relief. The parents increased the dose, and after 1 g had been administered over a nine-hour period, the child became lethargic and experienced six generalized seizures. Although the patient demonstrated toxic serum lidocaine levels, she recovered without sequela. In the next case, a 5-month-old boy was given another patient's viscous lidocaine for the relief of teething pain. This child also developed a seizure and had toxic levels of lidocaine. This child likewise had a benign course and was discharged without sequela.

The authors note that topical lidocaine has a relatively short duration of action, lasting only 30 to 60 minutes. The drug is absorbed from both the oral mucosa and the gastrointestinal system. Lidocaine absorbed from the oral mucosa bypasses the liver and is not detoxified as rapidly as a drug that is absorbed from the intestine and immediately passes through the liver. The authors emphasize the toxic potential of viscous lidocaine and also offer the caveat that seizures in a patient suffering from teething or gingivostomatitis should alert the physician of possible clandestine lidocaine overdose.

COMMENT: This article underscores my rule that viscous lidocaine should never be prescribed to outpatients. Not only do patients often take it incorrectly, they use it on friends and relatives that the physician never sees. The authors state that the duration of action is 30 to 60 minutes, although in my experience topically applied lidocaine does not last anywhere near that long. There is a great potential for it to be used every 15 to 20 minutes.

Teething or herpes stomatitis can be painful conditions, and I must admit that I have occasionally given parents a small test tube of viscous lidocaine to apply with a Q-tip to their infants as an outpatients. When this is done, however, the total dose is not more than a few milliliters. One should assume that the child will swallow any oral medication. Absorption from an inflamed mucosa will cause

PATIENTS RECEIVING PAIN MEDICATIONS

Total			Sickle Cell Crises		Lower Extremity Fractures		Second or Third Degree Burns	
	No.	%	No.	%	No.	%	No.	%
Total	108/268	40	46/53	87	31/84	37	31/131	24
Children	44/157	28	20/27	74	8/24	33	16/106	15
Adults	53/88	60	26/26	100	12/139	31	15/23	65

Source: Ann Emerg Med, *1990;19:1010-1013.*

lidocaine absorbed in the mouth or pharynx to bypass the protective effect of first-pass metabolism in the liver, so kinetics are similar to an IV bolus. A popular but unsubstantiated pediatric cocktail for the treatment of painful oral lesions is a combination of equal parts of viscous lidocaine, Benadryl elixir, and Maalox (so-called "magic mouthwash), used topically or as a rinse. I'm not convinced this works any better than popsicles/ice cream and acetaminophen (with or without codeine), but it's probably safe to make up small amounts of this mixture in the ED and give it to patients to take home. If one limits the quantity and carefully instructs the parents, I believe this is a reasonable way to approach this problem without totally eschewing viscous lidocaine. Other authors have suggested that viscous lidocaine is helpful for the treatment of stomatitis (*Cutis* 1978;22(2):183; *J Am Dent Assoc* 1980;101(5):803).

This article is not the first report of toxicity from viscous lidocaine. Seizures are common, and at least one case of cardiopulmonary arrest has been reported. Mofenson reports serum lidocaine levels of 10 μg/ml (toxic above 5 μg/ml) in a child given the preparation to treat teething (*Clin Pediatr* 1983;22(3):190). A popular over-the-counter teething product, Anbesol, may be toxic if used inappropriately. Anbesol contains up to 20 percent benzocaine, a local anesthetic that can cause methemoglobinemia from mucosal absorption. I have seen methemoglobinemia from benzocaine-containing Cetacaine spray used for NG tube passage and endoscopy.

Viscous lidocaine has gained popularity for other ED uses. I could never understand the rationale for coating an endotracheal tube with the lidocaine gel instead of K-Y jelly because it will take a few minutes for the anesthetic to be effective. Instead, it makes more sense to fill the nose 5-10 minutes prior to passing a nasal tube. For a difficult Foley catheter insertion, the compassionate physician will fill a 10 ml syringe with xylocaine gel and inject it directly into the penis prior to instrumentation. Simply coating the catheter at time of insertion is clearly worthless. I have used a viscous lidocaine gargle/swallow prior to nasogatric tube passage and think it's worthwhile but no better than

> "EXCESSIVE DOSAGE, OR SHORT INTERVALS BETWEEN DOSES, CAN RESULT IN HIGH PLASMA LEVELS AND SERIOUS ADVERSE EFFECTS. PATIENTS SHOULD BE INSTRUCTED TO ADHERE TO THE RECOMMENDED DOSAGE AND ADMINISTRATION GUIDELINES...."
>
> *Boldface warning about the use of viscous xylocaine,* Physician's Desk Reference, *44th edition, 1990, Medical Economics Co., Oradell, NJ.*

other anesthetic sprays. I personally don't use viscous lidocaine for symptomatic relief of acute pharyngitis because it is short-acting, gets absorbed quickly from an inflamed mucosa, and actually gives the patient an unpleasant sensation that he can't swallow. Despite the best intentions of medical students, viscous lidocaine provides no real anesthesia when applied topically to abrasions or burns, and it has no effect on the ear canal or tympanic membrane.

NOVEL METHODS OF EASING PAIN

Recent literature on pain has gone unnoticed, accenting how pain relief is relegated to secondary priority

Myriad ways to ease pain are available to the emergency physician, including the installation of medications into various spaces in the body, a novel way to produce analgesia in an injured knee, a method to ameliorate traumatic chest pain, and a treatment of acute gouty arthritis that does not include anti-inflammatory medication.

Some of this information has been reported within the past few months. I find it interesting, however, that many innovative analgesic techniques are not only poorly studied and poorly disseminated, but also that proven techniques are infrequently or slowly adapted to widespread clinical use. This further underscores the observation that clinicians and researchers often relegate pain relief to a secondary priority.

ANALGESIC EFFECT OF INTRAARTICULAR MORPHINE AFTER ARTHROSCOPIC KNEE SURGERY

Stein C, et al *N Engl J Med* 1991;325(16):1123

The authors of this report, anesthesiologists and orthopedic surgeons from Germany, evaluate the ability of low doses of intraarticular (IA) morphine to reduce pain following knee surgery. The basis for this study was the observation that opioid receptors have been identified in inflamed tissue in experimental animals, and the administration of opioids in the vicinity of peripheral nerve terminals produces "local" opiate analgesia.

Fifty-two postoperative patients undergoing arthroscopic knee surgery for diagnostic or therapeutic purposes were entered into the study. Subjects were randomized in a double-blind, placebo-controlled protocol containing four groups, each receiving one of the following treatments: 1 mg morphine/40 ml saline IA, saline IA and 1 mg morphine intravenously, 0.5 mg morphine/saline IA, or 1 mg morphine/0.1 mg naloxone/saline IA. Postoperative pain was assessed with a visual analogue pain scale and a questionnaire for a 24-hour period. Traditional supplemental analgesics were administered as needed.

Throughout the study, the pain scores were significantly lower in the group who received intraarticular (IA) morphine than those who received a similar dose of intravenous morphine. IA morphine also decreased the need for supplemental analgesics. Although the response was greatest with the 1 mg IA dose of the opiate, analgesia was also obtained with the smaller 0.5 mg IA dose. When naloxone

CHARACTERISTICS OF PATIENTS UNDERGOING ARTHROSCOPIC KNEE SURGERY

Variable	Group 1	Group 2	Group 3	Group 4
Sex (M/F)	11/7	8/7	7/3	5/4
Age (yrs)	40±13	37±15	38±12	40±12
Height (cm)	173±8	172±7	176±14	166±9
Weight (kg)	77±8	70±8	79±16	73±15
Duration of surgery (min.)	25±12	27±12	22±13	26±12

Source: N Engl J Med *1991;325:1123.*

was concomitantly administered IA, there was a reduction in the analgesic effect of the locally instilled narcotic.

The authors conclude that very low doses of intraarticular morphine provide significant postoperative analgesia via a peripheral site of action in the knee joint itself. Importantly, the analgesic effect was reversed by concomitant IA naloxone, suggesting that pain relief is mediated by local opioid receptors. Interestingly, the IA morphine had a slightly delayed onset of action and produced analgesia for a longer duration than traditional doses of intravenous morphine. The maximum analgesic effect of IA morphine was 3-6 hours.

The difference in pain relief between 0.5 and 1 mg morphine was not statistically significant, but there was a trend toward better pain relief with the higher dose. The authors emphasize the beneficial effect of an extremely small dose of IA morphine. They were not surprised, therefore, by the lack of significant systemic side effects. Systemic or spinal administration of morphine for postoperative pain can produce sedation, respiratory depression, pruritus, and urinary retention, none of which were seen in this study.

COMMENT: This is a fascinating study that could be a landmark report. The technique has widespread application to emergency medicine, particularly if it proves to be similarly effective for traumatic injuries to the knee, such as hemarthrosis, fractures, or soft tissue injuries (a good study for some interested reader to perform). It's

impressive that intraarticular morphine in doses as small as 1 mg produced significant pain relief. The reversal of analgesia by concomitant IA naloxone supports the theory that there are local opioid receptors and the mechanism of action is a local phenomenon. Because 1 mg intravenous morphine is worthless in adults with significant pain, there is little else to explain the effect of such low IA doses. One wonders about other applications of this technique, particularly IA nonsteroidal anti-inflammatory drugs (NSAIDs).

A frequently touted trick for facilitating an examination or providing analgesia in ED patients with painful traumatic knee injuries is to instill a local anesthetic into the joint following arthrocentesis. Despite the fact that many EPs use IA lidocaine, I was unable to find a controlled study evaluating the technique. IA lidocaine probably has some local analgesic effect, but in my experience it's not a magic cure. I find that IA lidocaine has minimal analgesic effect on extra-articular structures, such as collateral ligaments or soft tissue. Interestingly, the authors of this study instilled 40 ml saline into the joint with the morphine, but I have routinely been using only about 5-10 ml 1% lidocaine. Perhaps my lack of response is a volume issue. I would like to see a study that evaluates both IA morphine and perhaps IA bupivacaine for traumatic knee injuries seen in the ED. Perhaps the technique even has merit for acute gouty arthritis or a septic joint.

If one does opt for IA local anesthetics, I strongly suggest that one use a new bottle to avoid possible contamination of the joint. Multidose vials of local anesthetic that have been sitting open on the suture cart are clearly not appropriate for such injections. One danger of producing complete analgesia in an injured joint is that the patient will walk during the painless period and exacerbate an injury, so caution and careful patient selection are suggested.

INTRAPLEURAL BUPIVACAINE ANALGESIA IN CHEST TRAUMA: A RANDOMIZED DOUBLE-BLIND CONTROLLED TRIAL

Knottenbelt J, et al *Injury* 1991;22(2):114

This randomized double-blind study investigates the analgesic effect and safety of intrapleural (IP) bupivacaine for patients with thoracic injuries. The authors note that in addition to the obvious stress to the patient, severe chest pain following thoracic injuries interferes with chest wall movement and may adversely affect oxygenation, the ability to clear secretions, and eventually predispose to pneumonia.

In this study, 120 consecutive patients with a chest tube placed for a hemothorax or pneumothorax from blunt or penetrating chest injuries were studied. Six patients had blunt chest injury with fractured ribs and 114 had penetrating chest wounds. The protocol called for either 10 ml 0.5% bupivacaine/10 ml saline or 20 ml saline placebo to be instilled into the pleural cavity. Following drainage of any free-flowing blood or fluid, the test drug was instilled in the chest tube while the patient was lying on the contralateral side with the tube clamped for 5 minutes.

Pain relief was noted on a visual analogue scale before treatment and at 5 and 15 minutes after the test drug. If satisfactory pain relief was not obtained within 15 minutes, the patient received either standard analgesics or open label treatment with IP bupivacaine.

Pain relief was satisfactory for two or more hours in 62 percent of those given IP bupivacaine compared to 15 per-

blood levels were not studied. The authors suggest that because additional bupivacaine provided relief when the initial dose did not, the first dose may have been inadequate in some patients.

The authors conclude that the intrapleural instillation of 20 ml 0.25% bupivacaine (100 mg) is highly effective in providing analgesia in patients with chest injury. It is speculated that residual blood in the pleural cavity may further dilute the concentration to ineffective ranges, and an additional dose or higher initial dose may be required in some cases. These authors did not insert a chest tube merely to instill the drug for pain relief, but they do not discount this as a possible use for the technique.

COMMENT: Other authors have also touted intrapleural (IP) bupivacaine as an analgesic technique, but the procedure has not had widespread acceptance. Rocco et al (*Reg Anesth* 1987;12(1):10) administered IP bupivacaine via an intrapleural catheter in six patients with multiple rib fractures. When 20 ml 0.5% IP bupivacaine with epinephrine (1:200,000) was given e eight to 12 hours, complete pain relief and an improvement in arterial blood gases were noted in all patients. The procedure was without side effects, and intercostal or abdominal muscle weakness did not occur.

Some patients also received IP bupivacaine by continuous infusion for up to 10 days with similar success and without untoward effects. As a final perspective, Rosenberg et al (*Anesthesiology* 1987;67(5):811) were unable to provide adequate analgesia in post-thoracotomy patients with IP bupivacaine, so the procedure is not for one.

The philosophy behind this study is similar to the previous one in that the helpful analgesic/anesthetic is administered into the pain-producing area as opposed to attempting to provide pain relief via a central mechanism.

The authors of this study did not measure bupivacaine serum levels, but the patients experienced no untoward effects from the doses used. A potential problem could be paralysis of respiratory muscles, but this apparently does not occur. A maximal safe volume of bupivacaine in adults is in the vicinity of 70 ml 0.25% concentration (175 mg), although some physicians rec-

MEAN VISUAL ANALOGUE SCORES ADDRESSING PAIN IN PATIENTS WHO RECEIVED IA AND IV MORPHINE AFTER ARTHROSCOPIC KNEE SURGERY

Group	Hours After Surgery					
	1	2	3	4	6	24
	millimeters					
1	22±17	19±17	14±8	10±8	9±13	5±4
2	28±19	28±12	26±19	23±15	37±31	12±15
3	24±19	20±16	15±13	11±13	9±9	1±3
4	38±15	32±15	24±9	20±9	14±9	3±6

Source: N Engl J Med *1991;325:1123.*

cent of those given placebo. The duration of effective analgesia was about four hours. There were 74 early failures, 21 of whom were retreated with IP bupivacaine as the analgesic of choice by the attending physician. Subsequent relief was obtained in 20 of these 21 patients. There were no significant side effects related to the study. Bupivacaine ommend 400 mg as a maximum safe dose for the local infiltration of bupivacaine.

An older and more accepted technique for pain relief of traumatic chest injuries is the use of intercostal nerve blocks. In my opinion, intercostal nerve blocks are significantly underused in the ED, and the technique should be

DISADVANTAGES OF TRADITIONAL CHEST TRAUMA ANALGESIA

Rib blocks	• *Multiple punctures* • *Moderate expertise required* • *Not suitable for posterior fractures* • *Painful* • *Time-consuming*
Thoracic epidural analgesia	• *Expertise required* • *Hypotension*
Opiates	• *Respiratory depression* • *Cough reflex suppressed*
Paracetamol	• *Often not adequate*
NSAIDs	• *Bronchospasm gastrointestinal bleeding* • *Anti-platelet activity*

Source: Injury *1991;22(2):114.*

part of the emergency physician's therapeutic arsenal. Patients with fractured ribs can obtain remarkable relief from the procedure. These nerve blocks are most appropriate for patients with localized chest wall pain, by blocking the rib above and below the ones fractured, and the procedure can easily be done on outpatients.

The possible downside of an intercostal nerve block is the production of a pneumothorax, a well-known complication but one that should be minimized with careful technique. It's estimated that a collapsed lung results in less than 0.1 percent of cases of intercostal blocks, a lower incidence than noted with central venous pressure (CVP) catheter placement (*Clin Anesthesia* 1969;2:281). I personally do not routinely obtain a chest film following intercostal nerve block for asymptomatic patients who are discharged, although it's not unreasonable to do so.

Certainly if the patient gets short of breath, has an increase in pleuritic chest pain, or has a coughing spasm during the procedure (signifying lung contact), a post-procedure chest x-ray is in order.

Importantly, intercostal nerve blocks result in relatively high blood levels of local anesthetics when compared to the same dose used for soft tissue infiltration, so if multiple ribs are blocked, it's important to carefully calculate the total dose.

Finally, it's no fun to have a chest tube under any circumstances, but I believe that insertion can be relatively painless when done properly. The most common error that I note is the insufficient use of local anesthetics. The periosteum and pleura should be anesthetized when possible, and you just can't do a proper job with less than 10 ml local anesthetic. There is no reason to use lidocaine when the longer acting bupivacaine is available.

LIDOCAINE REGIONAL BLOCK IN THE TREATMENT OF ACUTE GOUTY ARTHRITIS OF THE FOOT

Haber GR, et al
J Am Podiatr Med Assoc 1984;79(9):492

This article explores the theory that a local anesthetic, when used to produce regional nerve block, may abort an attack of gout without the use of NSAIDs. The authors studied 16 patients with a diagnosis of acute gouty arthritis confirmed by aspiration of urate crystals or based on a clinical picture consistent with the disease. The duration of pain was less than 48 hours in all cases. Patients had no allergy to local anesthetics, no evidence of infection, or no involvement of joints other than those of the foot.

The treatment consisted of a posterior tibial nerve block or an entire ankle block if the dorsum of the foot was involved. The anesthetic was 2% lidocaine. Acetaminophen with codeine was prescribed for pain, but neither NSAIDs nor colchicine was given. Once the nerve block was deemed effective, patients were discharged and re-examined in 24 hours. If the pain had not been aborted by the local anesthetic at 24 hours, traditional anti-inflammatory therapy was prescribed.

Nine of the sixteen patients (56%) had complete resolution of pain, but six (38%) did not improve. Interestingly, even when pain was reported as improved, erythema and heat were not significantly affected.

The authors conclude that local anesthetics may successfully abort or moderate an attack of acute gouty arthritis in many patients. The proposed mechanism is an interruption of nerve conduction with resultant arterial dilation. Much of the therapeutic effect was attributed to increased blood flow to the affected area. The authors note that the temperature in the big toe is generally below 37°C, and many attacks of gout appear to be related to circumstances that decrease temperature, such as night time or strenuous exercise. Therefore, a vasodilation-medicated increase in temperature may be the actual mechanism of action. Increased blood flow will cause urate crystals to be soluble in the warmer extremity.

This attractive alternative for the treatment for acute gout of the foot may circumvent the side effects of NSAIDs and colchicine. This approach may be particularly beneficial for patients with ulcers, GI bleeding, or those with renal insufficiency, known complications of NSAID use.

COMMENT: This is a fascinating article that has received little clinical attention. I have never tried the technique or heard it mentioned elsewhere, despite the fact the paper was published in 1984. Although many people respond quickly to indomethacin or colchicine, adjunctive therapy aimed at both analgesia and resolution of the acute attack is attractive, especially for patients with contraindications for NSAIDs. Most physicians are happy making the diagnosis of gout and prescribing NSAIDs, yet skimp on narcotics for acute pain relief. Many rarely, if ever, use adjunctive treatment such as nerve blocks or even splinting. In my opinion, patients with gout of the wrist or ankle should never leave the ED without a plaster splint in place and a 24-hour supply of a narcotic.

Gout frequently coexists with many other chronic diseases so one routinely encounters patients who have contraindications to NSAIDs. The two most common contraindications are renal insufficiency, common in patients with congestive heart failure or diabetes, or a history of ulcer disease. The anti-prostaglandin effect of NSAIDs decreases renal blood flow and circumvents the body's basic defenses against gastric ulceration. There are no totally effective means to counteract these side effects, but there is some evidence that misoprostol, a prostaglandin analog, may decrease GI pathology when administered concurrently with NSAIDs. Misoprostol does not appear to have any major effect against NSAID-induced renal insufficiency.

Colchicine is a great drug for the treatment of acute gout, and I almost invariably use it in the ED, even if pain has been present for a number of days. My regimen is to give colchicine intravenously in a one-time 2 mg dose. I've occasionally used colchicine pills, but I think it is almost criminal to prescribe oral colchicine until patients experience nausea or diarrhea. Usually one overshoots the toxicity of colchicine because of the drug's delayed effect, and

USE OF INTRAPLEURAL BUPIVACAINE FOR TRAUMATIC CHEST PAIN		
	Placebo (60 patients)	*Intrapleural Bupivacaine (60 patients)*
Initial satisfactory pain relief for 2 hours or more	*9 (15%)*	*37 (62%)*
Failure of adequate pain relief	*51 (85%)*	*23 (38%)*
Mean duration of analgesia	*0.9 hrs*	*3.9 hrs*
Pain relief in 74 initial failures when treated with bupivacaine		*21 of 20*

Source: Injury 1991;22(2):114.

the diarrhea, nausea, and vomiting of colchicine is far worse than any gout attack. Therefore, if I use oral colchicine I give it only as a single dose in the ED (about 2-3 tablets). Although I prefer to give colchicine intravenously, one must be careful not to infiltrate the infusion because it can cause tissue slough.

I have occasionally used a local nerve block for pain relief from acute gout, but I have not used a nerve block for the sole treatment. I am unsure why the authors did not choose bupivacaine rather than the short-acting lidocaine. A posterior tibial block will anesthetize most of the big toe, but if the dorsum of the foot is involved, a complete ankle block is required. Anatomically, the superficial peroneal nerve may also require blocking to get complete toe anesthesia.

I find any nerve block at the ankle technically difficult and generally have only a 50-60 percent success rate. Although most physicians are keyed into gout causing acute podagra, the disease often involves the dorsum of the foot by producing an acute tenosynovitis of extensor tendons. A red, hot, swollen, tender dorsum of the foot usually prompts the uninitiated to diagnose and treat for cellulitis rather than gout. Because there is no joint involved, there is no fluid to aspirate for crystal analysis.

The theory that the beneficial effects of local anesthetics will cause uric acid crystals to go into solution because of increased heat from vasodilation suggests that heat rather than ice may be an appropriate topical treatment for acute gouty arthritis. In addition to a therapeutic nerve block, there is at least one other antigout therapy to consider in the patient with contraindications to NSAID use. Specifically, corticosteroids are potent antigout medications. Most patients can safely tolerate 60-80 mg prednisone for a few days and an intraarticular steroid injection (such as long-acting Depo-Medrol) can do wonders for acute gouty arthritis. (I wonder what effect intraarticular morphine would have on acute gouty arthritis). I believe high-dose, short-term prednisone is underused to treat refractory gout. I frequently prescribe it for two to three days and can't understand the reluctance to use this therapeutic medication when it's used with little prompting in higher doses and for much longer periods for asthma or poison ivy.

NSAIDs as Unique Analgesics

NSAIDs are particularly effective for treating biliary colic, renal colic, and dysmenorrhea

Nonsteroidal anti-inflammatory drugs (NSAIDs) have been used for many years as safe and effective analgesics for a variety of conditions. These drugs clearly quell the inflammation and pain of arthritis, but when NSAIDs are used as first-line analgesics for soft-tissue injuries, back pain, and headaches, they are probably only slightly more effective than aspirin or acetaminophen.

It appears, however, that NSAIDs have rather spectacular analgesic effects in at least three situations when one might not readily think to use these drugs. In these instances, specific antiprostaglandin activity directly attacks the pathophysiologic mechanisms responsible for pain, often elevating NSAIDs baseline pain-relieving properties to a level equal to narcotics.

This chapter discusses the use of NSAIDs as specific analgesics in biliary colic, renal colic, and dysmenorrhea, situations where the emergency physician is frequently called upon to render pain relief.

BILIARY COLIC TREATMENT AND ACUTE CHOLECYSTITIS PREVENTION BY PROSTAGLANDIN INHIBITOR

Goldman G, et al *Dig Dis Sci* 1989;34(6):809

This article appears in a rather obscure journal and seems to have been missed by many emergency physicians. It is a fascinating study with significant application to patients with abdominal pain secondary to gall bladder disease. The authors note that cholelithiasis leads to biliary colic when stones become impacted in the cystic duct. An impacted stone initiates a cascade of events that initially includes reflex gall bladder smooth muscle contraction, manifested as colicky pain. As a result, enzymes, including prostaglandins, are released and precipitate an inflammatory process that ultimately leads to acute cholecystitis.

Prostaglandins are felt to be important mediators in the inflammatory process, and, in synergism with bradykinins and histamines, this chemical mediator ultimately causes edema and acute inflammation. Therefore, antiprostaglandin medications play a double role in the treatment of gall bladder disease, preventing the mechanical process that produces biliary colic and halting the biochemical process that accounts for progression to acute cholecystitis.

Sixty patients (average age 61 years) with biliary colic secondary to ultrasonography-proven cholelithiasis were entered into the study. Treatment consisted either of 75 mg IM diclofenac (Voltaren), papaverine, or placebo, administered in a double-blind protocol. Patients were observed for 24 hours to assess pain relief and progression to acute cholecystitis. Subjects were excluded if they initially exhibited symptoms of acute inflammation, such as marked right upper quadrant guarding or rebound tenderness, fever, elevated serum amylase, or leukocytosis. Patients with a history of peptic ulcer disease were also excluded. A fourth group of patients with low back pain were included as diclofenac controls to evaluate the baseline analgesic effect of the NSAID.

The response to treatment, mean response time, and recurrence of pain in each group are listed in Table 1. Diclofenac produced rapid, impressive, and statistically significant analgesia when compared to placebo or papaverine. Only one patient who received the NSAID continued to have pain, and none progressed to acute cholecystitis during the observation period. About a quarter of the patients treated with placebo or papaverine ultimately required hospitalization because their biliary colic pro-

gressed to acute cholecystitis, evidenced by the appearance of fever, leukocytosis, and increased pain. Only 25 percent of patients with low back pain experienced complete pain relief with the NSAID.

The authors conclude that diclofenac is an effective analgesic in patients with acute biliary colic, and its use may negate immediate hospitalization or the need for emergency surgery by virtue of the fact that it prevents biliary colic from progressing to acute cholecystitis. It is speculated that the therapeutic value of Voltaren is secondary to the drug's antiprostaglandin effect, basically short-circuiting the subsequent cascade of pathologic events that result from a stone blocking the cystic duct. This is a specific effect in addition to the intrinsic systemic analgesic properties of Voltaren. Although the authors agree that the ultimate treatment for cholelithiasis is an operation, there is a clear benefit to this medical alternative in patients who are not candidates for immediate surgery.

COMMENT: It appears that prostaglandins are key mediators in the development of both the pain of biliary colic and the edema and inflammation of cholecystitis. Therefore, it makes sense to include an antiprostaglandin

Table 1.
EFFECTS OF INDOMETHACIN VS. PLACEBO FOR THE TREATMENT OF RENAL COLIC

	Average size of stone	Mean interval to passage	Recurrent episodes of colic after ED discharge	Recurrent episodes requiring narcotics	Hospitalization required for pain
Treatment groups					
Indomethacin* suppositories (13 subjects)	3.4 mm	82 hours	1 recurrence = 4 patients Multiple=8 patients	1	0
Placebo (13 subjects)	3.1 mm	89 hours	1 recurrence = 13 patients Multiple=8 patients	17	5

*50 mg every 8 hours

Source: J Urol 1989;141:1428.

in one's treatment strategy, particularly if the drug can short-circuit the pathology by blocking a specific patho-physiologic mechanism. Importantly, one can obtain anal-gesia without a concern for side effects common to nar-cotics — sedation, hypotension, or respiratory depression. This may be a tremendous benefit in the elderly or severe-ly ill patient. Results of this study are quite dramatic, not only in Voltaren's ability to relieve pain, but particularly the drug's ability to alleviate the need for immediate surgery. Importantly, there is no claim that Voltaren cures already established acute cholecystitis. I would be very skeptical of the claim that one injection of an NSAID pre-vents cholecystitis, but I have seen ketorolac give signifi-cant pain relief to simple biliary colic.

Other authors, almost exclusively from Scandinavia, have reported impressive results when NSAIDs (Voltaren and also indomethacin) were used to treat biliary colic. Svanik et al demonstrated that 50 mg IV Indocin provid-ed complete pain relief in 21 of 24 patients with biliary colic within 20 minutes (*Scand J Urol Nephrol* 1983; 17:55). Jonsson et al concluded that IV Indocin provides pain relief in biliary colic that is comparable to narcotics (*Acta Chir Scand* 1985;151(6):561). Obviously, a patient who is vomiting or otherwise unable to take oral medica-tion would benefit most from a parenteral NSAID. In this country, this would require the use of ketorolac (Toradol), the only NSAID currently available for parenteral use. Indomethacin suppositories may be a suitable alternative for outpatients. Curiously, Indocin is available as an IV preparation, but I have never seen it advertised, studied, or used in the ED. (The *Physicians' Desk Reference [PDR]* indication is for the treatment of patent ductus, and it only comes in 1 mg vials.)

The major advantage of an NSAID is that it does not significantly sedate patients, alter their mental status, cause respiratory depression or hypotension, or produce constipation. There are, in reality, only theoretical advan-tages for most patients. One is probably that IV/IM Toradol does not cause vomiting, a common side effect of most parenteral narcotics. For some reason, surgical house staff don't become upset when the emergency physician provides pain relief with Toradol but fall apart when an appropriate narcotic has been administered. Toradol does cause some sedation but not the degree encountered with narcotics. Any NSAID will also func-tion as an antipyretic, so one needs to be aware that the temperature — often an important clinical guide to more serious disease — has been pharmacologically manipulat-ed. My uncontrolled experience has been that Toradol is an effective analgesic for many but not all cases of biliary colic, and I use it initially in lieu of narcotics. If the first dose fails, narcotics should be used. The 30 mg dose IV seems to work as well as 60 mg. Toradol should not be given repeatedly in high doses, so most patients with gall bladder disease are quickly switched to narcotics as inpa-tients. In patients who are cured of their acute attack of biliary colic, I will frequently discharge them on an around-the-clock (not PRN) oral NSAID while awaiting outpatient studies or referral. Oral Toradol is very hard on the stomachs of most patients.

USE OF INDOMETHACIN SUPPOSITORIES IN A PROPHYLAXIS OF RECURRENT URETERAL COLIC

Kapoor DA, et al *J Urol* 1989;142(6):1428

This is a prospective, randomized, double-blind place-bo controlled study on the efficacy of indomethacin suppositories for the relief of acute pain and the preven-tion of recurring colic in patients with kidney stones. The authors note that the standard management for patients with acute renal colic has traditionally consisted of the administration of narcotics, and their use is often compli-cated by constipation, nausea, vomiting, or sedation. In addition, narcotics do not treat or prevent renal colic by any specific physiologic mechanism but merely alleviate pain by a generalized central analgesic effect. Basically, nar-cotics treat pain but do not prevent it.

This study appeared in 1989, but the association between renal colic and NSAIDs has been known since the early 1970s.

Forty-one ED patients were enrolled in the study and initially received meperidine (1 mg/kg) when an intra-venous pyelogram (IVP) demonstrated a ureteral calculi. Following initial pain relief, subjects received either place-bo or indomethacin suppositories (50 mg every 8 hours) as outpatients. Supplemental narcotics (acetaminophen plus oxycodone) were allowed as needed for additional pain control. Twenty-six patients were available for re-eval-uation at five days following the initial presentation.

The mean calculus size in both groups was compara-ble, ranging from 3.1 to 3.4 mm. (See Table 2.) The major-ity of stones were in the distal third of the ureter. All 13 patients in the placebo group experienced at least one episode of recurrent renal colic following discharge, and eight had more than one episode. Only four of 13 patients treated with indomethacin suffered a recurrent episode of colic, and only one required supplemental narcotics for pain control. No patient receiving indomethacin subsequently required hospitalization for uncontrolled pain.

Impressively, the ratio of supplemental narcotic use by the placebo group versus the Indocin group was approximately 8:1. Most patients eventually passed their stones without surgery. Many patients in both groups developed diarrhea, thought to be secondary to the glycerol component of the suppository.

The authors note that the probable cause of acute renal colic is distension of the ureter or renal capsule when urine flow is obstructed by an ureteral calculus. The distension of these structures effects a release of prostaglandins, which in turn increases renal blood flow and glomerular filtration. The diuretic reflex increases pressure and ureter wall tension, and, if some degree of ureteral obstruction is present, pain is produced. The administration of an antiprostaglandin limits this reflex physiological response to an impacted stone and blocks the basic pain-producing mechanism.

Although there were no significant differences in calculus size between the two groups, the interval to passage, or the number of patients requiring surgical intervention, there was a significant difference in pain relief in the indomethacin group. The authors conclude that indomethacin will prevent the recurrence of renal colic in patients with ureteral stones, and this analgesic effect is secondary to the NSAID's antiprostaglandin activity. The authors believe that indomethacin is well tolerated and has fewer side effects than narcotics, and this therapy can be an important adjunct for the outpatient treatment of renal colic.

COMMENT: I doubt that any practicing emergency physician has not heard about or used NSAIDs for the treatment of acute renal colic, often with amazing success. The drugs work so well that if success is not achieved, one questions the diagnosis or strongly suspects drug-seeking. There are at least a dozen similar articles in the medical literature and all have reached the same conclusion — Indocin relieves renal colic as well as narcotics and with fewer side effects.

Most EPs are turned onto the use of parenteral ketorolac (Toradol) for acute therapy, but the use of Indocin suppositories to prevent a recurrence in outpatients is less well known. Because of slow absorption, suppositories are probably more applicable for outpatient use, but I will frequently order 50-100 mg Indocin rectally as soon as I consider the diagnosis, often prior to obtaining an IVP. As

Table 2.

RESPONSE TO VARIOUS TREATMENT REGIMENS IN PATIENTS WITH BILIARY COLIC

Treatment groups (20 subjects each)	None	Response to Treatment Improved	Complete Relief	Mean Response Time	Pain Recurrence	Hospitalization and Urgent Surgery
Placebo	15 (75%)	4 (20%)	1 (5%)	35 min.	80%	5 (25%)
Papaverine	13 (65%)	7 (35%)	0	25 min.	86%	4 (20%)
Diclofenac	1 (5%)	2 (10%)	17 (85%)	15 min.	5%	0
Low back pain treated with diclofenac	8 (40%)	7 (35%)	5 (25%)	17 min.	-	-
P value		<0.002		<0.05	<0.001	

Source: Dig Dis Sci *1989;34(6):809.*

noted, there is an IV form of Indocin listed in the *PDR*, but our pharmacy has never carried it and it's impractical to use. Suppositories can be given in addition to parenteral Toradol, but like these authors, I will often initially use IV Demerol or morphine.

Most studies, however, demonstrate an equal efficacy of narcotics and NSAIDs. Note that at discharge the Indocin is prescribed on a regular basis, not used as a PRN therapy.

Side effects of Toradol are minimal, although I have been impressed that drowsiness is fairly common, and an occasional patient will experience minor GI upset. The GI ulcerations and renal dysfunction associated with long-term NSAID use are not a problem with the short-term ED use of Toradol. Indocin is one of the most potent inhibitors of prostaglandin synthesis so there are concerns about its long-term use. However, three to five days of Indocin suppositories should not be a problem. Aside from GI upset, the most serious side effect of Indocin I have seen is the occasional severe headache it produces, often miserable enough to prompt an evaluation for subarachnoid hemorrhage. Some patients experience dysphoria or a spaced-out feeling with Indocin. It is important to realize that NSAIDs do not promote the passage of urinary calculi. Likewise, there is no benefit to antispasmodics or fluid loading; neither will hasten the passage of a ureteral stone.

NSAIDs have narcotic-like potency for specific conditions where pathology is prostaglandin-mediated, and the drugs are certainly safe and suitable for patients with undefined pathology or unstable cardiorespiratory status. However, these drugs are not, in my opinion, suitable for most patients with severe generic pain. When treating the real pain secondary to such things as thermal burns or fractures, I strongly believe that narcotics are still the drugs of choice. The pain of a fractured femur should at least initially be attacked with morphine or Demerol.

Finally, it bothers me no end to see house staff reflexively forcing prescriptions for NSAIDs on patients with minor soft tissue trauma or low back pain when simple acetaminophen or aspirin would be equally effective. In our efforts to give patients the expected prescription, the knee-jerk reflex of treating all painful conditions with a $30-$40 prescription NSAID has become commonplace. Although the vast majority of healthy people may take NSAIDs for seven to 10 days without any complications whatsoever, there are significant gastrointestinal or renal side effects that are associated with long-term use, especially in the elderly.

In addition to the obvious increased cost of medical care, long-term NSAIDs are known to increase the incidence of serious or even fatal GI bleeding or exacerbate renal failure. Even though the well-meaning emergency physician writes an NSAID prescription that is intended to be used only for a short time, such prescriptions have a half-life much longer than initially intended, and once started, patients may be on these drugs for months. In addition, I have seen patients who have been prescribed three or four different NSAIDs by different physicians because of the propensity to dispense these drugs routinely for vague or minor symptoms. The overuse of NSAIDs is my particular bias, and because these drugs are now available over-the-counter, real medical problems are possible.

EFFECTS OF NAPROXEN SODIUM ON MENSTRUAL PROSTAGLANDINS AND PRIMARY DYSMENORRHEA

Chan WY, et al *Obstet Gynecol* 1983;61(3):285

This is one of many studies that demonstrates the ability of NSAIDs to provide prompt relief from the pain of primary dysmenorrhea and reduce the symptomatology of menstrual distress. This is a randomized, double-blind controlled study of 12 patients with primary dysmenorrhea who were studied for three menstrual cycles in a crossover design. The treatment consisted of naproxen sodium, 550 mg at the onset of menses followed by 275 mg QID for three days, or placebo. The amount of menstrual flow was determined by measuring tampon use and the amount of prostaglandins in the menstrual flow was quantitated by radioimmunoassay. Patients were asked to keep a record of the degree of relief from uterine cramps and also from other extrauterine symptoms.

Treatment with naproxen was associated with a 78 percent decrease in the release of menstrual prostaglandins and a 23 percent reduction in menstrual fluid volume. Placebo had no significant effect on either parameter. Severe cramping was reduced by 64 percent with the NSAID. The drug also significantly reduced dizziness, nausea, and vomiting. Importantly, the effect of the treatment was noted within one hour after the first dose, with a maximum effect at two hours. The authors conclude that naproxen provides prompt relief of the pain and also ameliorates other associated side effects of primary dysmenorrhea. The mechanism of action is mediated through a decrease in menstrual prostaglandin release.

COMMENT: This is one of many articles that demonstrate a beneficial effect of NSAIDs for the treatment of primary dysmenorrhea, and NSAIDs are clearly the drug of choice for this condition. The severity of dysmenorrhea has been correlated with the level of menstrual prostaglandin production in other studies. Other authors have shown similar improvement in both pain and other symptoms with mefenamic acid (Ponstel), ibuprofen (Motrin), indomethacin (Indocin), and piroxicam (Feldene). Theoretically, any NSAID should work, although aspirin has not been found effective. Parenteral ketorolac is a good choice for relief of pain in the ED.

Importantly, NSAIDs have both a prophylactic and therapeutic activity that is above and beyond a simple analgesic effect. No NSAID has been shown to be superior, but some theoretical benefits are touted. Mefenamic acid inhibits both synthesis and release of prostaglandins, whereas others just block the release so this drug is preferred by some. The patient-friendly once-a-day regimen of Feldene also has its supporters.

Interestingly, patients may have marked success with one NSAID and then become tolerant after a number of menstrual cycles. Because most patients with primary dysmenorrhea are healthy, there is no need to be concerned about GI or renal side effects with a three- to five-day regimen that is used on a monthly basis. Acute dysmenorrhea also lends itself to treatment with a parenteral NSAID. When symptoms are frequent, NSAIDs should be used prophylactically instead of only therapeutically.

There is little doubt that NSAIDs, when taken prophylactically, at the first sign of pain, or the beginning of menstrual flow are safe and effective for control of pain and to reduce the systemic symptoms of primary dysmenorrhea. Failure to respond is unusual and should suggest an alternative diagnosis, such as endometriosis, infection, ovarian disease, or other pelvic pathology.

LOCAL ANESTHETICS: INJECTION TECHNIQUES

Mastering the finer points of local anesthesia can be as easy as grabbing whatever is available

Emergency physicians administer local anesthetics every day, and they should be the hospital's experts in pharmacological principles, side effects, general usage, and injection techniques. It's easy to grab whatever anesthetic is on the suture cart and inject it, but it's just as easy to master the finer points of local anesthesia. In a continuing discussion about unique techniques for pain relief in the ED, this chapter highlights some tricks of the trade and concepts that should be familiar to all EPs.

BUFFERED VERSUS PLAIN LIDOCAINE AS A LOCAL ANESTHETIC FOR SIMPLE LACERATION REPAIR

Bartfield JM, et al *Ann Emerg Med* 1990; 19(12):1387

This is one of many studies that tout the benefit of adding bicarbonate to local anesthetics to reduce the pain of injection. The authors studied 91 adult ED patients with simple linear lacerations who were about to undergo suturing. Study solutions were either 1% plain lidocaine or buffered lidocaine. The buffered solution was freshly prepared just prior to use by adding 7.5% sodium bicarbonate to 1% plain lidocaine in a lidocaine:bicarbonate volume ratio of 9:1.

In a double-blind random fashion, wounds were injected with either buffered or nonbuffered lidocaine. The anesthetic was administered via a standardized technique of slow infiltration through the wound edge with a 25 gauge needle. Each patient was randomly assigned to receive two solutions in a varying sequence. Subjects could receive either plain or buffered lidocaine into the first wound edge, and subsequently receive the same or different solution in the second wound edge. Pain during injection was noted, and the adequacy of anesthesia was determined when sutures were placed. The same operator infiltrated both wound edges to ensure uniformity of technique.

Buffered lidocaine was consistently less painful upon injection than plain lidocaine. When the effectiveness of the solutions was analyzed, judged by the need for additional anesthesia, 11 percent of patients with buffered lidocaine and 15 percent with plain lidocaine required repeat injection. About five percent of patients in each group experienced some pain during suturing despite receiving additional anesthetic. Wounds of the face and scalp were more likely than other sites to require additional anesthetic.

The authors note that lidocaine is packaged in acidic pH (6.5) to enhance solubility and prolong shelf life. The anesthetic itself has a pH of 7.9 before HCl is added. Many other authors have similarly shown that buffered lidocaine causes significantly less pain during infiltration than does unbuffered lidocaine. A similar benefit has been found by buffering lidocaine with epinephrine, mepivacaine (Carbocaine), and bupivacaine (Marcaine, Sensorcaine). The mechanism by which buffering reduces injection pain is not established, but it is not merely a function of pH. The advantage of buffering is likely pH-related, but alkalinization probably changes the kinetics of lidocaine and enhances diffusion across cell membranes.

Lidocaine is largely uncharged (nonionized) in an alkaline milieu, so buffering increases lipid solubility and allows for the "immediate" diffusion of anesthetic into nerve cells. Buffering also tends to prolong the action of lidocaine, probably because the lipophilic substance remains tissue bound.

The authors conclude that infiltration of buffered lidocaine causes significantly less pain than does plain lidocaine, and alkalinization does not change anesthetic efficacy. It is recommended that buffered lidocaine be used routinely to minimize patient discomfort.

COMMENT: If you are a practicing emergency physician, you have to have been living under a rock not to be aware of the benefits of buffered lidocaine. Given the overwhelming data proving a significant decrease in injection pain and no loss of anesthetic effect when lidocaine is buffered with small amounts of bicarbonate, there is currently no rationale whatsoever for not using the buffered solution on every patient. If you inject slowly, buffered lidocaine is virtually painless! For those who are not believers, I suggest you have yourself injected in a blinded fashion by a colleague to prove to yourself that there is a clear advantage.

Local anesthetic solutions clearly hurt and the numbing procedure is often the worst part of anyone's ED visit. Once you hurt the already anxious or frightened patient with the anesthetic, any subsequent discomfort — even pain that could be otherwise tolerated — is magnified tenfold. Particularly when children are involved, you get only one chance to numb a laceration easily. Following a

> EVERY EP SHOULD BE AWARE OF THE BENEFITS OF BUFFERED LIDOCAINE

painful injection, even the minor sensation of pressure, which is often left intact despite loss of pain sensation, is interpreted by the patient as pain and there's a reflex withdrawal every time you touch the skin.

The rather high incidence of ineffective anesthesia in this study (about 5%) is somewhat confusing, but perhaps it was related to an inadequate initial volume. The operator should be generous with volume on the initial injection.

The amount of pain associated with local anesthetic infiltration is a complicated issue. Consensus holds that the more rapid the injection, especially with epinephrine solutions, the greater the degree of pain.

Injecting anything into a wound can be painful. Anesthetic agents themselves, however, appear to have inherently painful properties. Morris et al conducted an interesting study to determine the pain associated with injection of various local anesthetics (*Anesth Analg* 1987;66(11):1180), and found that lidocaine was the least painful — it actually hurt less than saline! Bupivacaine and mepivacaine were intermediate, and etidocaine (Duranest) was the most painful. Injection pain was not related to pH; in fact,

PATIENT GROUPS

Number	First Edge	Second Edge
24	Plain lidocaine	Buffered lidocaine
28	Buffered lidocaine	Plain lidocaine
24	Buffered lidocaine	Buffered lidocaine
15	Plain lidocaine	Plain lidocaine

Source: Ann Emerg Med *1990;19:1387-1389.*

the very acidic chloroprocaine (pH 3.4) hurt less than saline (pH 6.8).

The pH of standard lidocaine is not very acidic, ranging from 5.0 to 7.0. Lidocaine with epinephrine has a pH of 4.5 (3.3-5.5). I'm convinced that patients cannot feel a 25 gauge needle that is slowly inserted through a wound edge, and I don't buy the theoretical benefits of using smaller needles. It's the anesthetic, not the needle, that produces pain, and I believe it's barbaric to inject through intact skin when a wound edge is available.

Most EPs use either lidocaine or bupivacaine. There are those who advocate initially injecting all lacerations with the longer acting bupivacaine. Bupivacaine is one of the most painful local anesthetics so if it's used, buffering is clearly in order. I personally don't use bupivacaine on routine linear lacerations because post-suturing pain is not an overwhelming issue in most patients. I will, however, always use bupivacaine for digital block given for surgery on an ingrown toenail or paronychia or for draining a thrombosed hemorrhoid or abscess.

Adding bicarbonate to bupivacaine will also reduce injection pain, but if a 1:10 ratio is used, bupivacaine will precipitate. I have used cloudy buffered bupivacaine solutions and have not noted a significant reduction in anesthesia or other problems with wound healing, but authors always make a big deal about precipitated bupivacaine. When Cheney et al (*Am J Emerg Med* 1991;9(2):147) investigated buffered bupivacaine solutions, they noted that a minuscule amount of bicarbonate (only .05 ml bicarbonate in 10 ml bupivacaine, a 1:200 dilution) is required to reduce injection pain, and this amount does not produce precipitation. Others have suggested a 0.1:10 ml ratio. An easy way to buffer bupivacaine is to draw up a few mls of bicarbonate from a multidose vial and gently squirt out the

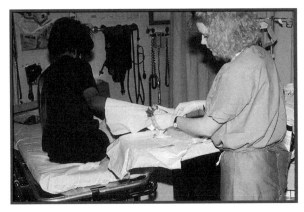

What's wrong with this picture? The medical student tried to repair this hand wound with the patient sitting upright. The patient did not want to lie down and seemed very brave and not troubled by the blood and needles. Soon after the picture was taken, the patient fainted and almost went head first onto the concrete floor. See color plate in center well.

visible solution from the barrel of the syringe. The bicarbonate that remains in the dead space of a 20 gauge needle — about 0.2 ml — will buffer 3-4 ml bupivacaine without causing significant precipitation. In my experience, buffering bupivacaine helps but does not make the injection totally painless, as it does with lidocaine.

Lidocaine with epinephrine is generally thought to elicit more pain on injection than plain lidocaine. Stewart (*J Dermatol Surg Oncol* 1990;16(9):842) added varying concentrations of bicarbonate to 1% lidocaine with epinephrine (1:100,000). The pH of the unbuffered lidocaine/epinephrine solution was 4.0, and the buffered solution pH ranged from 6.5 to 7.3. As with studies investigating plain lidocaine, bicarbonate also significantly reduced the pain of intradermal injection of lidocaine with epinephrine. The ratio in this study was 1 ml 7.5% bicarbonate to 20 ml 1% lidocaine/epinephrine.

I haven't studied it carefully, but my impression is that buffered epinephrine solutions are still moderately painful. More concentrated lidocaine solutions are not more painful on injection than diluted ones. Most EDs use 1% lidocaine, and I can see no advan-

CATEGORIZATION OF PODIATRIC EPINEPHRINE USERS	
Respondents using only 1:100,000 epinephrine solutions in the great toe and lesser toes	*551 (50%)*
Respondents using only 1:200,000 epinephrine solutions in the great toe and lesser toes	*135 (12%)*
Respondents using 1:100,000 and 1:200,000 epinephrine solutions in the great toe and lesser toes	*154 (14%)*
Respondents using other concentrations of epinephrine solutions in the great toe and lesser toes	*24 (2%)*
Respondents not using any epinephrine solutions in the great toe or lesser toes	*239 (22%)*
Total respondents reviewed	*1098 (100%)*

Source: J Am Podia Assoc *1981;71(4):189.*

tage at all of using 2%. Actually 0.5% will also provide excellent local anesthesia, and you can dilute 1% with equal part saline to reduce toxicity if you're concerned about total dose. Remember that intravenous regional anesthesia (Bier Block) uses 0.5% lidocaine. Larger nerve blocks probably require 1%. Likewise, there is no advantage of 0.5% bupivacaine over the 0.25% solution.

There has always been some concern about the potential for epinephrine-containing anesthetics to potentiate infection because the vasoconstrictor decreases tissue oxygen tension. This is probably a theoretical concern, but the clinical relevance is unknown.

In experimental animals, Tran et al (*Plast Reconstr Surg* 1985;76(6):933) demonstrated increasing bacterial counts with increasing concentrations of epinephrine in tissue sites injected with bacteria and epinephrine. The clinical significance of these findings are unclear, but it makes reasonable sense to eschew epinephrine whenever possible. Vasoconstrictors are occasionally appropriate to promote hemostasis, but I believe that epinephrine, especially in higher concentrations, should not be used routinely merely to prolong anesthesia. It's better to use bupivacaine. Probably the only common reasons to use epinephrine solutions are to decrease bleeding (such as in the scalp) or to limit anesthetic absorption when large volumes are used, especially in vascular areas, such as scalp and multiple rib blocks. Buffered lidocaine prolongs anesthesia in sciatic nerve blocks, but it does not significantly prolong anesthesia when injected locally.

Most investigators use freshly buffered lidocaine because of concern that alkaline solutions are unstable for extended periods. Our ED keeps 7.5% sodium bicarbonate solution in multidose 50 ml vials on the suture cart to add as needed. You can also use cardiac bicarbonate (8.4%) in similar doses.

Bartfield et al recently demonstrated that buffered lidocaine need not be prepared just prior to use (*Ann Emerg Med* 1992;21(1):16). When stored at room temperature for up to seven days, buffered lidocaine maintained adequate analgesic properties and continued to exhibit reduced pain upon injection. Over the study period, the lidocaine concentration decreased by about 10 percent, but this was not clinically relevant. No bacterial contamination was noted during the study period.

Another technique that is commonly referrred to is the use of warm lidocaine to reduce injection pain. Lidocaine is not kept in the refrigerator and is mostly used at room temperature. Warming it may offer slightly better injection

CATEGORIES IN WHICH PODIATRISTS WOULD NOT USE ANESTHETIC SOLUTIONS CONTAINING EPINEPHRINE IN THE GREAT TOE AND LESSER TOES

- *Peripheral vascular disease*
- *Diabetes mellitus*
- *Cardiac disease*
- *Geriatrics*
- *Hypertension*
- *Vasospastic disease*
- *History of allergy to local anesthetics*
- *Pregnancy*
- *Local infection or ulceration*

Source: J Am Podia Assoc *1981;71(4):189.*

properties, but it's probably not worth the trouble.

As a final note on technique, I suggest that one never inject local anesthetics into patients who are in any position other than supine. I have seen near disasters when seemingly brave and unfazed patients get injections while in a chair or sitting on the side of the bed, and the potential to unexpectedly faint and fall on the hard floor is real. I follow this "inject while supine" rule with tetanus shots, steroids injections and, above all, local anesthetics.

UTILIZATION OF EPINEPHRINE-CONTAINING ANESTHETIC SOLUTIONS IN THE TOES

Roth R *J Am Podia Assoc* 1981;71(4):189

This article attempts to define and clarify the role of lidocaine with epinephrine (L-E) solutions used for anesthesia of the toes. Data were obtained via a questionnaire sent to 839 podiatrists. The author attempted to develop standards of care for the use of these solutions, to define indications, and to document complications. Despite the fact that most textbooks vehemently condemn using L-E in digits, podiatrists have not abandoned its use for anesthesia of the toes. The concern is that epinephrine will produce prolonged vasoconstriction and gangrene of digits. The podiatry literature deemed epinephrine/lidocaine anesthetics safe for use for digital blocks in toes as early as 1971, but there are still misconceptions and myths about the incidence of untoward reactions.

In this detailed questionnaire, sent to all podiatrists listed as members of the American Podiatry Association in 1978, questions were asked about the general use of different concentrations of epinephrine, contraindications, adverse reactions, and frequency of use. The database consists of 1,098 returned questionnaires and an amazing 2,109,555 injections.

There was a consensus from the respondents that L-E should not be used to anesthetize toes in patients with peripheral vascular disease, diabetes, cardiac disease, hypertension, or vasospastic disorders. When epinephrine was used, approximately half of the respondents selected 1:100,000 solutions, 12% used 1:200,000 concentration, and 14% used both.

Amazingly, only 22 percent of respondents used epinephrine-free anesthetics when performing digital blocks. The average volume of injected anesthetic was 3 ml. In addition to adhering to general contraindications, respondents stated that they assessed pedal pulses, skin color, skin temperature, capillary filling time, and general medical history when determining whether to use epinephrine-containing solutions.

Significant tissue necrosis or gangrene was reported in 31 instances, or approximately 1 in 68,050 injections. There were 16 cases involving loss of part or all of the involved toe. It is not certain whether these complications were directly related to the use of L-E or to other compli-

cations of surgery. The incidence of complications was approximately 2.5 times greater when the more concentrated 1:100,000 epinephrine was used instead of the more diluted 1:200,000 concentration.

The author comments on the wide use of local anesthetics containing epinephrine in the toes by podiatric practitioners. Epinephrine is used by the vast majority of podiatrists despite voluminous literature that states that such solutions are contraindicated.

Based on more than two million injections, the author concludes that patients without significant medical, neurological, or vascular problems can safely receive epinephrine-

COMPLICATIONS REPORTED BY PODIATRISTS USING EPINEPHRINE ANESTHETICS

	Epinephrine Concentration Used		
	1:100,000	1:200,000	1:100,000 and 1:200,000
Total injections into great toe and lesser toes	1,395,306	313,258	400,991
Cases with significant tissue necrosis or gangrene	23	2	6
Cases resolving with adequate therapeutic measures	12	1	2
Cases resulting in loss of part or all of the involved toe or more radical amputation	11	1	4
Loss of part or all of toe	8	1	2
Radical amputation	3	0	2
Amputation within the foot	2	0	2
Above or below knee amputation	1	0	0

Source: J Am Podia Assoc 1981;71(4):189.

containing solutions for digital block of the toes. It's further concluded that complications are well within the acceptable limits of safety. The incidence of serious complications is 1 in 68,000 injections, and significant tissue loss occurs in 1 in 132,000 injections. It is concluded that there are no data to support the widely held contention that epinephrine is absolutely contraindicated in surgery of the toes.

COMMENT: There are a number of articles in the podiatry literature supporting the use of L-E for digital anesthesia. At least two other authors have proclaimed as myth, exaggeration, or outright fallacy the widely held contention that these solutions are contraindicated. Kaplan and Kashuk presented the first extensive work to debunk the epinephrine myth. They reported no significant problems in 65,000 digital surgical procedures where anesthetic solutions with 1:100,000 concentration of epinephrine were used. Steinberg (*JAMA* 1971;61:341) reported similar success with more than 200,000 injections. Throughout the podiatry literature, the consensus is that epinephrine-containing anesthetics are safe for digital nerve block in patients without significant vascular or neurological pathology.

From a methodology stance, the data upon which authors base their conclusions are drawn from questionnaires and retrospective analysis, and it's possible that many complications were never reported. I'm not sure if I would report my disasters with all of the warnings in the literature. The diatribe against the use of epinephrine probably arose from complications that resulted when epinephrine used to be added just before surgery in a concentrated form. Because the relatively dilute 1:100,000 and 1:200,000 solutions are now commercially available, the actual amount of epinephrine injected is significantly less.

I could not find a hand surgeon as brave as our podiatry colleagues, although I suspect that the toe data could be extrapolated to fingers. Johnson (*JAMA* 1967;200(11): 990) took a brave position almost 30 years ago when he stated that epinephrine was a "very useful adjunct to hand surgery (that) has been maligned." Although he condemned L-E for digital nerve blocks, he reported no complications in 421 hand surgery cases when 0.5% lidocaine with 1:200,000 epinephrine was used for local infiltration in the hand (exact details not explained). He points out that a tourniquet, commonly used during hand surgery, certainly produces a degree of ischemia equal to or greater than locally injected L-E.

I can find no support for the use of L-E for digital blocks in the emergency medicine literature. In fact, almost every review of local anesthesia vehemently warns against its use in digits, the ears, penis, and nose. This warning is repeatedly seen despite lack of documentation of significant morbidity, and I suspect most authors merely quote package inserts, other physicians, previous unreferenced texts, or

> THERE IS NO SUPPORT FOR L-E FOR DIGITAL BLOCKS IN THE LITERATURE.

a prejudice they hold from medical school.

Although I believe L-E is generally safe to use in the hand or feet in patients without underlying vascular or neurological problems, I can think of no good reason to use it — ever. I have spent a few anxious moments following the injection of even plain lidocaine into fingers and toes when the distal digit became pale or cyanotic, probably because of excess volume compressing vascular structures, or from transient vasospasm. I have also seen medical students inadvertently inject L-E into digits with no side effects whatsoever or only transient vasospasm that clears in a few minutes.

Given the fact that tourniquet ischemia for an hour is tolerated by hands and feet during surgery, I can't imagine that a few minutes of ischemia from epinephrine results in certain disaster. The argument for the use of epinephrine is that it prolongs anesthesia and causes a bloodless operating field. I prefer to prolong my anesthesia by using bupivacaine and to obtain a bloodless field with a tourniquet. In my opinion, one should never repair a nail bed, search for a tendon laceration, or try to remove a foreign body in an extremity without an ischemic tourniquet. You're quickly branded as an amateur by the hand surgeons if they see you spending more time sponging to obtain a bloodless field than you spend on your surgical repair. The bottom line is that one need not be overly paranoid about the use of L-E in digits, but there are no compelling reasons to use it, and there are certainly better alternatives when it comes to obtaining local anesthesia. If you use it, opt for the 1:200,000 concentration.

THE REVERSAL OF THE ISCHEMIC EFFECTS OF EPINEPHRINE ON A FINGER WITH LOCAL INJECTIONS OF PHENTOLAMINE

Markovchick V, Burkhart K
J Emerg Med 1991;9(5):323

This is a single case report documenting the reversal of epinephrine-induced ischemia by the injection of the alpha blocker, phentolamine. This patient developed ischemia following a puncture wound of the thumb from an automatic epinephrine injector used to treat allergic reactions, but one could extrapolate a similar scenario should local anesthetic with epinephrine be injected in an area that subsequently becomes ischemic.

The patient experienced blanching and numbness in the finger immediately after the inadvertent epinephrine injection. The amount was not stated, but 0.3 ml of a 1:1000 solution is a standard dose in anaphylaxis kits (EpiPen). Note, however, that this is much more concentrated than the 1:100,000 solution used as a local anesthetic. The 1:1000 solution is the same concentration used for subcutaneous injections in asthma.

Sensation and capillary filling returned within 10 minutes following the injection of 2.5 mg phentolamine diluted in 2.5 cc saline. The antidote was injected locally along the course of the digital arteries of the thumb. A small amount of phentolamine was also injected directly into the tip of the thumb where the epinephrine had been injected. The vasoconstriction did not return, and there was no subsequent morbidity.

The authors note that experimental data has demonstrated the beneficial effect of phentolamine in preventing skin sloughs when laboratory animals are injected with vasoconstrictive drugs (dopamine, norepinephrine). Phentolamine (Regitine) is a pure alpha blocker, and it's used to treat hypertension from pheochromocytoma or cocaine. Although the authors note that there is no proof that this epinephrine injection would have produced significant morbidity, they did note rather impressive response to the antidote.

COMMENT: Most textbooks emphasize the caveat that epinephrine should not be used in areas of end arteries, such as the fingers, toes, ears, and nose. I do not believe that it's a foregone conclusion that small amounts of epinephrine in local anesthetics necessary spell doom for the injected part, and I think the danger is over-rated. As noted, our podiatry colleagues preferentially use epinephrine-containing solutions around the toes for digital nerve blocks. Nevertheless, it is best to avoid epinephrine-containing solutions when anesthetizing these areas.

Should blanching or ischemia develop, it probably should be reversed by Regitine. I know of no downside to using phentolamine, and I also recommend that it be used routinely if a dopamine or Levophed infusion infiltrates, even prior to obvious ischemia. The *PDR* recommends local injection to prevent skin necrosis after infiltration of Neo-Synephrine. Intraarterial Regitine has been used to reverse severe vasoconstriction in an extremity when, during a cardiac arrest, epinephrine was inadvertently injected into an antecubital artery (*Ann Emerg Med* 1989;18(4):424). In a similar scenario, Maguire et al (*Am J Emerg Med* 1990;8(1):46) reported that a phentolamine/lidocaine digital injection reversed epinephrine-induced vasospasm in a finger; again, the culprit was a self-injecting bee sting kit. Apparently, either direct phentolamine injection into the blanched area or a nerve block in the vicinity of arteries will reverse ischemia of a digit. For large areas, intraarterial phentolamine should be given. I have personally treated children who have injected their fingers with an EpiPen by injecting the Regitine:saline into the same spot where the epinephrine was injected. It works in about 3-4 minutes, but I have always wondered if any harm would occur if the area was left alone. It's difficult, however, to look at a white finger for very long when an antidote is readily available. (see also, "Myths and Misconceptions about Epinephrine," Section X, Chapter 6.)

REACTIONS TO LOCAL ANESTHETICS

Most emergency physicians will never see a patient with a true allergy to local anesthetics; most are confused with a vagal or epinephrine reaction or acute anxiety

Most emergency physicians will never encounter a patient with a true allergy to local anesthetics. The more likely scenario is the patient who claims an allergy based on a poorly remembered — and never documented — unpleasant childhood or distant experience. The alleged allergy is usually confused with a vagal or epinephrine reaction or acute anxiety, but the patient is convinced that they can never again have a tooth drilled or a laceration repaired using a local anesthetic.

The occasional patient may wear an identification bracelet placed by a physician who witnessed true anaphylaxis, but it's virtually impossible to separate historic allergic reaction from psychomotor, vagal, or epinephrine-related side effects, or even from problems due to excessive dosage. This chapter addresses the problem of patients with alleged allergies to local anesthetics, a reasonable ED approach with some alternatives, and a discussion of a very bizarre procaine reaction.

AN APPROACH TO THE PATIENT WITH A HISTORY OF LOCAL ANESTHETIC HYPERSENSITIVITY: EXPERIENCE WITH 90 PATIENTS

deShazo RO, Nelson HS
J Allergy Clin Immunol 1979;63(6):387

Although this article is almost 20 years old, it still has significant application to the current practice of emergency medicine. The authors, allergists at Fitzsimons Army Medical Center, Aurora, CO, describe their approach to patients who were referred to them with alleged allergy to local anesthetics. The aim of the referral was to identify hypersensitivity to specific local anesthetics and to recommend a suitable alternative that could be safely used during minor surgical procedures. This report details the authors' experience with a progressive skin testing and subcutaneous challenge protocol.

A careful and detailed history was first taken with attention to the specific characteristics of the adverse reaction and an attempt to identify the specific agent involved.

Importantly, the time relationship between anesthetic administration and onset of the reaction was carefully investigated. The exact method of skin testing and the progressive subcutaneous challenge is shown in Table 1. Diluted and full-strength lidocaine were most often used as testing agents because of low incidence of antigenicity.

Anesthetic with and without the methylparaben preservative was used to help distinguish between anesthetic or preservative hypersensitivity. Skin testing was done with controls and under the supervision of a physician in a facility capable of treating untoward reactions. Patients were observed for one hour following completion of the full-strength subcutaneous challenge. If the test was negative, patients were considered not to be at risk for the therapeutic use of the agent tested.

It was difficult to reach a conclusion about immediate hypersensitivity based on the patient's history. Only 38 of the 90 subjects had a history that was specific enough to allow classification of the type of reaction they experienced. Fourteen patients were classified as having manifested immediate hypersensitivity because they experienced urticaria, laryngeal edema, or hypotension. Twenty-four patients were labeled as having a nonallergic reaction because their facial edema, transient syncope, or some other reaction occurred more than six hours after anesthetic use.

In more than half the cases, it was impossible to ascertain whether an immediate hypersensitivity reaction had occurred. Usually the reaction happened in the remote past and details were lacking, or the patient could only remember a caution against the future use of local anesthetics.

None of the 14 patients who gave a history compatible with immediate hypersensitivity had a positive skin test to the local anesthetic tested. Lidocaine was used most frequently, but mepivacaine (Carbocaine) was also tested. Five of the seven patients who stated they were specifically allergic to lidocaine were given the drug without difficulty. Two patients were not given lidocaine but tested negatively to the chemically similar mepivacaine. The remaining patients were challenged with a local anesthetic other than the one incriminated by history, and none had a positive reaction even though the selected drug was from the same chemical class.

All of the remaining patients with an incompatible or uncertain history for allergy underwent the full challenge, usually with lidocaine. In only 10 cases was a positive skin test noted, and in four cases these subjects tolerated a subcutaneous challenge with the same drug, indicating a false positive skin test. One local anesthetic was cleared for use in every patient. One patient, with a history of sensitivity to many local anesthetics, was found to have rubbed the skin test site in order to create a false positive reaction. No patients had a positive skin test to a paraben-containing agent if they did not also have a positive skin test to local anesthetic without the preservative.

The authors emphasize that the majority of clinical responses thought to be allergic reactions are actually psychomotor events. Toxic blood levels can occur from excessive doses, but this is rarely the case with outpatient procedures. Although epinephrine is often blamed for nonallergic reactions, the amount of epinephrine administered with local anesthetics is actually quite low, and probably not a major factor. They estimate that true immediate hypersensitivity accounts for considerably less than one percent of all alleged allergic reactions.

In this review of 90 patients who believed they were allergic, not a single case of immediate hypersensitivity was documented. In five cases, the alleged culprit was not tested, but the patient displayed no sensitivity to an alternative anesthetic.

The authors conclude that skin testing for local anesthetic hypersensitivity has a low but significant incidence of false positive reactions, especially when full-strength anesthetic is used. False positive skin tests may be due to histamine release from needle trauma or a primary irritant effect of the intradermal administration of undiluted solutions. The lack of sensitivity to parabens would challenge

Table 1. SKIN TESTING AND PROGRESSIVE CHALLENGE WITH LOCAL ANESTHETICS	
Method	*Drug dose/route*
Prick test	*1% drug, diluted 1:100*
Prick test	*1% drug, full strength*
Intradermal skin test	*0.02 ml 1% drug, diluted 1:100*
Intradermal skin test	*0.02 ml 1% drug, full strength*
Subcutaneous injection	*0.1 ml 1% drug*
Subcutaneous injection	*0.5 ml 1% drug**

Drug was administered at 20-minute intervals unless history suggested a delayed reaction. *If history suggests delayed onset of symptoms, wait 24 hours before proceeding.

Source: J Allerg Clin Immunol *1979;63(6):387-394.*

contentions that many allergic reactions are actually hypersensitivity to preservatives. The authors believe that their study establishes the usefulness and safety of a progressive challenge test for the management of patients with suspected local anesthetic allergy.

COMMENT: Immediate hypersensitivity to local anesthetics is extremely rare, and the majority of patients who have been labeled as allergic are not. It's still prudent, however, always to ask about hypersensitivity and believe the patient's history until proven otherwise. Local anesthetics used today are generally divided into two specific groups, benzoic acid esters and amides (see Table 2).

Identifying specific drugs in these two groups is a question on almost every board examination. The reason to know the chemical class of anesthetics is that it is generally regarded as safe to administer a local anesthetic from a chemical group that is different from the one causing hypersensitivity. Therefore, if you know that the patient reacted to an ester such as procaine when he had a tooth pulled 20 years ago, he can safely be given lidocaine, an amide. In general, reactions to esters are more common, and it is extremely rare for amides, especially lidocaine, to produce hypersensitivity. There is cross reactivity among members of the same class — especially the esters — but no cross reactivity between esters and amides.

Procaine (Novocain) was used extensively in the past, but it is rarely administered today. The only common current application for procaine is as a local anesthetic to decrease the pain of an intramuscular injection of penicillin G (Bicillin C-R, Wycillin). It is likely that adults who were truly allergic to a local anesthetic as a child had received procaine, usually for dental procedures.

The authors of this study believe that allergy to methylparaben is unusual. Paraben allergy does exist so some authors emphasize that crash cart lidocaine or "pure lidocaine" without preservatives may be used more safely in patients with an alleged lidocaine but actually paraben allergy. Clinically it's impossible to differentiate historically between lidocaine and methylparaben allergies when faced with a patient in the ED, so I don't buy this argument and would not feel comfortable merely using the preservative-free anesthetic if a specific lidocaine allergy were claimed.

Paraben preservatives are structurally related to ester anesthetics and can produce immediate hypersensitivity, but there are little hard data on the allergic potential of this preservative. Interestingly, metabisulfites are used as preservatives in epinephrine-containing anesthetics, and the

allergic potentiality of sulfites is well documented. It would be prudent to inquire specifically about a sulfite allergy before these anesthetics are given.

Swanson (*Ann Emerg Med* 1983;12(5):316) relates a case where a woman with a history of allergy to local anesthetics was referred for general anesthesia for minor surgery. The history consisted of urticaria and shortness of breath following injections of an unnamed local anesthetic. She

Table 2.

GENERAL CLASSES OF LOCAL ANESTHETICS

Esters

• *Procaine (Novocain)*

• *Cocaine*

• *Tetracaine (Pontocaine)*

• *Benzocaine*

Amides

• *Lidocaine (Xylocaine)*

• *Bupivacaine (Sensorcaine, Marcaine)*

• *Mepivacaine (Carbocaine)*

• *Prilocaine (Citanest)*

Source: James R. Roberts, MD

received a 0.1 cc test dose of 2% lidocaine (from the crash cart) and because she had no reaction within 30 minutes, the surgery was performed using 1 cc of the preservative-free lidocaine. The authors conclude that she was allergic to either an ester type anesthetic or possibly methylparaben. The conclusion may be valid, but it was not supported by this limited investigation.

Unless the patient has a medical alert bracelet or a specific knowledge of the previous reaction, I believe that it's reasonable to attempt to ferret out true allergy to local anesthetics in the ED when the only options are no anesthesia or general anesthesia. Most emergency physicians do not have the time to perform the entire progressive challenge test noted in this article, but a shortened version is not impractical.

It would seem reasonable to use a tuberculin syringe and first administer a dilute concentration of preservative-free lidocaine as an intradermal skin test, with saline as a control (like giving a TB skin test). Skin testing is not an exact science, but a definite reaction to a dilute concentration probably means hypersensitivity. When the specific allergen is unknown, lidocaine is the most reasonable drug to use because it has such a low allergic profile. If a lidocaine allergy is specifically stated, I would opt for testing with bupivacaine. Although they are chemically similar, cross reactivity among members of this group is not thought to occur. If there is no reaction to the skin test, proceed with subcutaneous testing. It would take approximately an hour to administer this sequence in the ED. Of course, it should be done under proper monitoring and with the facilities to treat anaphylaxis should it occur.

Most authors emphasize the unreliability of skin testing for drug hypersensitivity. Some, in fact, think it's a waste of time because of false positive and false negative reactions. Using a dilute solution will do away with many false positives due to needle trauma or an irritant effect, but the physician should be aware of the limitations of skin testing. If the dilute skin test is obviously positive, I personally would stop and consider an alternative course. I have not been able to find data on desensitization or the prophylactic use of steroids/antihistamines. There is no need to go into the specifics of anxiety or vasovagal reactions because most emergency physicians are well aware of these issues.

I would emphasize, however, that no patient should be given a local anesthetic while sitting; it is better to have them lie flat. I have seen some near disasters when a neophyte medical student attempts to anesthetize a hand while an already anxious patient, sitting on the side of the stretcher and watching, begins to fall.

Most lacerations in the ED will require far less than the toxic dose of local anesthetics, but it is, of course, important to know how to calculate dose based on volume of anesthetic. This is particularly important when repairing multiple lacerations or performing rib blocks. I'm continually amazed that many physicians are unable to do this because they don't know the math. If one wants to calculate

---

Table 3.

CALCULATION OF ANESTHETIC DOSES

Anesthetic solutions are marketed with drug concentration expressed as percentages (e.g., bupivacaine 0.25%, lidocaine 1%). To ascertain the strength of a solution, in milligrams per milliliter, consider:

A 1% solution is prepared by dissolving 1 gm of drug in 100 ml of solution. Therefore, 1 gm/100 ml = 1000 mg/100 ml = 10 mg/ml. To calculate the strength from the percentage quickly, simply move the decimal point one place to the right. For example:

0.25% = 2.5 mg/ml	*(bupivacaine)*
0.5% = 5 mg/ml	*(tetracaine)*
1% = 10 mg/ml	*(lidocaine)*
2% = 20 mg/ml	*(viscous lidocaine)*
4% = 40 mg/ml	*(cocaine)*
5% = 50 mg/ml	*(lidocaine ointment)*
20% = 200 mg/ml	*(benzocaine)*

When combined in an anesthetic solution, epinephrine is usually in a 1:100,000 or 1:200,000 dilution.

1 ml of 1:1000 epinephrine = 1 mg.

0.1 ml of 1:1000 epinephrine in 10 ml anesthetic solution = 1:100,000 dilution = 0.010 mg/ml.

0.1 ml of 1:1000 epinephrine in 20 ml anesthetic solution = 1:200,000 dilution = 0.005 mg/ml.

Examples of epinephrine content:

	1:100,000	*1:200,000*
5 ml	*0.050 mg*	*0.025 mg*
10 ml	*0.100 mg*	*0.050 mg*
20 ml	*0.200 mg*	*0.100 mg*

Therefore, 50 ml of 1% lidocaine with epinephrine 1:200,000 contains 500 mg lidocaine and 0.25 epinephrine.

Source: Clinical Procedures in Emergency Medicine, 2nd. Ed., Roberts JR and Hedges HR, editors, Philadelphia, PA, W.B. Saunders Co., 1991.

mg/ml based on percent concentration, merely move the decimal point over one place to the right. Therefore, 1% lidocaine has 10 mg/ml, and 0.25% bupivacaine has 2.5 mg/ml. Table 3 explains the calculation for drugs and dose of epinephrine. It's obvious that one administers extremely small amounts of epinephrine with local anesthetics, much less than used subcutaneously for the treatment of asthma. Epinephrine reactions are probably overrated, and I question whether supposed reactions to vasoconstrictors are actually anxiety reactions.

USE OF DIPHENHYDRAMINE FOR LOCAL ANESTHESIA IN CAINE-SENSITIVE PATIENTS

Pollack CV Jr., Swindle GM
J Emerg Med 1989;7(6):611

This is one of only a few articles that critically evaluate the common suggestion that diphenhydramine (Benadryl) can be used as an alternative anesthetic in patients with an allergy to ester or amide anesthetics. Most physicians will quote this trick yet few have actually used it. The authors describe three patients who gave a history of "caine" allergy and required local anesthetics for laceration repair. The authors note that the actual incidence of true allergy to local anesthetics is not known, but it's quite low. Patient's perception of an allergic history is often wrong or, at best, difficult to interpret, but true anaphylaxis to local anesthetics can occur.

In this report, parenteral 5% diphenhydramine (Benadryl) was diluted with saline (1:4 volume) to produce a 1% solution that was then used for local infiltration. Complete anesthesia was obtained, and the wounds appeared normal at follow-up. In one case, 0.1 cc of 1:1000 epinephrine solution was added to the antihistamine solution to produce hemostasis. In all three cases, the duration of anesthesia was approximately 30 minutes.

Although dermatologic, dental, and podiatry procedures have been performed in the past using diphenhydramine as a local anesthetic, this alternative agent has not found its way into the emergency medicine literature. There is a topical anesthetic effect of diphenhydramine, and the drug is often used in solutions to control the pain of gingivitis, stomatitis, eczema, or external hemorrhoids.

The actual anesthetic mechanism is unclear, although antihistamines are structurally similar to many local anesthetics. Anesthesia comes from something other than local pressure or edema of the diphenhydramine injection

because saline placebo does not appear to have anesthetic properties. A membrane stabilization mechanism has been suggested.

The authors emphasize that Benadryl is available in a 5% solution, and this preparation should be diluted in a 1:4 ratio with saline to provide a 1% concentration. It is noted that the onset of action of Benadryl may be longer and the duration of anesthesia may be shorter than lidocaine. The authors do note that local irritation, vesicle formation, and skin slough have been reported with higher concentration of Benadryl so there's a potential downside to its use. They do conclude, however, that patients who are sensitive to caine anesthetics can be given 1% diphenhydramine as an acceptable local anesthetic.

COMMENT: I have used Benadryl as a local anesthetic on only a few occasions, and it has been satisfactory, although I could not always obtain anesthesia to the extent I could with lidocaine. An alternative is to use heavy parenteral sedation or general anesthesia. A caution with this technique is in order. The 1997 *Physicians' Desk Reference (PDR)* states that "because of the risk of local necrosis, Benadryl should not be used as local anesthesia." This is not referenced or further explained, and this caution does not occur for the IM route. It's difficult to defend a tissue slough or necrosis — directly related to Benadryl or not — with this straightforward warning in the "Bible" (the *PDR*) for malpractice lawyers. If it's used, I suggest obtaining written informed consent and using only a dilute 1% solution. Benadryl should be reserved for local infiltration only, not nerve blocks.

I have not seen anaphylaxis reported with tetracaine, epinephrine, and cocaine (TAC) solution, or from lidocaine, benzocaine topical sprays, or viscous lidocaine, but such an event is theoretically possible. Likewise, it's possible to experience anaphylaxis from the tetracaine found in topical eye anesthetics.

PSYCHOSIS AND SEIZURES FOLLOWING THE INJECTION OF PENICILLIN G PROCAINE. HOIGNE'S SYNDROME

Silber TJ, D'Angelo L
Am J Dis Child 1985;139(4):335

This is a pediatric citation detailing a problem previously reported in the adult literature — an acute non-allergic reaction to the IM administration of procaine penicillin G. The authors describe the case histories of four patients, ages 10 to 18, who were treated for sexually transmitted diseases — usually gonorrhea — with 4.8 million units of procaine penicillin G IM.

None had a known allergy to penicillin or had experienced a previous reaction. Within a few minutes following the IM injection, the patients became restless, agitated, confused, hyperactive, delusional, incoherent, and frankly psychotic. Some hallucinated or had a feeling of impending death. There were only minimal autonomic findings such as mild hypertension and tachycardia, but two patients had a single, self-limited grand mal seizure. Within half an hour, all patients had recovered and were back to their normal state.

The authors are describing Hoigne's syndrome, a clinical manifestation of central nervous system toxicity to procaine. The syndrome is characterized by auditory and visual disturbances, psychiatric manifestations, and occasionally seizure activity.

Patients do not show evidence of immunologic hypersensitivity, such as hives, wheezing, hypotension, or angioedema. The general consensus is that this reaction is not caused by penicillin but by high serum levels of procaine, a drug that has good penetration into the cerebrospinal fluid. Direct intravascular injection is unlikely, and perivascular deposition is postulated. The reaction is self-limited and generally lasts only 15 to 30 minutes. Procaine has a very short serum half-life and is metabolized by serum cholinesterase. Specific therapy was not required in these patients, but it is postulated that a variety of sedatives, such as phenobarbital, may be helpful. There is no known link to underlying psychiatric disorders.

COMMENT: As stated previously, physicians rarely use procaine anymore except as an adjunctive anesthetic to decrease the pain with IM administration of penicillin G. This nonallergic procaine reaction is probably familiar to physicians who used to treat venereal diseases with high doses of this medication, and it happened with surprising frequency. The reaction occurs in up to two percent of patients given 4.8 million units procaine penicillin.

I have personally seen this reaction at least three times, and it is rather bizarre. Within a few minutes of injection, even when the nurse has discounted intravascular injection by aspiration, the patient rapidly becomes acutely psychotic. They may be active physically and emotionally and can be quite difficult to control. Commonly, patients anxiously express that they are going to die, and have a variety of visual hallucinations or transient blindness. I had to chase at least one patient around the emergency department to give him an intravenous bolus of Valium. Within half an hour, subjects are back to normal, usually with little recollection of their strange behavior.

Because of this reaction, public health departments in many cities stopped giving IM procaine penicillin for venereal diseases in the 1970s and switched to oral amoxicillin/probenecid. There is usually some tachycardia and hypertension with the mental status changes, but it's a relatively mild reaction from a cardiovascular standpoint.

The syndrome is idiosyncratic in nature. From a clinical standpoint, it's most important to recognize this reaction for what it is: a self-limited, nonimmunologic phenomenon. At least one author has demonstrated a low serum cholinesterase level in patients experiencing this reaction. The aim of therapy is to keep patients from hurting themselves, and it seems very reasonable to give a short-acting benzodiazepine, such as intravenous midazolam. Certainly patients given an injection of procaine penicillin should be observed for 15-20 minutes to ensure that this, or any allergic reaction, will not occur.

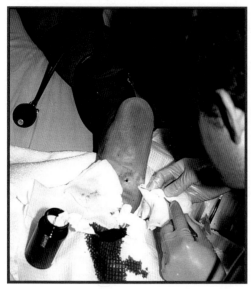

To examine a puncture wound of the foot properly, have the patient lie prone on a stretcher, get a
good light and an ischemic tourniquet, and then
set aside a few minutes. Examining the patient in
a wheelchair in the hall is an amateur move that
invites trouble. See page 5.

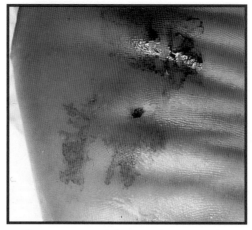

In this case, material from a sock was imbedded in
a relatively superficial wound. The overlying skin
was debrided, and the patient did well without
antibiotics. See page 6.

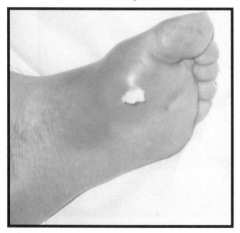

This patient stepped on a nail while wearing
tennis shoes and presented 72 hours later with
an obvious soft tissue infection. When the puncture tract was examined by lifting up a flap of
skin, a small piece of rubber was found and
excised by a coring technique. A gauze pack was
placed for 24 hours. Although a setup for
Pseudomonas osteomyelitis, this patient
responded well to a cephalosporin and had no
further problems. See page 7.

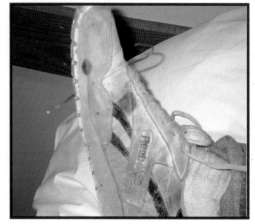

This patient stepped on a wire while wearing
sneakers. Despite aggressive coring, a drain, and
anti-staphylococcal antibiotics, he developed a deep
soft tissue infection that required prolonged IV
antibiotics. Long-term sequelae did not occur, but
pseudomonal osteomyelitis, especially in this high-
risk area of the foot, is a potential complication.
See page 11.

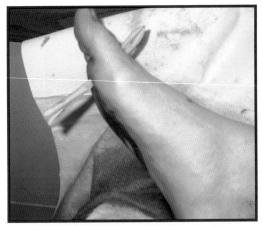

When treating a through-and-through puncture wound, it is difficult to get adequate debridement or irrigation. An option is to place a small Penrose drain through the puncture track. It should be left in place for only 24-36 hours. See page 12.

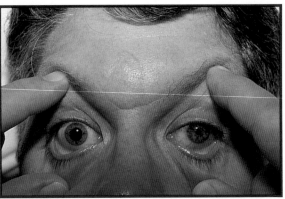

If this fixed and dilated pupil is caused by the intraocular instillation of an anticholinergic medication (prototype is atropine), it will not constrict within 15-20 minutes after the local instillation of 1% pilocarpine eye drops. A pupil that is dilated because of a neurologic cause, such as cerebral herniation or a lesion of the oculomotor nerve, will constrict. Pilocarpine is a direct-acting cholinergic agent, like acetylcholine, that causes miosis by stimulating the neuromuscular junction of the sphincter of the eye. Pilocarpine may not constrict a pupil that is dilated with an adrenergic agent. (See Thompson et al, Sur Ophthal 1976;21(2):45.) See page 52.

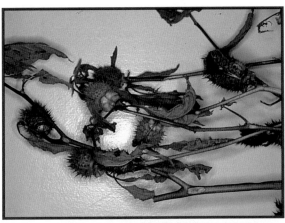

The jimson weed plant (Datura stramonium) is ubiquitous in the United States. The seeds, leaf, and stem contain atropine/scopolamine alkaloids with potent anticholinergic effects. When ingested to get high, systemic anticholinergic effects can be seen, including bilateral dilated pupils. If parts of the plant inadvertently come in contact with the eye, a unilateral fixed and dilated pupil can result. See page 53.

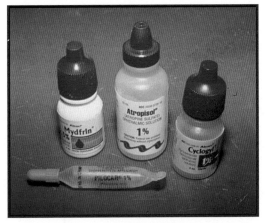

The screw-off caps of ophthalmologic drops are color-coded. Drops with red caps will dilate the pupil, those with green caps will constrict the pupil. Antibiotics and other preparations have a clear, white, or another color-coded cap. See page 54.

ACUTE NARROW-ANGLE GLAUCOMA, P. 66

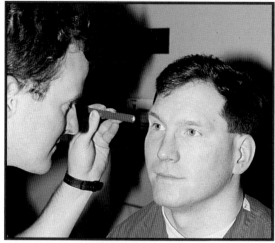

To assess the depth of the anterior chamber and hence the potential for pupillary dilation to precipitate acute glaucoma, a penlight is held laterally and a light beam is directed medially. To avoid false testing, the light beam should be exactly perpendicular at the line of sight when the patient looks forward (parallel to the coronal plane of the face). The light beam should pass through the medial and lateral canthus simultaneously and the amount of iris that is illuminated is observed. See page 66.

FISH BONES IN THE THROAT, P. 76

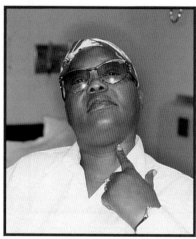

Some fish bones can be easily removed in the ED, and most patients can localize the general area where a fish bone has lodged. This patient consistently pointed to the left submandubular area, and a fish bone was found impaled in the left tonsil, almost exactly where the patient indicated. See page 76.

ACUTE ANGLE-CLOSURE GLAUCOMA, P. 68

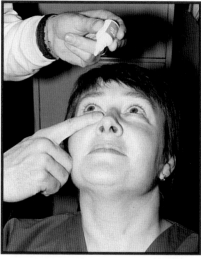

Prior to the instillation of eye drops, the medial punctum is occluded with gentle finger pressure and held closed for a few minutes. This will limit the systemic absorption of medication by decreasing the amount of drug drained by the nasolacrimal duct. Some eye drops, such as beta blockers (Timolol) can cause significant systemic effects, especially after the repeated administration required to treat acute glaucoma. Some authors suggest tightly shutting the eyes as an alternative to finger pressure. See page 68.

FISH BONES IN THE THROAT, P. 79

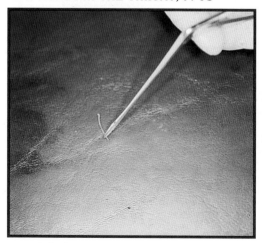

Bones lodged in the throat are difficult to see and can resemble strands of saliva. Be careful when exploring with your hemostat. See page 79.

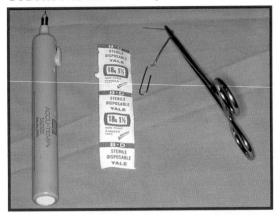

A number of devices are available to trephine the nail. The heated paper clip is an inexpensive and disposable apparatus. See page 96.

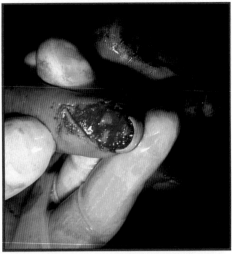

Under digital block with bupivacaine, the essential bloodless field is obtained by a tourniquet, and the extent of the nail bed laceration is determined. The nail may be gently removed by spreading small scissors placed between the nail and nail bed, allowing the nail bed to be anatomically repaired with 6-0 absorbable sutures. See page 102.

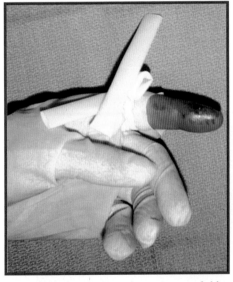

An easy way to obtain a clean operative field is to put a sterile glove on the patient and cut out the involved finger. This does away with annoying paper drapes. Note a Penrose drain used as a tourniquet. A tight-fitting glove allows one to roll back the latex to the base of the finger for use as a tourniquet. See page 102.

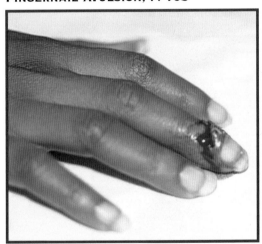

In a very common scenario, this patient slammed a car door on her finger, avulsing the base of the nail. The root of the nail lies on top of the eponychium and must be implanted back to its original position under the eponychium (cuticle). This injury is also commonly associated with an avulsion of the extensor tendon (mallet finger), a nail bed laceration that needs repair, or a tuft fracture. See page 103.

FINGERNAIL AVULSION, P. 104

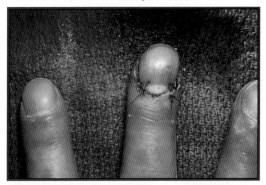

Without trimming or debriding, the base of the avulsed nail is carefully replaced in the nail fold (between the eponychium and the nail bed). This step is critical to avoid synechia formation and a resulting split nail. Although it was not done in this case, it would be desirable to put a few holes in the replaced nail to allow drainage of the nail bed. The replaced nail may be sutured in place, but avoid putting sutures in the nail root. In two weeks the sutures are removed. The nail may grow normally or be pushed out by the new nail. See page 104.

PARONYCHIA, P. 107

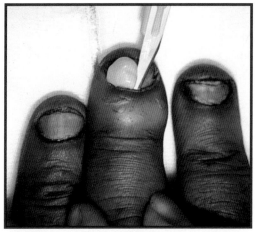

A paronychia is a collection of pus under the cuticle, not a cutaneous abscess per se. Instead of incising the skin, simply lift up the cuticle with a blade or scissors, spread the eponychial space with a blunt instrument, and pack the space open for 24-36 hours to promote drainage. Removing the nail or incising the overlying skin should be avoided whenever possible, which is most of the time. See page 107.

INJECTION TECHNIQUES, P. 138

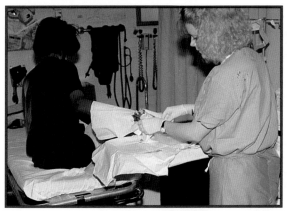

What's wrong with this picture? The medical student tried to repair this hand wound with the patient sitting upright. The patient did not want to lie down and seemed very brave and not troubled by the blood and needles. Soon after the picture was taken, the patient fainted and almost went head first onto the concrete floor. See page 138.

ACHILLES TENDON RUPTURE, P. 212

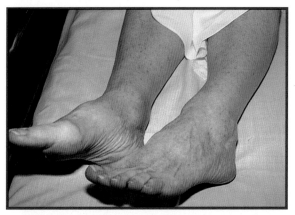

This elderly woman came to the ED complaining of pain in the ankle after stepping up to a curb. The triage note stated sprained ankle. She was able to walk with a limp and had minimal pain. Note the soft tissue swelling about the ankle. X-rays were negative, and she was able to weakly plantar flex the foot. Such an injury could be mistaken for a simple sprain. See page 212.

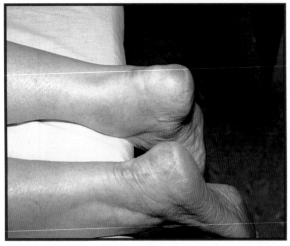

In addition to swelling about the malleoli, there is ecchymosis and swelling posteriorly, but this was not appreciated until the patient got out of the wheelchair and onto the stretcher. A palpable defect in the Achilles tendon could not be appreciated due to swelling. See page 213.

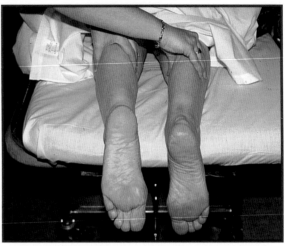

To perform the Thompson test, the patient is prone on the stretcher with the legs overhanging. The calf is squeezed briskly and motion of the foot is noted. In this case, one foot does not plantar flex. At operation, she had complete rupture of the Achilles tendon in the non-flexing foot. See page 214.

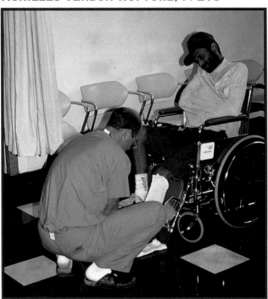

The best way to miss an Achilles tendon rupture is to examine a patient in the hallway in a wheelchair. This patient had a complete rupture, could plantar flex the foot while sitting, and was sent home with the diagnosis of a sprained ankle. See page 215.

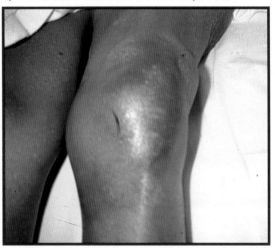

This elderly man tripped on a sidewalk but caught himself before he hit the ground. When he tried to walk, the leg consistently gave way. In the ED, the diagnosis was knee strain and hemarthrosis (note prep for arthrocentesis). The x-ray was normal except for soft tissue swelling. If one looks for it, the classic soft tissue defect superior to the patella is obvious, but in this case it was not initially appreciated. He could not lift his heel off the stretcher, but when put in a knee immobilizer and given crutches, he could walk quite well. See page 217.

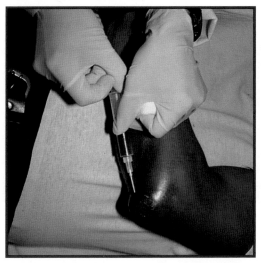

The preferred treatment for nonseptic olecranon bursitis is aseptic needle aspiration and instillation of long-acting steroids. To drain the bursa, hold the barrel of a 10 cc syringe parallel to the forearm and advance until fluid is aspirated via a 20 gauge needle. Note the classic serosanguinous fluid. With the needle still in the bursal sac, the syringe containing steroid is substituted for the aspirating syringe. See page 221.

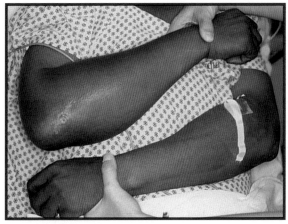

This patient has septic olecranon bursitis (cultures positive for S. aureus). Note the skin defect from a previous trauma, the obvious diffuse cellulitic appearance, and the lack of a distinct fluctuant mass. The area was painful and tender. The patient was febrile. He failed outpatient treatment and required seven days of intravenous antibiotics for complete resolution. See page 222.

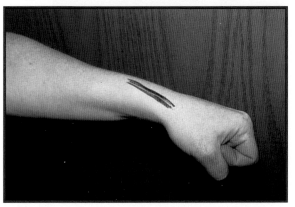

de Quervain's tenosynovitis produces pain in the radial aspect of the wrist due to inflammation of the abductor pollicis longus and extensor pollicis brevis tendons. Pain may radiate up the forearm or into the thumb, but it is maximal at the radial styloid (area marked). See page 226.

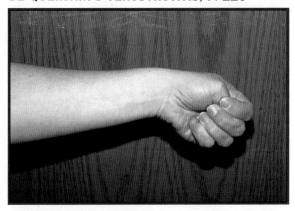

Finkelstein's test involves grasping the thumb in the palm and ulnar deviation of the wrist. When the pain is reproduced, this test is sensitive for de Quervain's disease, but it's probably not very specific. See page 226.

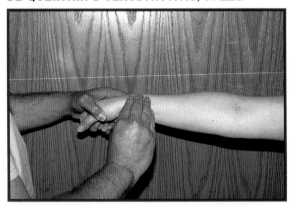

When inflammation is severe, crepitus may be felt under the skin by the examiner's fingers when the inflamed tendons are moved. See page 228.

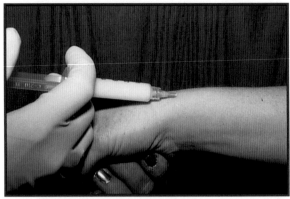

The definitive therapy for de Quervain's disease is injection of the tendon sheaths and peritendinous area with a long-acting corticosteroid. If the steroid is mixed with lidocaine, the accuracy of the injection is immediately known. The lidocaine also gives additional volume so injections do not have to be so anatomically precise. Although it's difficult to appreciate clinically, the steroid should be placed in the tendon sheath (but not the tendon itself) for best results. See page 228.

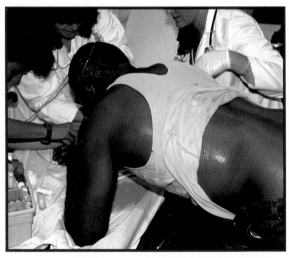

This diaphoretic, hypoxic asthmatic is near respiratory arrest. Despite a very high blood pressure, a pulse of 160 bpm, and being 64 years old, epinephrine was given (0.3 mg subcu every 20 minutes), and all parameters improved. Intubation was not required. See page 262.

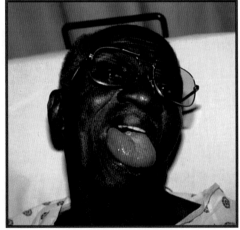

This 76-year-old man, who was hypertensive (170/110) and tachycardiac (110/bpm), was stung in the tongue by a bee while licking an ice cream cone. He noted immediate swelling of the tongue. The treatment alternatives were blind nasotracheal intubation, a retrograde wire or cricothyroidotomy, or medical therapy (including epinephrine). He responded to antihistamines, steroids, and two doses of 0.2 mg subcutaneous epinephrine (20 min apart) with a decrease in blood pressure and pulse. He recovered completely in a few hours without the need for artificial airway. See page 263.

THE ECLECTIC NATURE OF ED PAIN CONTROL

Unique uses of anesthesia in the emergency department range from preparing for lumbar puncture to treating post-herpetic neuralgia

The everyday practice of emergency medicine requires the physician to be well versed in all forms of pain control and symptomatic relief, and the collage of articles reviewed here demonstrates the eclectic nature of our specialty. This chapter continues the discussion of unique or special uses of anesthetics and analgesics in the emergency department.

A CONTROLLED CLINICAL TRIAL OF LOCAL ANESTHESIA FOR LUMBAR PUNCTURE IN NEWBORNS
Porter FL, et al *Pediatrics* 1991;88(4):663

The authors of this study attempted to define the role of local anesthesia prior to lumbar puncture in critically ill newborns. Their aim was to document the value of anesthesia in reducing unwanted or detrimental physiological responses to the painful procedure. They note that any change in normal physiological parameters, which they term "physiologic instability," may herald clinical deterioration in already unstable acutely ill neonates. There is evidence that the response to pain in newborns results in adverse changes in blood pressure, heart rate, and respiratory rate, and these physiologic parameters better reflect distress than does crying or other pain responses common to adults. The premise is that physiologic instability secondary to environmental stimuli, invasive procedures, and pain should be avoided because they may have significant medical consequences in critically ill patients.

Prior to routine lumbar puncture, 77 neonates randomly received either nothing (placebo was thought to be unjustified) or local anesthesia with the subcutaneous injection of 0.1 ml/kg of 1% lidocaine. The heart rate, respiratory rate, transcutaneous oxygen saturation, and carbon dioxide tensions were measured at baseline, during handling and preparation for the procedure, and monitored continuously throughout the procedure. The lumbar puncture (LP) was performed in a lateral position with hips and neck flexed, using a 22 gauge spinal needle.

The use of lidocaine did not minimize physiologic instability or otherwise affect physiological parameters during the lumbar puncture. Although the lidocaine was not associated with any adverse effects, using local anesthesia did lengthen the duration of the entire procedure. There were significant physiological changes from baseline noted during the preparatory procedures of positioning and handling, but the LP itself was apparently tolerated equally well in both treated and untreated groups. The authors emphasize that local anesthesia did not decrease the need for repositioning during the puncture nor did it affect the maximum number of attempts required to obtain CSF.

It is concluded that simply preparing and positioning a neonate for lumbar puncture measurably increases heart rate and heart rate variability, and causes a significant decrease in respiratory rate while reducing oxygenation. Once the infant is prepared and positioned, few additional adverse changes are noted in response to the actual introduction of the spinal needle. The authors could find no beneficial effect of local anesthesia prior to lumbar punctures in this study.

They were somewhat surprised by the data because the results of this study are in marked contrast to previous reports of significant, even dramatic, physiological changes during unanesthetized circumcision in full-term healthy neonates. It is suggested that in premature sick newborns, seemingly innocuous pre-procedure activities such as handling, positioning, and cleaning have a more destabilizing effect on vital signs than does the administration of local anesthetics or the lumbar puncture itself.

The authors stop short of concluding that local anesthesia is worthless prior to lumbar puncture in the ill neonate. They offer the following explanations: Perhaps the maximal physiological response had already been elicited by the preparatory procedures and could not be further increased by painful stimuli; the dose of anesthetic was inadequate, or some yet unidentified parameter more accurately reflects a newborn's pain. It is suggested that pretreatment with parenteral sedation, rather than local anesthesia, may be more helpful.

COMMENT: Hopefully all medical personnel have rejected the myth that neonates do not feel pain (*N Engl J Med* 1987;317(21):1321). It would be inconceivable to perform a cut down or lumbar puncture or insert a chest tube in an adult or even a young child without the use of local anesthesia, and the same holds for even the smallest newborn. Although it is doubtful that the physiologic stress of an LP has any significant medical effects in chil-

Table 1.

PHYSIOLOGIC CHANGES DURING LUMBAR PUNCTURE

Physiologic parameter	Baseline to Preparatory		Preparatory to Puncture	
	Mean ± SD	P value	Mean ± SD	P value
Mean heart rate, bpm	12.9±15.3	.0001	-7.5±15.6	.0001
Standard deviation of heart rate, bpm	4.8±6.2	.0001	0.1±8.5	.9810
Interquartile range of heart rate, bpm	8.2±14.3	.0001	-0.2±17.8	.9362
Mean respiratory rate, bpm	-2.2±7.7	.0164	-0.6±7.2	.4707
Mean tcPO2, mm Hg	-11.8±19.6	.0001	-10.1±19.9	.0001
Mean tcPCO2, mm Hg	-0.2±5.6	.8195	3.3±12.2	.0311
Minimum tcPO2, mm Hg	-17.3±29.2	.0001	-9/1±18.6	.0002
Maximum, tcPCO2, mm Hg	-0.4±12.8	.8129	6.2±12.1	.0001

Source: Pediatrics, 1991;88:663-669.

dren and adults, it's logical to consider the other advantages of performing one painlessly.

Given the tremendous amount of unfounded anxiety about and fear of spinal taps in the general population, even the smallest amount of pain from a spinal needle can be perceived as a major discomfort, making further attempts at obtaining CSF more difficult. If it does nothing else, local anesthesia makes the procedure easier for the physician. It's logical to reduce pain and anxiety whenever possible, and despite physician and nurse bias, I could find no data that prove a painful experience in the ED as a young child emotionally scars one for life.

With proper local anesthesia, lumbar puncture can and should be virtually painless, but merely raising a skin wheal does not accomplish this objective. For LP anesthesia, I prefer to use a 1½ inch 25 gauge needle and draw up additional lidocaine — the prepackaged kits usually contain only a few milliliters — and inject subcutaneously along the entire tract of the envisioned spinal tap. Such deep subcutaneous infiltration is required if the procedure is to be totally painless.

I believe local anesthesia makes LP easier in the struggling child although some physicians also routinely use sedation for the procedure. I do not usually sedate infants for lumbar puncture although the technique has advocates. In children older than 6-8 months and in adults, I now routinely administer some form of parenteral sedation/analgesia. Most neonates can be held adequately by a good assistant — proper holding is certainly the key for success — but it may be impossible to do the procedure with any ease without parenteral sedation in older children. If one does choose sedation, a number of alternatives are available, although intravenous midazolam (0.1 mg/kg) is the clear winner in my opinion.

This benzodiazepine is also well absorbed intramuscularly (especially a deltoid injection) if one does not choose to start an IV. Prolonged sedation or altering the mental status with IV midazolam should never be an issue due to the drug's short half-life and the availability of flumazenil. Chloral hydrate, phenobarbital, or narcotics are occasionally used, but all have some theoretical downside. Chloral hydrate, in particular, is a clinical dinosaur given its prolonged sedation and relatively low safety margin.

Fentanyl is also a popular agent for neonatal use (*Anesthesiology* 1987;66(6):433). In my experience, pediatricians seem to have philosophical problems with sedating children in the ED for an LP — groundless objections as far as I can discern — but they seem eager to give chloral

hydrate to sedate kids for CT scans and other procedures. The authors of this study do suggest that sedation prior to preparatory procedures may be the ideal way to minimize the physiological instability associated with handling.

One should make a clear distinction between procedures performed on neonates/newborns and older children. I would be quite cautious about sedating neonates for pro-

Table 2.

ADEQUACY OF ANESTHESIA 25, 40, AND 50 MINUTES AFTER APPLICATION

A=Acceptable; U=Unacceptable

	25 min.		40 min.		50 min.	
Anesthesia	A	U	A	U	A	U
Xylocaine 10%	9	0	6	3	2	7
Placebo spray	0	9	2	7	0	9
Lidocaine 4%	10	1	8	3	7	4
Lidocaine hydrochloride 5%	7	4	4	7	4	7
Placebo liniment	4	7	3	8	4	7

Source: ORL *1990;52:168-173.*

cedures in the ED. My reluctance is a safety concern. Although one may be concerned about minor changes in heart rate and oxygen tension from procedures in the neonatal ICU, this is usually not a major issue in healthy full-term neonates brought to the ED. Sedation is always an option if the procedure cannot be accomplished without it, but it is extremely easy to make a mistake with dose calculations. Many emergency nurses and physicians are not familiar with using drugs in such small children. It's axiomatic to use supplemental oxygen, pulse oximetry, and ECG monitoring routinely when intravenous drugs are used for sedation in children and adults.

With specific reference to the actual mechanics of lumbar puncture in a sick neonate, one should be very careful about patient positioning. It's critical to avoid excessive flexion of the neck in neonates or fail to appreciate apnea during a prolonged or difficult procedure. I had one nonsedated child with meningitis suffer a respiratory arrest during an LP, probably the result of prolonged restraint with excessive neck flexion in an already unstable patient. Lumbar puncture in any sick child is a three-person procedure: one to do the tap, one to hold the child, and one to ensure that the patient's vital signs are not compromised.

Gleason et al (*Pediatrics* 1983;71:31) made interesting observations in an attempt to define the optimal position for LP in preterm infants. The authors studied the effect of three positions on transcutaneous PO_2 and PCO_2, minute ventilation, heart rate, and blood pressure in 10 infants positioned for an LP. They note that such a procedure in preterm infants is occasionally accompanied by clinical deterioration, and it is generally accepted that some decompensation may be the result of improper positioning.

In their study, 17 healthy preterm infants were held in one of three positions for five minutes: lateral recumbent position with full neck flexion, lateral recumbent with partial neck extension, and a sitting position with head support and spinal flexion. Infants were placed in these positions for monitoring purposes only, and no actual procedures were performed. Hypoxia was seen in all three positions and the decrease in oxygenation was greatest in the commonly used lateral recumbent/neck flexed position; the PO_2 dropped an average of 28 mm Hg. The PCO_2 also rose slightly (3 mm Hg). Heart rate increased in all three positions, but blood pressure remained virtually unchanged.

The data suggest that LPs performed in the standard lateral recumbent flexed position have the highest risk of potential morbidity, especially hypoxia, and the authors caution that if a patient is placed on his side, the neck should be extended. It is also suggested that the ideal position for the LP in the neonate is the upright sitting position. Other authors have noted a decrease in PO_2 as much as 45 mm Hg when supine infants are placed in a tight knee chest position for three minutes. It appears that the position that most of us use to perform LPs in neonates is the most detrimental to oxygenation.

Clearly LPs in obtunded or otherwise compromised small children should be done with extreme caution. Perhaps we should be using supplemental oxygen and pulse oximetry ECG monitoring during all LPs on neonates, even if sedation is not used. The authors believe that ventilation-perfusion imbalance is the prominent mechanism

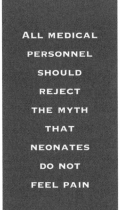

ALL MEDICAL PERSONNEL SHOULD REJECT THE MYTH THAT NEONATES DO NOT FEEL PAIN

to account for the decrease in oxygen saturation. One should use extreme caution with something as simple as positioning sick neonates who have respiratory or cardiovascular instability.

TOPICAL ANESTHESIA OF THE NORMAL TYMPANIC MEMBRANE: A CONTROLLED CLINICAL TRIAL OF DIFFERENT SUSPENSIONS OF LIDOCAINE

Moller A, Grontved A
ORL J Otorhinolaryngol Relat Spec 1990;52(3):168

The authors of this Scandinavian study attempted to find an effective method for topical anesthesia of the tympanic membrane (TM) for minor surgical procedures. Twelve healthy human volunteers were subjected to a randomized, double-blind crossover trial of topically applied lidocaine aerosol 10%, lidocaine 4%, lidocaine HCl 5%, and placebo. The lidocaine aerosol was first sprayed into a syringe and shaken to evaporate the propellant, and the tempered aerosol and other solutions were then dropped directly into the ear canal. Sensation in the TM was tested 25 minutes post installation by a series of painful stimuli. Results demonstrating the adequacy of anesthesia are presented in Table 2.

Acceptable anesthesia was noted in those given 10% lidocaine aerosol and in most of the subjects given 4% lidocaine. Those receiving placebo or the 5% lidocaine HCl — the formulation used for infiltrative anesthesia — had unacceptable anesthesia. Importantly, the duration of anesthesia was quite transient, lasting only about 20 minutes. The authors concluded that topical anesthesia of the tympanic membrane can be achieved with lidocaine aerosol 10% and lidocaine 4%, but 5% lidocaine HCl is ineffective.

The mechanism of action of topical anesthetics is thought to be related to the ability of nonionized particles to permeate membranes. At a pH of 8.2, the lidocaine aerosol is largely nonionized and consequently more readily diffusible across the tympanic membrane. Lidocaine HCl, which has a pH of 4.2, is predominantly ionized and therefore very poorly diffusible. Alkalinization of anesthetic solutions decreases stability and shelf-life but apparently increases topical potency.

COMMENT: Even the most cooperative patient cannot hold still for an ear procedure when the unanesthetized tympanic membrane or ear canal is even lightly touched. Unfortunately, complete anesthesia of the ear is not readily achieved in the ED. Note that it required 25 minutes for the topical anesthetic to become effective, and anesthesia only lasted 15-20 minutes. Importantly, anesthesia in this case was only of the tympanic membrane and not of the ear canal itself.

I have been quite frustrated in my attempts to obtain topical anesthesia for removal of foreign bodies of the ear. The sensitivity of the ear canal is readily appreciated by the patient with otitis externa. Because the canal is so sensitive, I rarely debride otitis externa even though it's recommended (but never studied) by many textbooks. The skin of the canal is innervated by sensory nerves from surrounding pinna. One can obtain anesthesia of the skin of the external canal ringing the external ear meatus with subcutaneous lidocaine. Be sure to infiltrate the junction between the bony and cartilaginous parts of the anterior wall of the auditory canal. However, this is quite painful and often worse than the procedure itself.

Absolutely key to the successful removal of foreign bod-

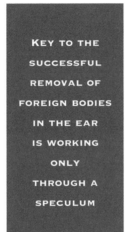

KEY TO THE SUCCESSFUL REMOVAL OF FOREIGN BODIES IN THE EAR IS WORKING ONLY THROUGH A SPECULUM

ies (FBs) in the ear is to work only through a speculum, which protects the skin of the ear canal by limiting contact by the instrument. One should also have uninterrupted time to carry out such procedures, analgesia/sedation are usually called for, and the procedure should not be attempted without the proper equipment and light source. Many of these requirements are not readily available in a busy ED. Personally, I would rarely attempt removal of a foreign body in the ear without at least some parenteral medication; my favorite is a combination of IV fentanyl/midazolam. I can understand the frustration of an ENT consultant who is called to retrieve an ear FB after the emergency physician creates a swollen, bloody ear canal and a hysterical patient. The bottom line: Don't persist in unsuccessful attempts to remove a complicated FB lodged deep in the ear.

I have personally attempted anesthesia of the TM with the 10% lidocaine aerosol and can attest to the fact that it is initially rather irritating when put in the ear, particularly if the bubbles are not dissipated. I have also been less than thrilled with its ability to produce anesthesia of the tympanic membrane, although part of the problem is probably that the canal itself is still sensitive. Some of my colleagues swear by the use of tetracaine,

	Physician's global response: improved[1]			Categoric pain severity changes[2] (%)			Pain (mm) per VAS[3]			Pain relief per VAS[4]		
Group	Wk 2	Wk 4	Wk 6	Wk 2	Wk 4	Wk 6	Day 0	Wk 2	Wk 6	Wk 2	Wk 4	Wk 6
Capsaicin	62	77	77	25	31	46	71.0	56	50	46	54	54
Vehicle	31	31	31	6	19	6	71.5	67.5	72.5	19	19	6

Table 3.

RESPONSES OF PATIENTS TREATED WITH CAPSAICIN CREAM OR ITS VEHICLE

VAS=Visual analogue scale.
[1] Pain gone, much better, or slightly better.
[2] Pain severity compared with baseline.
[3] Decrease equals improvement.
[4] Percentage of patients with >40% relief of pain on VAS.

Source: J Am Acad Dermatol *1989;21:265-270.*

epinephrine, and cocaine (TAC) solution in the ear, but I have not seen it studied. The traditional method of topical anesthesia of the TM is with phenol, a substance rarely found in the ED.

TOPICAL CAPSAICIN TREATMENT OF CHRONIC POSTHERPETIC NEURALGIA

Bernstein JE, et al
J Am Acad Dermatol 1989; 21(2):265

The article describes a rather unique and largely unknown treatment for the post-herpetic neuralgia (PHN) that frequently follows herpes zoster (shingles) infections. The authors used a topical preparation of capsaicin, a substance that enhances the release of and inhibits the reaccumulation of substance P. Substance P is a neurotransmitter released from nerve terminals in the peripheral nervous system, and it is thought that pain perception in the skin is mediated by this chemical. In a double-blind study of 32 elderly patients with chronic PHN, either topical capsaicin 0.25% or its cream vehicle were applied three to four times per day for six weeks.

All subjects had either poorly or incompletely controlled pain with traditional oral analgesics, antidepressants, or neuroleptic agents, and all had symptoms that interfered with sleep or daily activities. Additional measures to control pain were not allowed during the study period. Most patients had trunk or abdominal involvement, but about one-third had a cranial distribution of PHN pain. After the first two weeks of therapy, 62 percent of the capsaicin-treated patients and 31 percent of vehicle-treated patients report a significant reduction in symptoms. By four weeks, 70 percent of the treated patients had beneficial results. The clinical improvement with capsaicin was statistically significant at all time points during the study.

There were minimal adverse effects of the topical preparation, and complications were limited to burning, stinging, or irritation at the site of application. The authors believe that topically applied capsaicin is a safe and effective treatment for post-herpetic neuralgia. Drawbacks to therapy are the minimal local side effects, and the fact that the drug must be applied three or four times a day for maximum results. It may take two to four weeks for stubborn cases to respond. Because partial or complete relief of pain was obtained in nearly 80 percent of patients with previously intractable pain, the authors believe that the risk to benefit ratio of other therapeutic modalities makes capsaicin an ideal choice.

COMMENT: Capsaicin is a unique substance that has only recently been studied in a scientific manner. Capsaicin is the naturally occurring ingredient in red peppers and other members of the nightshade family of plants. Capsaicin is thought to achieve its pharmacologic activity by decreasing the neurologic activity of sensory neurons because of the depletion of neurotransmitters from these fibers. The compound affects small diameter pain-evoking afferent nerves in the skin. Capsaicin is currently marketed under the trade name Zostrix (0.025%) or Zostrix-HP (0.075%), and both are listed in the *Physicians' Desk Reference (PDR)*. The manufacturer, GenDerm Corporation (Lincolnshire, IL 60069), will send physicians reprints and an informative monograph. In addition to PHN, capsaicin has been used for the treatment of rheumatoid arthritis, diabetic neuropathy, postmastectomy pain syndromes, and reflex sympathetic dystrophy. Capsaicin is not a local anesthetic, and it only blocks impulses carried on type C neurons.

Scheffler et al (*J Am Podiatr Med Assoc* 1991;81(6): 288) conducted a double-blind vehicle-controlled eight-week study of the effect of capsaicin cream in relieving the pain of diabetic neuropathy. Treated subjects demonstrated a significant benefit, with 90 percent of those given capsaicin reporting improvement. Diabetic neuropathy is an extremely frustrating problem that frequently sends patients to the ED with burning, numbness, hypersensitivity, or radiating pain in a symmetrical stocking-glove distribution. The problem is often worse at night, so it usually awakens the patient. The symptoms may be extremely disabling. A number of medications have been tried, including tricyclic antidepressants, carbamazepine, and neuroleptics, but none have had prolonged success. Capsaicin appears at least to be worth a try for patients who present with either diabetic neuropathy or painful post-herpetic neuralgia. One caveat to remember is that the compound can be rather irritating to the skin and it takes time to work. I am somewhat skeptical about this product, but it will be interesting to note the evolution of this rather unique topical preparation. I have not seen alcoholic peripheral neuropathy studied, but perhaps capsaicin may also help this distressing condition.

EFFECTIVE SEDATION IN THE ED

Fentanyl has a pharmacologic niche in the emergency department, alone or with benzodiazepines

Previous chapters have focused on unique and special uses of anesthetics and analgesics in the emergency department, with an emphasis on generic pain control. Emergency physicians are also frequently called upon to perform painful or difficult procedures where significant sedation is required for patient comfort or cooperation or to facilitate or expedite medical care. In addition to being the hospital's expert on the use of local anesthetics and pain medications, the practicing EP must likewise be at clinical ease with the multiple agents used to produce adequate sedation. The days are over when one can merely physically restrain the terrified child or otherwise ignore the pain of an agitated or uncooperative patient.

Aggressive chemical restraint/sedation is one of the hottest areas in emergency medicine today. The term "conscious sedation" is often used to describe procedures that border on general anesthesia, and EPs today are administering drugs or embracing techniques that were previously only used by anesthesiologists. Many scenarios are now under the purview of emergency medicine — from sedating the head-injured patient for a CT scan to gaining control over the frightened child in need of meticulous laceration repair to paralyze the wildly agitated and hyperthermic cocaine overdose. This chapter will detail the use of a potent narcotic, fentanyl, a drug that seems to have found a particular pharmacologic niche in the ED. It may be used alone or with benzodiazepines. If you are not currently using fentanyl on a daily basis, I urge you to carefully consider the following discussion.

USE OF IV FENTANYL IN THE OUTPATIENT TREATMENT OF THE PEDIATRIC FACIAL TRAUMA

Billmire DA, et al *J Trauma* 1985;25(11):1079

This interesting paper is a retrospective review of 2,000 children with facial trauma who were treated over a four-year period at the Children's Hospital of the University of Cincinnati. The authors note that pediatric patients with facial lacerations are a special breed, and their age mandates specific management techniques. Even a minor laceration may require sedation, physical restraint, or even occasionally general anesthesia to obtain a satisfactory or cosmetic surgical closure. The authors report their experience in repairing facial lacerations under IV sedation with fentanyl.

SAFE AND EFFECTIVE ED SEDATION GUIDE TO USING FENTANYL/MIDAZOLAM

Note:

1. For predominantly analgesia, with moderate sedation, increase the dose of fentanyl.

2. For predominantly deep sedation, muscle relaxation, and amnesia, increase the dosage of midazolam.

For Average 70kg Adult, Obtain 4 ml Fentanyl/2mg Midazolam

Preparation:

1. This is a two-person procedure. An assistant continually monitors vital signs. Once medication is given, the patient is not left alone until completely awake.

2. Secure free-flowing IV access. (Heparin lock is an alternative.)

3. Connect patient EKG, pulse oximetry, and blood pressure monitor.

4. Have naloxone, flumazenil, and Ambu bag at the bedside.

5. Administer nasal oxygen at 4-6 L/min. (Don't wait for hypoxia.)

Drug Administrations:

1. Administer fentanyl, 1µg/kg/minute, until proper sedation is achieved or for a total of 5 µg/kg. Note: Standard concentration: 50 µg/ml. Most adults require 3-4 ml (2-3 µg/kg) for adequate sedation.

2. Administer midazolam 1 mg/minute until proper sedation achieved. Decrease usual dose of midazolam because of potentiation by fentanyl.

3. Wait five minutes after final drug administration before performing procedure.

4. Administer local anesthetic if required.

Post-Operative Period:

1. Reverse drugs if necessary from clinical standpoint. Generally it is best to allow gradual recovery.

2. Observe patient for full hour after awake. Prohibit driving for 12 hours.

Source: James R. Roberts, MD

The majority of injuries were routine facial lacerations repaired in the ED on an outpatient basis, but injuries included complicated dog bites and trauma from a motor vehicle accidents. Approximately 20 minutes prior to suturing, intravenous fentanyl, in a dose of 2-3 µg/kg, was given by slow IV infusion over three to five minutes. In the authors' experience, younger children required slightly higher doses than older children, but a maximum dose of 3 µg/kg is recommended. When sedation was achieved and traditional local anesthesia administered, lacerations were cleaned, debrided, and sutured. Supplemental fentanyl was used as necessary, and naloxone was also available for immediate use because respiratory depression is a well known side effect of excess fentanyl.

The average case required 20-30 minutes of surgical time, approximately the effective duration of action of IV fentanyl. Minimal physical restraints were used as necessary. Of the 2,000 cases, three children experienced short-term apnea and required reversal with naloxone and temporary bag-mask ventilation. Tracheal intubation was never required. No patient was hospitalized for fentanyl-associated problems. Nausea and vomiting were not a problem, and there were no episodes of delirium or muscular rigidity.

The authors believe that their three-and-a-half-year experience in more than 2,000 cases has shown fentanyl to be a safe and effective adjunct for the treatment of pediatric facial trauma. The authors cite as particularly desirable the drug's rapid onset, short duration of action, and rapid recovery. They believe that IV fentanyl negated the use of general anesthesia in some instances, and the drug made the procedure easier and certainly less stressful for the child, parent, and physician. The powerful narcotic effect of fentanyl is stressed, particularly the potential for respiratory depression. The unique muscular rigidity that had been rarely described with rapid IV injection of high doses is emphasized. A minor drawback of this technique is the need to start an IV.

COMMENT: The judicious use of powerful intravenous medications for sedation and to gain rapid control of the uncooperative patient is one of the most intriguing topics in emergency medicine today. Certainly emergency physicians should be at the forefront of such a crusade, and we should be the leaders in the hospital in this endeavor. Any EP who is not familiar with a number of options for conscious sedation — and using them on a daily basis — is still practicing in the Dark Ages. Although this particular article is a general overview of the authors' experience and contains no real hard data, the mere fact that it appears in the surgical literature is important.

Emergency physicians generally believe they have cornered the market when it comes to being kind or gentle to patients and therefore such support from our surgical colleagues is indeed welcome. For some reason the plastic surgeons have been particularly pharmacologically enlightened, while the orthopods still rely heavily on "Brutane" anesthesia (*Plast Reconstr Surg* 1981;67(6):799). It is certainly laudable that consulting surgeons — primarily busy house staff — have outpatient sedation in mind, but a bizarre fact of this article is that surgeons repaired 2,000 lacerations in the ED in a short three-year period. Clearly these cases should have been done by the EPs. Politics aside, however, this is a welcomed article.

Although it is easy to get a consensus on the need for effective sedation in emergency patients, it's impossible to gain a consensus on the ideal agent or regimen. Each physician has his own favorite oral, intramuscular, rectal, intranasal, or intravenous drug or cocktail, and it's always best to use a regimen with which one is most familiar and comfortable. On a milligram for milligram basis, fentanyl is 100-200 times more potent than morphine. Fentanyl has been used orally as a lollipop, as a sustained-release transdermal patch, and as an inhaled analgesic.

For my practice the intravenous use of a short-acting easily titrated medication is most ideal. I cannot overemphasize my bias and underscore the ideal characteristics of intravenous fentanyl. Except for the slight downside of having to start an IV, this potent narcotic possesses ideal characteristics for ED use: a rapid onset, short duration, relatively accurate dosing, immediate reversibility, and overall safety. The dose of 2-3 μg/kg extrapolates into a reasonable starting dose for adults as well. I have used fentanyl hundreds of times and urge all physicians who have not had experience with it to consider it. The authors of this paper used fentanyl alone, but I almost always use it in conjunction with benzodiazepines, particularly midazolam (Versed). If pain relief with light to moderate sedation is paramount, go heavy on the fentanyl; if heavy sedation or amnesia is your main goal, opt for more Versed. When these two drugs are used together, they are extremely effective and also quite potent. To avoid problems, this combination must be used quite carefully, with strict attention to detail. (See table.)

A few caveats about the everyday clinical use of fentanyl should be emphasized. The drug has an initial onset of action in one to two minutes but takes a few more minutes to reach its peak effect. As with many drugs used in the ED, a common error is to attempt a painful procedure before the drug has had enough time to be fully effective. It's best to wait about five minutes after completing the initial infusion before operating or giving more drug. One should be patient and not rush the procedure or excessive sedation will occur or the majority of analgesia will occur in the postoperative period. If you are using fentanyl alone, a reasonable starting dose is 2 μg/kg. Additional 1 μg/kg supplemental doses may be given as needed, up to a total of 5 μg/kg. I aim to put the patient in a light sleep (eyes closed, snoring) and unresponsive to voice. Fentanyl is available in a 50 μg/ml concentration, and the average adult gets a good response from 3-4 ml. Approximately one hour post-injection, the patient is back to the original clinical state.

I prefer to observe all patients for a full hour after they wake up and prohibit driving for that day. Unless the sedation is excessive, I do not routinely reverse fentanyl with naloxone, allowing for a gradual recovery that smooths out the hospital stay while charts are completed, post-reduction x-ray taken, splints and dressings are applied, or abscesses are packed.

Aside from its short duration of action, fentanyl has other advantages over morphine and meperidine. Fentanyl is used for anesthesia in cardiac surgery in doses totaling 100 μg/kg with minimal detrimental hemodynamic effects. Unlike other traditional opiates, fentanyl does not cause significant histamine release and therefore rarely produces hypotension. This characteristic makes it safer than morphine or meperidine in trauma patients where alcohol intoxication, drug use, or unsuspected hypovolemia are possible. Reported in the literature is a vagal effect similar to morphine, but bradycardia is rarely seen. Nausea and vomiting, common to morphine and meperdine, are virtually absent with fentanyl. It's the best drug to give any patient in whom vomiting is undesirable. A rather strange but well publicized phenomenon noted fentanyl is a peculiar muscle rigidity of the chest wall and trunk. This is described with rapid bolus injections of high doses, but should not be a problem with the slow injection of the doses used in the ED. The rigidity can be very distressing to both patient and physician should it occur; I have never personally seen it. Naloxone reportedly reverses it.

Apnea is the major serious side effect of all narcotics, including fentanyl, but it should be rare with proper dosing and if the drug is given slowly. As with any potent drug, the physician should not give a bolus and then leave the room to fill out paperwork or finish up another patient. The general rule for administering fentanyl is to use a maximum infusion rate of 1 μg/kg/min, a technique that should be extremely safe. Another unusual yet characteristic effect of fentanyl is that it produces pruritus, particularly around the face, and as noted by the authors of this paper, patients frequently scratch their nose during the initial injection, contaminating a sterile field.

Fentanyl is a great drug, perhaps an ideal one, and its use should be familiar to every E.P. However, as with any powerful agent, this drug must be respected and used with extreme caution, especially when combined with even small doses of benzodiazepines. Michelson (*Anesth Plast Surg* 1987;11:207) touts the benefits of diazepam/fentanyl when used to supplement local anesthesia for inpatient surgery, but also comments on the potency of the combination. The major benefit of concomitant benzodiazepines is muscle relaxation, deep sedation, and potent amnesia, but remember that a few milligrams of midazolam go a long way when fentanyl is on board.

Wright (*Ann Emerg Med* 1992;21(8):925) emphasized that patients receiving intravenous benzodiazepines and narcotics can become hypoxic during conscious sedation and respiratory depression may not be clinically obvious. Patients receiving IV fentanyl often desaturate, with pulse oximetry in the high 80 to low 90 percent saturation range, and apnea may go unnoticed by the physician intent on a complicated laceration repair. Fentanyl, in relatively modest doses and especially when combined with benzodiazepines, depresses the protective ventilatory drive triggered by hypoxia and blunts the respiratory stimulation of elevated PCO_2. Curiously the patients may seem grossly normal and even somewhat awake while they are becoming more hypoxic. Tactile or verbal stimulation often reminds the patient to breathe, and pharmacologic reversal of fentanyl is usually not required if you have an assistant available to stimulate the narcotized patient.

I routinely use ECG monitoring, pulse oximetry, and administer nasal oxygen (4-6 L/min) to all patients receiving sedation for a procedure with intravenous fentanyl, with or without benzodiazepines. Importantly, intravenous sedation must be a two-person procedure; it's a technique not to be done alone or in a back room without help. An assistant should always be in the room to monitor vital signs, particularly respirations, allowing the primary physician to concentrate on the actual procedure. One cannot be expected to place meticulous sutures and also count the patient's respiratory rate. I always have naloxone available at the bedside, not locked up in a cart somewhere, although I do not routinely draw it up or use it to reverse narcotic effect. The Ambu bag should also be at the patient's bedside, and the IV must be flowing freely. If oxygen is used routinely, hypoxia is not a problem.

THE SAFETY OF FENTANYL USE IN THE EMERGENCY DEPARTMENT

Chudnofsky CR, et al *Ann Emerg Med* 1989;18(6):635

This is a retrospective study that also originated from the University of Cincinnati Medical Center, and it retrospectively reviewed the charts of 841 adult patients who received fentanyl over a three-year period. The narcotic was administered in the ED for orthopedic procedures, abscess irrigation and drainage, sedation for CT scans, burn debridement, chest tube placement, and as an adjunct to intubation. It was also given as a general sedative in patients with multiple trauma, including those with head injuries. The average dose of fentanyl was 180 μg (approximately 2.6 μg/kg), and the drug was given intravenously in all cases. Approximately half the patients received medications in addition to fentanyl, most commonly a benzodiazepine.

The safety profile of fentanyl in this unselected population of seriously ill patients was extremely positive. One patient reported nausea, two vomited, and one had urticaria. Respiratory depression developed in only six patients and three experienced hypotension. All three patients with hypotension had other factors that contributed to the hypotension, such as blood loss or excessive alcohol use. No case of respiratory depression required intubation. No patient experienced the peculiar muscular rigidity associated with fentanyl use. As noted in other studies, mild facial pruritus was commonly seen.

The authors conclude that fentanyl is a safe drug for sedation and analgesia in an unselected ED population. No significant downsides were identified, but the authors emphasize standard safety caveats: Initially start with a small dose (1 μg/kg/min and titrate for effect), use careful patient monitoring, have immediately available naloxone and resuscitation equipment, and use extreme caution in patients with excessive alcohol levels or in those who may have ingested other CNS or respiratory depressants.

COMMENT: This is also a retrospective study, but it includes hard data absent in the previous paper. The strongest clinical point in this paper is that the drug is safe to use as an initial medication in a relatively unselected ED population. Given the likelihood of unrecognized pathology or the presence of other drugs and/or medical conditions, the safety of fentanyl was downright amazing! Fentanyl's major benefit is as an analgesic for the performance of painful procedures, and although the drug has sedating properties, rapid sedation is not recommended for the widely agitated or psychotic patient. Fentanyl alone appears to be a reasonable sedative in head injured patients, and is usually safe to use for multiple trauma. The sedation is magnified by adding even small amounts of a benzodiazepine. A benzodiazepine alone is preferred to sedate the widely agitated psychotic patient, especially those encephalopathic from cocaine, amphetamine, or PCP toxicity. However, I would champion fentanyl's use in the multiple trauma patient who clearly requires pain control along with mild short-term sedation.

DURATION OF ANTAGONISTIC EFFECTS OF NALMEFENE AND NALOXONE IN OPIATE-INDUCED SEDATION FOR EMERGENCY DEPARTMENT PROCEDURES

Barsan WG, et al *Am J Emerg Med* 1989;7(2):155

The authors of this study evaluated the efficacy of two narcotic antagonists to reverse meperidine-induced sedation given in the ED for the treatment of painful procedures. The authors note that physician fear of hypotension and respiratory depression often limits the use of adequate doses of parenteral narcotics in the ED. The authors studied the experimental long-acting narcotic antagonist nalmefene (Revex), but the data are reviewed here because the authors used intravenous meperidine for the performance of a painful procedure. The dose administered was 1.5-3 mg/kg, to a maximum of 300 mg, given as a slow intravenous bolus.

The narcotic was given to adult ambulatory patients who were undergoing painful procedures, such as I&D of abscesses and painful orthopedic procedures. Vital signs and scores of alertness were followed for four hours. Interestingly, the mean dose of meperidine for all patients was 2.5 mg/kg, equivalent to 175 mg for the average 70 kg patient. Two patients were rescued with naloxone because of excessive respiratory depression, but the dose

given to these patients was not noted. Both nalmefene and naloxone effectively reversed the narcotic effect, but naloxone had a much shorter duration of action, being virtually ineffective in 30 minutes. Nalmefene was significantly superior in reversing sedation from 60 to 150 minutes post-administration. There were no significant differences in side effects. The authors conclude that nalmefene is useful in eliminating prolonged observation or prolonged sedation of patients who received high doses of long-acting narcotics for outpatient procedures.

COMMENT: I included this article because there are still physicians who have not yet embraced the use of fentanyl. Many physicians are still more comfortable providing short-term sedation with intravenous morphine or meperidine, but the obvious downside of these drugs is hypotension, nausea, and vomiting, and a prolonged

INDICATIONS FOR ED FENTANYL USE

Indication	No. (%)
Orthopedic procedure	336 (40.0)
Incision and drainage	246 (29.3)
General sedation	73 (8.7)
Radiography-CT sedation	60 (7.1)
Wound/burn care	39 (4.7)
Chest tube placement	22 (2.6)
Diagnostic procedures[1]	21 (2.5)
Airway/ventilatory control	20 (2.4)
Pain control	17 (2.0)
Miscellaneous procedures[2]	7 (0.7)
Total	841 (100)

[1] Diagnostic procedures such as lumbar puncture, peritoneal lavage, and anoscopy.

[2] Miscellaneous procedures such as burr hole, rectal disimpaction, hemorrhoid thrombectomy, etc.

Source: Ann Emerg Med 1989;18:635-639.

duration of action. Although this prolonged clinical effect is desirable for patients who are admitted to the hospital, it's undesirable for patients who are discharged following a relatively short but painful ED procedure. I particularly liked this paper because it emphasizes that doses of meperidine which are considered excessive by most physician are actually very safe. Note that the patients received an average of 175 mg of intravenous meperidine, a dose considered extremely high by some standards. Those who reluctantly give 25-50 mg of meperidine IV for extremely painful conditions or procedures — and consider themselves generous or aggressive — should take this dosing regimen to heart.

Meperidine in adequate doses is an excellent sedative and analgesic. The subjects of this study were healthy ambulatory patients without significant blood loss or concomitant alcohol or sedative drug use, and the authors note that hypotension was not seen. Interestingly, the respiratory rate was relatively unaffected by administration of these doses of meperidine. Although nalmefene may be effective, its long duration of action would preclude the subsequent use of narcotic analgesics for outpatient pain relief. Nalmefene has most utility as an antidote for narcotic overdose.

SEDATING THE PEDIATRIC PATIENT

*Chloral hydrate and DPT
are clinical dinosaurs for sedating children*

There are myriad regimens available to emergency physicians who sedate patients in the ED, with many variations on this theme and as a number of acceptable alternatives.

For general sedation (such as LP or cardioversion), I prefer midazolam. For painful procedures (such as irrigation and drainage, reductions), my particular routine is to use a combination of intravenous fentanyl and midazolam. Both agents possess ideal properties for short-term use and are applicable for the majority of situations encountered in the ED. Both drugs are titrated intravenously, have a rapid onset of action and a relatively short duration, produce significant analgesia or amnesia, and can be readily reversed with antagonists. When these drugs are titrated IV, the physician knows within minutes if more sedation is required, and the patient usually returns to a normal premedicated state within one hour.

I stress, however, that these agents are powerful CNS and respiratory depressants that should be used with caution. Some degree of respiratory depression commonly occurs when effective doses are used so certain safeguards should always be in place. Another person should be in the room to monitor the patient's condition, pulse oximetry and supplemental oxygen are routine, and naloxone, flumazenil, and an Ambu bag/intubation equipment are at the bedside. I also suggest the selected use of ECG monitoring, although arrhythmias are not a major concern.

Although a combination of intravenous fentanyl and midazolam can also be used for the pediatric patient, this chapter reviews agents that have been particularly popular for sedating children. Medications such as chloral hydrate and Demerol, Phenergan, and Thorazine (DPT) have been replaced by superior regimens, but their use is familiar to many clinicians. A relative newcomer is midazolam, particularly when it is used by the oral, rectal, or intranasal route. Although many combinations or single agents are acceptable, most physicians will choose a protocol with which they are comfortable and familiar. Although it would be impossible to get a consensus on the use of any particular sedation protocol, the "comfortable and familiar" rule is probably the best one to adopt. All physicians should master at least one of the commonly accepted techniques.

A PROSPECTIVE ANALYSIS OF
INTRAMUSCULAR MEPERIDINE,
PROMETHAZINE, AND CHLORPROMAZINE
IN PEDIATRIC EMERGENCY
DEPARTMENT PATIENTS

Terndrup TE, et al *Ann Emerg Med* 1991;20(1):31

This is a prospective study of 63 children sedated with the popular DPT cocktail. The three agents are mixed in a single syringe and given IM to children undergoing painful or stressful procedures. This concoction has been used since the 1950s and has been generally regarded as safe and effective. DPT has a few theoretical downsides, such as delayed onset and long duration of action, but the protocol has not been well studied in a prospective manner. The authors of this report examined various safety and efficacy parameters in an unblinded analysis.

Children younger than 16 years of age (average age 3.6 years) undergoing sedation at two medical centers received a single IM injection of DPT in the standard 2:1:1 mg/kg dose. Respiration, heart rate, arterial blood pressure, oxygen saturation, and Glasgow Coma Scale status were monitored and recorded. Only children who were considered hemodynamically and neurologically stable underwent the procedure. Exclusion criteria included a history of a seizure disorder or head trauma. Outcome parameters included onset and duration of action, efficacy, frequency of complications, and recovery time.

The patient's cooperation and degree of sedation were monitored by two observers using a visual analog scale. Parents were also asked to rate the procedure via a questionnaire, and they were contacted within 48 hours to assess problems after discharge. Indications for DPT sedation were laceration repair (76%), fracture reduction (18%), foreign body removal (5%), joint aspiration (5%), and I&D of abscess (1%). The mean laceration length was 2.3 cm (range 0.5-9.5 cm).

Minor and clinically insignificant changes in physiological variables followed DPT administration. No child experienced serious complications or required resuscita-

tion, and none had oxygen desaturation of less than 91 percent. Interestingly, it required an average of 27 minutes to produce sleep, 103 minutes for the child to recover to a sitting upright position, and total ED time was 4.7 hours. Overall there was moderate variation and unpredictability of this combination. When efficacy was analyzed, 71 percent were moderately or well sedated, but 29 percent experienced insufficient sedation. The parents reported that it required 11 hours for normal eating and drinking, and 19 hours for the child to appear totally normal. There were a few cases of pain at the injection site, emesis, prolonged sleepiness, or bad memories of ED experience, but the authors did not feel that side effects were medically significant.

The conclusion was that DPT produces safe and generally effective sedation for children undergoing procedures in the ED. The rather prolonged duration of action and time to recovery were noted, but they were judged to be comparable to other forms of IM sedation. The authors reference a number of previous studies on the effectiveness

Table 1.
CLINICAL USE OF DPT

Dose of Demerol: Phenergan: Thorazine = 2:1:1 mg/kg intra-muscularly		
Mean Time to:	*Sleep*	= *27 minutes (±24 minutes)*
	Sitting upright	= *103 minutes (±87 minutes)*
	ED discharge	= *4.7 hours (±2.4 hours)*
	Eating	= *11 hours (±7.9 hours)*
	Normal behavior	= *19 hours (±15 hours)*
Percentage of patients being moderately to well sedated = 71%		
Percentage of patients with "insufficient sedation" = 29%		

Source: Ann Emerg Med *1991;19:31.*

of DPT used for cardiac catheterization, endoscopies, dental procedures, and sedation for CT scans.

COMMENT: The authors conclude that DPT is a safe and effective combination for ED procedures, basing their opinion on a prospective study of only 63 patients. Given the downside of an injection and a 30 percent incidence of inadequate sedation in this study, I would not have reached a similar positive conclusion. Although this sample size is rather small, the same authors previously reported a retrospective analysis of 487 patients who received DPT in the ED (*Ann Emerg Med* 1989;18(5):528). I suspect that their retrospective study spawned this prospective evaluation. In the larger retrospective study, eight patients required repeat sedation, and three patients had significant respiratory depression requiring IV naloxone, but overall DPT was considered safe. That retrospective analysis failed to address the efficacy issue adequately, and DPT was not compared with other options. Children with acute or underlying neurological or cardiovascular abnormalities are more likely to experience complications from any potent medication, and all the children in the prospective study were healthy and undergoing semielective procedures. Certainly children with multiple injuries or those neurologically impaired would be more likely to react differently or unpredictably to these potent medications.

I was very surprised that the authors were pleased with an average ED stay of 4.7 hours and an average 19 hours to normal behavior. Importantly, these rather prolonged times occurred in children with minor lacerations, some as small 0.5 cm. As a parent I would be upset if my child were in the ED for almost five hours when requiring only a few sutures for a forehead laceration, and was not "normal" until the next day.

Although I will agree that DPT is an effective and relatively safe regimen for sedating children in the ED, I believe it is a clinical dinosaur for most outpatient procedures. I would not even use the combination for children who are to be admitted or who require prolonged ED stays. I believe DPT is impracticable for the majority of my patients. It just takes too long to work and too long to go away, and it makes no sense to use these medications when we have powerful, short-acting, reversible narcotics and benzodiazepines available. Most obviously, the IM route is painful, difficult to titrate, and unpredictable, and it usually takes 30 minutes before you know whether you gave too much or too little. If you opt for more drug, the ED time is further extended so most would tend to proceed with the procedure under less than ideal sedation.

The entire concept of sedating children for minor procedures is one of significant personal bias, controversy, and individual preference. Some EPs do it routinely, others rarely. I cannot believe that physically restraining a one- or two-year-old child to suture a facial laceration under local anesthesia scars that child emotionally for life. Therefore, I rarely sedate children for routine minor laceration repair. Most children are terrified of any doctor or ED and unless

Table 2.

EFFICACY GROUPS AFTER MPC (DPT*)

	VAS Group			
	0<5	*5<7.5*	*>7.5*	*P*
Patients (%)	18(29)	13(21)	32(51)	-
VAS score (mean ± SD)	2.8±1.8	5.9±0.7	9.1±1.0	<.05
Age (yrs)	3.4±1.7	3.2±1.8	3.9±2.3	NS
Indications N(%)				
Laceration	13(72)	9(69)	26(81)	NS
Fracture	2(11)	1(7.7)	5(16)	NS
Other	3(17)	3(23)	1(3.1)	NS
RR (mean ± SD)	24±3.8	27±4.8	22±4.8	NS
HR (mean ± SD)	116±30	110±24	111±22	NS
Systolic BP	103±9.4	99±15	102±17	NS
Decreased RR (N)(%)	4(22)	3(23)	6(19)	NS
Decreased HR (N)(%)	1(5.5)	0	3(9.4)	NS
Decreased BP (N)(%)	2(11)	0	2(6.3)	NS
Minimum OS (%)	96.4±1.9	95±2.6	95±1.9	NS
Minimum GCS	12.3±2.4	10.6±3.5	11.2±3.4	NS

Demerol/phenergan/thorazine

Source: Ann Emerg Med *1991;20:31-35.*

you provide near-general anesthesia from the time they are in the parking lot until discharge; they will "have a bad experience," even if only having their ears examined.

It's paramount, therefore, to evaluate carefully what one actually does by sedating the child for the few minutes it takes to suture a simple laceration. In my mind, sedation is often for the convenience of the doctor or to allay parental anxiety, although I find many parents afraid of outpatient sedation. Sedation is frequently required to close a complicated laceration properly, perform an LP, or obtain a CT scan, and I strongly support sedation for these scenarios. Routinely sedating children for minor laceration repair if merely to reduce stress or anxiety, however, seems to be massive overkill. Even if you must physically restrain a child and administer a painful local anesthetic, the entire incident seems forgotten by the time the parents reach the nearest ice cream store.

The other problem with IM DPT is that you must heavily sedate the child in order to achieve a stationary target for suturing. When I used to give DPT, the child was either in a deep sleep for three to four hours (requiring frequent checks), or woke up as soon as I started prepping the laceration and still required restraint. When I was finished, the child would quickly go to sleep for the next few hours. The best point to take from this paper is that 2 mg/kg of Demerol is a safe dose of narcotic to use for pain control (if not sedation), and this should be especially noted by the physician who considers himself courageous or generous when ordering a 1 mg/kg injection.

Importantly, one must be careful not to confuse analgesia and pain control with sedation for procedures. Certainly no child with a thermal burn, sickle cell crisis, or fracture should remain in the ED for more than a few minutes before the issue of pain control is at least addressed. These patients require genuine pain control, not merely sedation. Fracture reduction and abscess drainage are distinctly different from laceration repair, and these prolonged or painful procedures should probably always be accompanied by sedation/analgesia.

Finally, Nahata's experience with DPT was not as positive as that of other investigators (*Clin Pediatr* 1985; 24:558). In a prospective series of 95 patients receiving

the combination for various procedures, four developed respiratory depression and one had a respiratory arrest with a rather modest dose.

Phenothiazines such as promethazine and chlorpromazine have been used for years in an effort to potentiate narcotics. However, these drugs are major tranquilizers,

Table 3.

EFFECTIVENESS OF SEDATION WITH CHLORAL HYDRATE

Study	No. of Patients	No. Sedation Failures	Sedated (%)	Mean Dose (mg/kg)
CAT Scan	25	5	80	62
MRI	10	2	80	54
EEG	6	0	100	48
Bone Scan	3	0	100	68
Others*	6	0	100	59
Total	50	7	86	58

*Echocardiogram, two brain stem auditory evoked response tests, removal of skin lesion, removal of lip stitches, and ophthalmologic exam.

Source: South Med J *1990;83,9;1040-1043.*

not analgesics. There are many theoretical and practical reasons to avoid phenothiazines for pain control. Stambaugh (*J Clin Pharmacol* 1981;21(4):140) notes that the meperidine/chlorpromazine combination may be a toxic one. Subjects given both drugs were noted to have marked and prolonged (often debilitating) lethargy and a greater depression in systolic and diastolic blood pressure than when meperidine alone was used. Also, data from the late 1950s and early 1960s demonstrating that promethazine actually has an anti-analgesic effect have largely been lost in the medical literature. Those data by Dundee (*Br J Anaesth* 1961;35:597) are frequently quoted by pain specialists but largely ignored by the majority of clinicians. The bottom line is that phenothiazines have no substantial analgesic effect and can produce significant hypotension and deep sedation. Many authors suggest that phenothiazines not be used in minor surgical procedures in combination with meperidine and other opiates (*Goldfrank's Toxicologic Emergencies*, 4th Edition, Goldfrank L, et al, Appleton & Lange; 1990:419).

EFFICACY OF SEDATION OF CHILDREN WITH CHLORAL HYDRATE PD

Rumm PD, et al *South Med J* 1990;83(9):1040

This is a prospective study of 50 children sedated with chloral hydrate prior to CT scan, MRI imaging, bone scan, and EEG. The authors, from Brooke Army Medical Center, note that chloral hydrate has the advantage of being given orally and has compiled an excellent safety record, making it the first agent chosen for pediatric sedation at their institution. Many previous studies have failed to document any life-threatening side effects when chloral hydrate is routinely used to sedate children.

The children in this study ranged in age from two months to 14 years. Half an hour prior to the procedure, they were administered a mean dose of 58 mg/kg of chloral hydrate. A sedation checklist was maintained prior to the procedure and for half an hour afterward. Of the 50 patients, 43 were sedated effectively, giving an 86 percent success rate with a single dose. There were no significant complications or side effects in any patient although seven children with an underlying neurological abnormality were sedation failures. Many authors have noted that there is a subgroup of patients that may be difficult to sedate, particularly those with known neurological deficits. The authors conclude that chloral hydrate is a safe and effective oral sedative for children, but those with neurological disorders may need alternative drugs or a larger dose.

COMMENT: Pediatricians love chloral hydrate, and it is a drug that has been used safely for many years. It is still the standard outpatient prescription for children undergoing elective procedures, such as CT scanning. When used for this indication, and given in the proper dose, the drug is a rather effective and safe agent.

Like DPT, however, it is less than ideal for sedating children for ED procedures. Once again, one must be careful not to confuse sedation with analgesia. If one only wants the child to sleep during a CT scan, chloral hydrate may be a good choice, but the drug lasts a few hours, cannot be reversed, and is certainly not an analgesic. As with DPT, it requires half an hour for the doctor to know whether the dose will be successful although the 50-75

mg/kg range is almost universally effective. Chloral hydrate would probably be a poor choice for sedating a child with a laceration or for the patient requiring a lumbar puncture. It would be of little use if the main goal is pain relief. I have little personal experience with chloral hydrate and view it as another clinical dinosaur in the context of its use in the ED.

A few words on the pharmacology of chloral hydrate are in order. The liquid drug tastes terrible, and it's available only as an oral agent. It is somewhat irritating to the GI tract and has been associated with nausea and vomiting. The drug is quickly metabolized to trichlorethanol, a highly lipid soluble metabolite that is responsible for the prolonged hypnotic effect. The combination of alcohol and chloral hydrate, commonly known as a "Mickey Finn," is quite sedating and makes overdose with the two agents particularly dangerous. Large ingestions of chloral hydrate have been associated with serious or fatal cardiac arrhythmias, and this can be a rather nasty overdose. Cardiac arrhythmias are not a problem in children with the 50-75 mg/kg dose used for sedation.

THE EFFECT OF ORAL MIDAZOLAM ON ANXIETY OF PRESCHOOL CHILDREN DURING LACERATION REPAIR

Hennes HM, et al *Ann Emerg Med* 1990;19(9):1006

This study, from the department of pediatrics at the Children's Hospital of Wisconsin, evaluated the efficacy of midazolam to alleviate anxiety during laceration repair in children younger than 6 years of age. The anxiety level of 55 children presenting to the ED was assessed by a scoring system derived from anxiety rating scales. Children with high anxiety levels received a single oral dose of placebo or midazolam (0.2 mg/kg). Lacerations were then sutured with the addition of tetracaine, epinephrine, and cocaine (TAC) solution and local anesthetic infiltration. The anxiety was again assessed during laceration repair, and respiratory depression and complications were noted.

The anxiety level of 70 percent of the children given midazolam and 12 percent of the patients administered placebo decreased significantly. There were no significant changes in heart rate, respiratory rate, or systolic blood pressure during the average 20-minute laceration repair time. All patients were discharged within 15 minutes of completion of the procedure. The authors conclude that a single dose of oral midazolam is a safe and effective method to relieve anxiety in young children undergoing laceration repair in the ED.

COMMENT: This is one of a few studies that carefully evaluates the effect of anxiety control in pediatric ED patients. Note that the authors were attempting only to relieve anxiety and not relieve pain or sedate patients to a point of unresponsiveness. This is slightly different from previous studies which attempted to put patients to sleep. One could argue about the overall need to provide routine anxiety control for minor procedures, and the actual ben-

Table 4. MEANS AND STANDARD DEVIATIONS OF VITAL SIGNS TO MEASURE ANXIETY LEVEL DURING LACERATION REPAIR				
	Midazolam Group		*Placebo Group*	
Vital sign	*Before*	*After*	*Before*	*After*
Heart rate (min⁻¹)	*114±19*	*117±26*	*120±20*	*120±25*
Respirations (min⁻¹)	*26±5*	*28±8*	*25±6*	*26±5*
Systolic blood pressure (mmHg)	*100±11*	*99±9*	*100±11*	*106±13*

Source: Ann Emerg Med *1990;19:1006-1009.*

efit of this intervention is difficult to decipher. Importantly, midazolam did not negate the need for standard local anesthesia. The advantages of an oral medication over an injection are obvious, and the short action of midazolam negates many of the downsides of chloral hydrate. Midazolam appears to be ideal for minor surgical procedures, meeting all important criteria: rapid onset, short duration, immediate reversibility, and a minimal complication rate.

Although I strongly prefer intravenous agents, if I were to give an oral sedative in the ED, I would opt for midazolam. The nonparenteral use of this drug has had increasing popularity, and a number of studies have championed its use. There is no special oral preparation; one merely uses the same solution that would be used for IM or IV use. It does, however, taste quite bitter, and there is no mention of non-parenteral use in the 1997 *Physicians' Desk Reference (PDR)*. There is no question that midazolam will reduce anxiety, but it does not sedate patients heavily enough to be used as a sole agent for painful procedures. Midazolam may be nice for preoperative use or for CT scans, but importantly, it is not an analgesic.

The standard IM/IV dose of Versed for sedation of children is 0.1 mg/kg. Oral, rectal, or intranasal use requires a significantly higher dose. Feld (*Anesthesiology* 1990;73(5):831) administered placebo or oral midazolam to 124 children (ages 1-10) undergoing short elective surgical procedures. The dose was 0.25, 0.5, or 0.75 mg/kg, given 30 minutes prior to induction of anesthesia. The authors noted acceptable sedation, decreased tearfulness and combativeness, and improved quality of induction of anesthesia in the children receiving the higher doses. The 0.25 mg dose, however, was no different from placebo. It is interesting to note that a relatively high oral dose (0.75 mg/kg) was well tolerated and that the smaller dose effective in the Hennes study was no better than placebo. Roelofse et al (*J Oral Maxillofac Surg* 1990;48(8):791) administered rectal midazolam via a feeding tube as premedication to 80 children undergoing dental extraction under general anesthesia. The dose ranged from 0.25 to 0.45 mg/kg. They also noted decreased anxiety, easier induction of anesthesia, and less agitation when compared to placebo, and suggest midazolam be employed as a preanesthetic agent.

A novel use for midazolam is the intranasal route (*Anesthesiology* 1988;69(6):972). Walbergh (*Anesthesiology* 1991;74(12):233) demonstrated that intranasal midazolam (0.1 mg/kg) had significant pharmacological advantages over rectal or oral administration in children undergoing elective surgery for congenital cardiac abnormalities. When the children were asleep, they administered midazolam, either IV or intranasally, and studied serial plasma levels. Peak plasma levels occurred 10 minutes following intranasal installation, compared with a previously reported 53 minutes after oral administration or 16-30 minutes after rectal administration. Intranasal use resulted in blood levels approximately 60 percent of that noted with intravenous administration. Only blood levels were measured, not a clinical effect. I have not personally used intranasal midazolam, although I have heard positive support from colleagues. One problem I can imagine is that awake, children may have trouble tolerating nose drops. I have personal unsuccessful experience trying to get my children to accept even simple nose sprays, particularly when they are ill or anxious. I understand that the Versed solution may be quite irritating to the nose of an awake child.

The bottom line is that oral, rectal, or intranasal mida-zolam in doses one to seven times the IV dose are reasonable alternatives to the intravenous or IM route. I'm not sure that some of these alternatives are less stressful than a single injection although the routes may be more acceptable to parents. I intuit that these fancy routes of administration may treat the parent or physician more than the child. One logistical problem should be anticipated: Because the drug has a short duration of action, be prepared to do the procedure during a relatively short therapeutic window, or re-dosing may be required.

KETAMINE IN THE ED

Ketamine is not used often in the emergency department, despite its excellent safety profile and numerous advantages for emergency medicine practice

In previous chapters, I discussed the pros and cons of various anesthetics and analgesics used in the emergency department, and most of the drugs have been quite familiar to practicing clinicians. Ketamine, a parenteral anesthetic, however, has enjoyed relatively little use in the ED despite its excellent safety profile and numerous advantages for emergency medicine practice.

There are probably few emergency physicians in this country who have had extensive experience with ketamine, but one wonders if perhaps this drug should receive more scrutiny and perhaps be used more widely. The drug has some drawbacks for use in adults, but its unique properties make it an excellent agent for short-term sedation of children undergoing painful procedures. Ketamine's potential use in selected asthmatic patients is especially interesting.

KETAMINE SEDATION FOR PEDIATRIC PROCEDURES: PART 1, A PROSPECTIVE SERIES

Green SM, et al *Ann Emerg Med* 1990;19(9):1024

This fascinating report should be read by all physicians who routinely sedate children during painful or stressful ED procedures. The specifics of the clinical protocol and the patient response are described in detail. An accompanying article (*Ann Emerg Med* 1990;19(9):1033) is an informative in-depth review. The authors describe the use of IM ketamine to facilitate a variety of procedures in 108 children ranging in age from 14 months to 13 years. The study was prospective but unblinded and uncontrolled.

The authors begin by describing their frustration in treating children with medical conditions that require patient cooperation, such as the repair of complex facial lacerations, and they note the shortcomings of some routinely used sedation protocols, such as the traditional meperidine, promethazine, and chlorpromazine (Demerol, Phenergan, and Thorazine, a DPT cocktail). They note that ketamine has many ideal properties for ED use: easy IM administration, rapid onset, effective analgesia and amnesia, adequate immobilization, minimal cardiac or respiratory effects, and a rapid smooth recovery.

In the study, ketamine sedation was considered for any patient who required a painful or tedious procedure, and where success of the procedure depended upon patient cooperation or immobilization, the child was hysterical or excessive pain was anticipated. Approximately 75 percent of the children were sedated for laceration closure, but children also received ketamine for reduction of dislocations or fractures, sedation for CT scanning, foreign body removal, abscess drainage, or nasal packing. Inclusion and exclusion criteria were the standard ones and are listed in the table.

The dose of ketamine was a modest 4 mg/kg, combined with atropine 0.01 mg/kg, given in a single IM injection. Adjunctive local anesthetics and physical restraint were generally not required. Available in the treatment room were pediatric intubation equipment, suction, oxygen, and crash cart medications. A physician or nurse provided one-on-one observation until recovery was established. Parents of the child received a follow-up telephone call from the authors. Interestingly, no monitoring equipment, such as pulse oximetry or ECG was mandated by the protocol, although many physicians choose to use these devices. An IV line was not routinely placed. The room was kept quiet and the lights were dimmed to avoid any excess audiovisual stimuli.

The child typically cried after the IM injection but appeared deeply sedated within minutes. A wide-eye glassy stare and nystagmus were usually noted, and muscle tone was slightly increased. The drug had a rapid onset; in 87 percent of the cases the procedure was performed within five minutes of the injection. Although vital signs were not routinely measured, the authors mention that ketamine occasionally caused a mild increase in pulse rate but no appreciable change in blood pressure. When monitoring equipment was used, there was no significant change in pulse oximetry or ECG patterns.

Attesting to the efficacy of the drug, 86 percent of the children demonstrated adequate sedation, analgesia, and immobilization with a single injection. Only three children required a repeat dose because of inadequate sedation, but an additional 2-4 mg/kg were allowed for longer procedures. The IM injection usually provided 15 to 20 minutes of adequate analgesia. By 120 minutes, almost all patients were recovered enough to be discharged. No allergic reactions were noted,

but a curious hyperemic flush was seen in about 18 percent of the children. Despite atropine, hypersalivation was noted in 13 percent, but it was not a clinically significant problem.

Although airway patency was maintained without intubation in every case, two children developed persistent vomiting associated with laryngospasm. Two children had insignificant transient stridorous breathing, but there was no evidence of aspiration in any subject. Six patients did vomit following discharge, but no untoward effects were noted.

The recovery period was described as "quiet and uneventful" in 80 percent, "mild agitation" in 17 percent, "moderate agitation" in three percent, and one child experienced "pronounced agitation." Some children had bizarre mentation during their recovery period, but there were apparently no unpleasant or terrifying hallucinations and

SPECIFIC USE OF KETAMINE ANESTHESIA

Dose:	*Ketamine (4 mg/kg) plus atropine (0.01 mg/kg)* *Single IM injection*
Setting:	*Quiet separate room with minimal verbal, tactile, auditory stimuli.* *One-on-one observation post procedure.* *Resuscitation equipment/pulse oximetry/EKG available* *IV access not routinely required*
Onset of action:	*Usually 5-8 minutes*
Duration of action:	*15-20 minutes*
Time to full recovery:	*1 to 1 1/2 hours*
Clinical characteristics:	*Blank, glassy-eyed stare and nystagmus (most)* *Non-purposeful movements (occasional)* *Muscle hypertonicity (48%)* *Hypersalivation (13%)* *Delayed vomiting (6%)* *Transient hyperemic rash (18%)*
Uncommon Events:	*Vomiting during anesthesia (rare)* *Laryngospasm (rare, often self limited and intervention not required).*

Source: James R. Roberts, MD

amnesia was consistent. No recurrent nightmares were reported on telephone follow-up. Transient ataxia or impaired coordination after discharge was reported in about 30 percent of cases. Overall, 96 percent of the parents were satisfied with the sedation procedure, and 100 percent were pleased with the concept of procedural sedation. Only one parent verbalized a negative response, and only eight exhibited some anxiety over the procedure. Ninety-five percent of the parents stated a desire to use ketamine again under similar circumstances.

The authors note that physician acceptance of ketamine was excellent, and consultants, such as plastic and orthopedic surgeons, frequently requested that they be allowed to enlist their patients in this study. Although

PROCEDURES USING KETAMINE IN 108 PATIENTS

Procedures	No. of patients (%)
Head and facial lacerations	57 (52.8)
Trunk lacerations	2 (1.9)
Extremity lacerations	24 (22.2)
Orthopedic procedures	10 (9.3)
Diagnostic evaluations	4 (3.7)
Miscellaneous procedures*	11 (10.2)

*Included abscess I&D, foreign body removal, lumbar puncture, nasal packing, and wound exploration.

Source: Ann Emerg Med 1990;19:1024-1032.

there was initial skepticism on the part of the anesthesia department in the participating institutions, these objections were overcome through dialogue.

The occurrence of laryngospasm in two children is discussed in detail. The incidence of laryngospasm and vomiting, even on a full stomach, is extremely low with ketamine, approximately 0.017 percent. The authors strongly recommend that physicians be prepared to treat vomiting and laryngospasm should they occur. Interestingly, both patients with vomiting/laryngospasm had a history of asthma or easy gagging or previous vomiting spells.

Patients with such history were subsequently given special precautions (IV access and pulse oximetry). Because neonates and young children have a higher incidence of laryngospasm, the suggested cut-off age was one year.

It appeared that 4 mg/kg was the minimum dose to expect consistent or adequate sedation. It was noted that because of occasional random movement, ketamine is not an ideal drug for sedation for CT scan. The authors suggest the use of one-on-one observation, a specified quiet area for administering ketamine, parental education prior to the procedure, and an awareness of and preparation for possible laryngospasm.

COMMENT: Like any powerful drug, ketamine must be respected and used carefully. Your first experience should not be when you're providing single coverage and the nursing staff is stretched thin or you've got multiple critical patients to worry about. A good first experience is to find a friendly anesthesiologist and observe the drug being given in the operating room. It would be politically unwise to unilaterally begin using ketamine without input from your anesthesia department, but expect significant opposition on your first planning session.

Given the safety, efficacy, and ease of administration of ketamine, especially in the pediatric patient, I'm somewhat puzzled about why it has not gained wide acceptance as a sedative in the ED. The incidence of side effects is actually much less than noted with most of the protocols used daily across the country, such as DPT, fentanyl/midazolam, or chloral hydrate. Ketamine is probably safer to use in the ED than large doses of parenteral narcotics and benzodiazepines.

Ketamine usually gets stellar reviews as an outpatient sedative and amnestic/analgesic agent for children that does not depress breathing or pulmonary reflexes. The ease of IM administration and preservation of cardiorespiratory function has made ketamine popular for burn debridement, oral surgery, and for field operations in developing countries. This article seems to echo the accolades when it comes to sedation for pediatric procedures.

When I asked my colleagues about their experiences with ketamine, most knew little about the drug and had never used it, but all voiced the same misconception. It's commonly believed that ketamine is associated with a high incidence of unpleasant hallucinations and delirium that may persist for days or weeks following the procedure. This is clearly not correct and has given ketamine unwarranted bad press. There is certainly a well described emergence reaction that can persist for a few hours, even up to a day, after sedation has worn off. The condition is not uniformly distressful and is usually described as pleasant, dreamlike, or a state of confusion. Some patients, however, exhibit irrational behavior and have bizarre or frightening hallucinations. These effects last for a short time only, and no residual or lasting psychologic effects are reported.

Emergence phenomena are more common in adults — about 10 to 30 percent experience it and this high incidence has turned off many anesthesiologists — but it's quite unusual in children under age 10. Curiously the problem is lessened with concomitant benzodiazepine use and with the IM route. Keeping the recovering patient in a quiet, dark room with minimal stimuli also seems to decrease the incidence. If I were to use ketamine in an adult, adding a benzodiazepine would be routine.

The only shortcoming of this otherwise superb paper is that the authors did not compare it with another protocol. Clearly they come across as advocates of ketamine. Although I'm a staunch advocate of judicious sedation for children, one should be careful not to overuse potent drugs for minor problems. The majority of young children probably don't require any form of sedation for the repair of minor lacerations. In this study most children received ketamine for laceration repair — six for scalp lacerations — and one patient received it for suture removal. This may have been overkill. Ketamine seemed to be ideal for some unusual cases where cooperation is always difficult — repair of a tongue laceration, removal of multiple cactus spine foreign bodies, a pelvic examination on an 8-year-old with a sexual assault, and to explore a complex abdominal wound in an hysterical child.

The overwhelming parental acceptance of ketamine is certainly impressive. Although only 70 percent of the parents were contacted by phone for follow-up, it is amazing that 96 percent were satisfied with the ED visit and even more interesting that 100 percent were pleased with the concept of procedural sedation. This brings up the concept of whether parents want their children sedated. From my experience, some parents are anxious or fearful of sedation outside the operating room, but may be reluctant to voice their concerns under stressful circumstances. Although many would accept narcotic or benzodiazepine sedation, seeing their child in a bizarre dissociated state induced by ketamine requires good communication and explanation prior to the procedure. I always discuss sedation with parents prior to giving it, and I don't use it if I detect genuine fear and cannot give enough reassurance.

INFORMATION AND OPINIONS FROM PARENTS ON 77 FOLLOW-UPS

Vomited after discharge	5 (6.5%)
Ataxia or impaired coordination after discharge	24 (31.2%)
Satisfied with results of ED procedure	74 (96.1%)
Pleased with concept of procedural sedation	77 (100%)
Would want ketamine in repeat situation	73 (94.8%)

Source: Ann Emerg Med *1990;19:1024-1032.*

In its 100 mg/ml concentration, only a few mls of ketamine are required for the 4 mg/kg starting dose. The drug may also be given intravenously at 2 mg/kg, but almost all reports of outpatient ketamine use suggest the IM route. An IV need not be routinely used but if one is already in place, it's reasonable to opt for IV use if the procedure is short. With this route, a 2 mg/kg dose wears off in only 10-15 minutes. Operative sedation lasts 15-30 minutes with a 4 mg/kg dose. The 4 mg/kg dose is actually quite modest. Some authors advocate continuous IV infusion for long-term sedation of children in intensive care units.

A few notes about the pharmacology of ketamine should be emphasized. Ketamine has only been available since 1970. It was derived from phencyclidine (PCP), the potent street hallucinogen. Although the drug has an outstanding safety record, the physician should have in-depth familiarity with it prior to use. Ketamine produces a trance-like cataleptic state which has been termed dissociative anesthesia. The eyes usually remain open with an undirected stare, and nystagmus is frequent. It is bizarre to have a child seemingly watch you reduce his fracture, or debride a burn, yet fail to even flinch.

The onset of action of ketamine is quite rapid due to its excellent lipid solubility and entrance into the brain. Although the specific mechanism is unclear, ketamine dissociates the cortex from the limbic system and essentially prevents the higher pain centers from perceiving painful stimuli. Narcotics and inhaled anesthetics suppress the reticular activating system.

Spontaneous breathing and protective airway flexes are maintained and endotracheal intubation is unnecessary with ketamine. Coughing, sneezing, and swallowing are not depressed. The drug does produce excess salivation in some patients, and it's reasonable to add atropine to counteract this effect. Ketamine has sympathomimetic activity by inhibiting the re-uptake of catecholamines, and a mild to moderate increase in blood pressure, heart rate, and cardiac output are common.

This sympathomimetic effect is generally not clinically significant with the doses used for outpatients. Ketamine

SIDE EFFECTS DURING KETAMINE SEDATION ON 108 PATIENTS

Reaction	Mild, No Intervention	Required Intervention
Hypersalivation	14 (13%)	0
Muscular Hypertonicity	52 (48.1%)	0
Transient clonus	2 (1.9%)	0
Transient stridor laryngospasm	2 (1.9%)	1 (0.9%)
Emesis while sedated	0	1 (0.9%)
Emesis well into recovery	6 (5.6%)	0
Transient rash	19 (17.6%)	0
Unpleasant agitation	1 (0.9%)	0
Nightmares	0	0

Source: Ann Emerg Med 1990;19:1024-1032.

would not, however, be a good drug to sedate the wildly agitated drug overdose or psychotic patient. The random movements of the head and extremities unrelated to painful stimuli are a well-known characteristic of ketamine anesthesia. Because of this, and the observation that ketamine increases intracranial pressure, the drug is not ideal to sedate trauma patients or head injured patients for CT scans.

I would avoid ketamine if the child had just eaten a large meal, but food in the stomach is not a consistent contraindication in the literature. Most of the vomiting

occurs well into the recovery period. Stridor/laryngospasm are mentioned in all reviews of ketamine — possibly due to salivation and a hypersensitive laryngeal reflex — but intubation was only required in two of 11,500 cases, according to one review. Laryngospasm is more common in neonates; the ideal ages for ketamine use are 1-10 years. I expect most physicians would think that two cases of laryngospasm in 108 patients is an unacceptable risk, but when I spoke with an author of this report, he informed me that this series is up to almost 800 cases without another report of laryngospasm. If laryngospasm did occur, I would suggest oxygen, suctioning, jaw thrust or bagging, perhaps IV lidocaine, and preparation for succinylcholine-assisted intubation. No drug will immediately reverse ketamine.

THE USE OF KETAMINE FOR THE EMERGENCY INTUBATION OF PATIENTS WITH STATUS ASTHMATICUS

L'Hommedieu CS, Arens JJ
Ann Emerg Med 1987;16(5):568

This is a short case report in which ketamine was used to treat five patients with status asthmaticus. Four patients had ketamine-assisted intubation, and all received ketamine after intubation for its bronchodilatory effect. The authors note that intubation itself may be associated with increased acidosis and bronchospasm. It is well known that intubation can produce increased airway resistance due to vagal stimulation, and from a physiologic standpoint, intubation often transiently worsens acidosis and bronchospasm.

The patients' ages ranged from 15 months to 12 years. The authors apparently used ketamine to facilitate bronchodilation rather than as a single drug for intubation. Succinylcholine was also administered. In four cases, patients who deteriorated after intubation were given ketamine, with a marked improvement in pulmonary function. The dose of ketamine for intubation and relief of bronchospasm was 1.5-2 mg/kg intravenously.

The documentation in this report is somewhat incomplete, but all subjects exhibited a decrease in PCO_2 (average 25 mmHg), a decrease in wheezing, and a rise in pH after ketamine administration. The authors note that the relief in bronchospasm occurs within a few minutes of IV administration, but the effect is transient, lasting only 20-30 minutes.

These anesthesiologists believe that the rapid of onset of sedation and associated bronchodilation make ketamine an ideal agent for the emergency intubation of asthmatic patients in respiratory failure. Because ketamine does not produce muscle relaxation, it is common to add a muscle relaxant, such as succinylcholine, to facilitate intubation.

COMMENT: The ability of ketamine to diminish bronchospasm and reduce airway resistance in patients with asthma has been known for some time. The mechanism of action is multifactorial but probably related to an increase in circulating catecholamines. It also directs smooth muscle relaxation and inhibition of vagal outflow. The ability of ketamine to clear wheezing consistently in asthmatics during anesthesia is well reported in the anesthesia literature (*Anesth Analg* 1972:51(4);588).

Ketamine can be used in three ways for patients with severe asthma: as an adjunct to intubation, as a bronchodilator for patients already on a ventilator, or to sedate anxious asthmatics to gain control (IV access, delivery of aerosols). There are numerous reports in the literature of ketamine being used as a bronchodilator to either avoid intubation in severe asthmatics (*Anesthesia* 1986;41(10): 1017) or given to ventilated patients in refractory bronchospasm, occasionally with life-saving results (*Anesth Analg* 1972;51(4):588).

I recently gave Ketamine (2 mg IM) to a mentally retarded 8-year-old with severe asthma. She was so strong, agitated, and hypoxic that she would not accept a face mask, nasal oxygen, or an IV. After the ketamine, an IV was started and inhaled bronchodilators and oxygen were administered with ease. My only other option would have been to paralyze and intubate her, and given her short fat neck, the intubation surely would have been difficult. It would make sense for the emergency physician to keep ketamine in his armamentarium for refractory asthma, not only as a tool for the facilitation of intubation but also as a bronchodilator in patients who are deteriorating despite being mechanically ventilated. It would be nice to see a prospective study on the use of ketamine in the ED for asthmatics.

SECTION VII

STREPTOCOCCAL PHARYNGITIS

THE BAFFLING CLINICAL FEATURES OF STREPTOCOCCAL PHARYNGITIS

A sore throat combined with cough, rhinitis, laryngitis, high fever, tender adenopathy, and severe pain equals strep? Not likely.

If one is not concerned with true science, treating a sore throat is quite straightforward. Although you would think a disease that affects almost one percent of the population per year would be totally sorted out by now, the entire concept is extremely complicated and even the most basic issues are vague or controversial. Using the premise that emergency physicians ought to do what is safe, simple, and reasonable, I will attempt to put the entire spectrum of streptococcal pharyngitis into perspective over the next few chapters. This chapter explores the epidemiology and clinical aspects of this common infectious disease, focusing on how patient presentation affects the clinician's approach to clinical decisions.

In medical school we were taught that you could trust your clinical acumen — specifically that a sore throat combined with cough, rhinitis, and laryngitis equaled a viral infection, but you could bet on strep if the patient looked toxic, and exhibited high fever, tender adenopathy, and severe pain. A bacterial diagnosis was clinched if you spotted pus on the tonsils. In the old days, one would simply treat all patients with this irrefutable evidence of streptococcal pharyngitis with penicillin to alleviate symptoms, decrease transmission, and prevent sequelae, especially rheumatic fever. The purist, especially the pediatrician or office practitioner, would often take a culture, but rarely could adequate follow-up be obtained from ED patients so most of us treated on the initial visit and eschewed traditional laboratory confirmation because we were sure of our diagnosis. Clinical dogma stated that if the patient was not better in 24-36 hours, the symptomatology was due to a nontreatable viral infection. Occasionally mononucleosis or gonorrhea could be diagnosed, but most of the time it was assumed that a slow resolution was due to one of the many respiratory viruses, none of which could be identified except at the federal Centers for Disease Control and Prevention or the National Institutes of Health.

Over the past 10 years, rigorous investigation has elevated the lowly sore throat to new clinical heights and has made most emergency physicians wonder what planet their professors came from and what exactly we have been treating all these years. Importantly a number of other organisms has been implicated as culprit, gold standards for the bedside diagnosis of strep have become tarnished, and rapid antigen testing has streamlined although not revolutionized laboratory evaluation. It is now clear that you cannot diagnose strep throat with a tongue blade and flashlight, and penicillin may not be the drug of choice for all comers.

FEBRILE EXUDATIVE TONSILLITIS: VIRAL OR STREPTOCOCCAL?

A Putto *Pediatrics* 1987;80(1):6

This is a well done prospective clinical study of children with acute febrile exudative tonsillitis. It was designed to answer the following question: Can one distinguish a viral vs. bacterial etiology for an acute sore throat in children based on clinical findings? The answer was a simple and resounding NO! In this study from Finland, 110 consecutive children treated as outpatients at a university hospital were evaluated for the chief complaint of sore throat. All patients had an exudate on the tonsils and an axillary or rectal temperature greater than 38°C. Those who received prior antibiotics were excluded as well as those with evidence of peritonsillar abscess, but about 20 percent of the subjects had experienced more than five similar previous episodes. The ages ranged from 6 months to 18 years (mean age 7 years) and 25 percent of the children were age 3 years or younger. Noted in the clinical evaluation was the presence or absence of pharyngeal edema or redness, cervical lymphadenopathy, otitis media, conjunctivitis, the degree of pain, and the presence of headache, abdominal pain, rhinitis, or cough. Laboratory tests included CBC, sedimentation rate, and numerous serological studies designed to identify bacterial or viral etiologies. The patients were followed up as outpatients with the use of a questionnaire that included documenting symptoms and temperature on a daily basis.

Using an immunoassay technique from nasopharyngeal mucus obtained by suction catheter and various serum viral antibody titers, the authors attempted to diagnose adenovirus, parainfluenza virus, influenza, and respiratory syncytial viruses. Sera were also collected for Epstein-Barr virus (mononucleosis). Each patient also had a throat culture taken by vigorously swabbing both tonsils with culture techniques designed to isolate beta-hemolytic streptococci and *Mycoplasma pneumoniae.* Serum was also tested for anti-streptococcal antibodies (anti-streptolysin O [ASO] titer and anti-streptococcal DNAseB). All children were treated with oral penicillin for 10 days.

Despite extensive laboratory evaluation, no etiology was identified in 35 percent of cases, and more than one agent was identified in 14 percent, the majority being mixed viral/bacterial infections. Exudative tonsillitis was attributed to a viral etiology in 42 percent of the children, beta-hemolytic streptococci in 31 percent (only 12 percent

had group A streptococci), and *M pneumoniae* in five percent. (Note that *Chlamydia* was not tested for.) The most common viruses were adenovirus (19%), Epstein-Barr (9%), and parainfluenza (7%). In 31 percent of the cases, a virus was the sole pathogen isolated. Only half of the cases of serologically proven mononucleosis had a positive rapid mononucleosis spot test.

Interestingly 11 percent of the children without complaints who served as controls also had positive strep cultures, although none was of the group A beta-hemolytic

MICROBIOLOGIC FINDINGS IN 110 CHILDREN WITH FEBRILE EXUDATIVE TONSILLITIS

Agent*	No. (%) of Children
Viruses	*46 (42)*
Adenovirus	*21 (19)*
Epstein-Barr	*10 (9)*
Parainfluenza	*8 (7)*
Influenza A	*3 (3)*
Herpes Simplex	*2 (2)*
Respiratory syncytial	*2 (2)*
Bacteria	41 (37)
β-Hemolytic streptococci	36 (31)
Group A	13 (12)
Group C	10 (9)
Group G	8 (7)
Group B	3 (3)
Group F	2 (2)
Mycoplasma pneumoniae	5 (5)
No pathogen	*39 (35)*

*More than one agent recorded in 15 children.

Source: Pediatrics 1987,80(1):6-12.

strain. Only 45 percent of subjects with a positive culture for group A streptococci had a rise in the ASO or anti-streptococcal DNAse B titer. A rapid antigen technique detected strep in 11 of 13 with positive cultures. The sensitivity of the rapid antigen technique was 85 percent, with a specificity of 99 percent when compared to culture. None of the patients with proven viral tonsillitis had a positive rapid test for group A beta-hemolytic streptococcal infection (GABHS), suggesting a very low false negative rate for this screening tool.

The age of the patient was the best correlate with etiology. Older patients tended to have bacterial sore throats while the younger children were infected with viruses. For patients age 6 years or younger, a virus was the etiologic agent of the exudative febrile tonsillitis in 53 percent of cases. Strep became more common in the older age group, and only 28 percent of those older than 6 had an identifiable viral etiology. Strep was found in 46 percent of the children older than 6 years, and an impressive 92 percent of the positive cultures were seen in this older age group. Importantly, not a single child younger than 3 years of age had a GABHS infection.

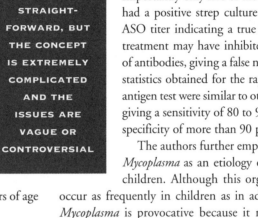

TREATING A SORE THROAT SEEMS STRAIGHT-FORWARD, BUT THE CONCEPT IS EXTREMELY COMPLICATED AND THE ISSUES ARE VAGUE OR CONTROVERSIAL

When other clinical findings were examined, it was noted that cough and rhinitis were more often associated with a viral tonsillitis, although 10 percent with cough or rhinitis had a culture positive for strep. The color or extent of the exudate did not distinguish a viral from bacterial sore throat. Although tender cervical nodes were recorded more often in children with a positive strep culture, this finding was seen in only 64 percent, and 17 percent of those with tender nodes had adenovirus infections. The highest temperatures recorded were in children with adenovirus tonsillitis. Half with a viral etiology had a temperature greater than 40°C. The WBC counts exceeded 15,000/μl in 55 percent of the children with beta strep and in 61 percent of the children with adenovirus. More children with viral tonsillitis (65%) than strep (40%) had a sedimentation rate greater than 30 mm/h.

The authors note that 82 percent of the children (all were treated with penicillin) with a positive strep throat were afebrile within 24 hours, and all were afebrile within 48 hours. As expected, fever persisted longer than 48 hours in 42 percent of the children with viral tonsillitis.

The authors emphasize the prominent role of viruses in the etiology of febrile exudative tonsillitis in children and note the correlation of age with etiology. In this and other studies adenovirus was the most common cause of non-streptococcal tonsillitis. In no case, however, did strep and adenovirus coexist, so clearly the clinical scenario was due solely to the virus. It is emphasized that GABHS is not a common cause of acute exudative tonsillitis in children; only 12 percent had this etiology and no patient younger than 3 years had a positive culture. Even in the presence of pus, fever, and tender adenopathy, children under 6 years were unlikely to have streptococcal tonsillitis. Importantly only five of the 11 children who had a positive strep culture had an elevated ASO titer indicating a true infection. (Early treatment may have inhibited the formation of antibodies, giving a false negative test.) The statistics obtained for the rapid streptococcal antigen test were similar to other investigators, giving a sensitivity of 80 to 90 percent with a specificity of more than 90 percent.

The authors further emphasize the role of *Mycoplasma* as an etiology of pharyngitis in children. Although this organism does not occur as frequently in children as in adults, the role of *Mycoplasma* is provocative because it responds to erythromycin, not penicillin. It's probable that many of the 35 percent of cases where no cause was found were due to other viruses not tested for.

It's clear from this study that clinical findings have little diagnostic value in differentiating bacterial from viral etiologies. Although children with symptoms of upper respiratory infection (rhinitis, cough, conjunctivitis) are more likely to have viral disease, the statistics are poor enough that they are of no significant clinical value. Importantly, higher temperatures and higher leukocyte counts were most often associated with adenovirus tonsillitis than with a strep throat. However, fever defervesced more quickly with penicillin if strep were present.

SEROLOGIC EVIDENCE OF CHLAMYDIAL AND MYCOPLASMAL PHARYNGITIS IN ADULTS

Komaroff AL, et al *Science* 1983;222(46236):927

This is a frequently quoted article that was one of the first reports to establish serologic evidence of *Chlamydia* and *Mycoplasma* as causes of adult pharyngitis. The authors from Harvard University and the University of

California, San Francisco, prospectively studied 763 adults with pharyngitis using extensive culturing techniques and serologic studies. The following etiologies were identified: *Chlamydia* (21%), *Mycoplasma* (18%), GABHS (11%), and mononucleosis (2%). None of the patients had concomitant ocular or genital chlamydial infection. The authors conclude that strep may not be the most common treatable cause of pharyngitis in adults and that *Chlamydia* or *Mycoplasma* organisms not sensitive to penicillin are relatively common.

COMMENT: This is one of the most frustrating columns I have attempted to write. The literature on strep throat is confusing, and it's amazing how different authors interpret exactly the same data when developing clinical guidelines. These two articles should be read by all emergency physicians because they critically evaluate clinical dogma used to make important decisions about treating a sore throat. They dispel many of the existing myths about etiology and physical examination. Both studies thoroughly confused me and made me wonder what I have actually been treating when I routinely prescribed penicillin for patients with fever, pus on the tonsils, and tender adenopathy.

Allow me to summarize the voluminous data in the first pediatric study. Even in the presence of fever, adenopathy, and visible pus on the tonsils, children under age 3 years rarely have streptococcal pharyngitis. Not a single case was documented in this study, but others have placed the incidence in this age group in the 5-10 percent range. It's still difficult to accept the fact that pus and leukocytosis do not equal a bacterial source. Others have also noted that adenovirus, probably the most common cause of non-streptococcal tonsillitis, often mimics the classic description of a strep throat in children (*JAMA* 1967;202:455; *J Pediatr* 1968;73:51; *J Pediatr* 1984;104:725).

Clearly GABHS is not a common cause of sore throat in younger children; only 12 percent in this study had this etiology. Even those with a positive culture could have been strep carriers with a viral etiology for the symptoms because only half had an ASO titer rise. This observation has been repeatedly confirmed by others, and it is clear that strep pharyngitis is not a disease of toddlers but primarily of school age children and young adults (prime ages 7 years to early 30s). Confirming this observation is the fact that common sequelae of strep throat — peritonsillar

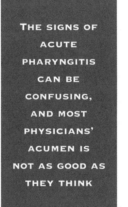

THE SIGNS OF ACUTE PHARYNGITIS CAN BE CONFUSING, AND MOST PHYSICIANS' ACUMEN IS NOT AS GOOD AS THEY THINK

abscess and rheumatic fever — are essentially absent in children under age 3 years (*Laryngoscope* 1988;98(9):956). Over the age of six years, the incidence of strep throat is higher, but it's still significantly less than viral causes. The data are all over the map, but as a summary of other studies, strep causes a sore throat in 20-30 percent of children with acute pharyngitis (mostly in the 6-14 year age group) and in 10-15 percent of symptomatic adults. Substantiating the observation that physicians overdiagnose strep in older adults, Komaroff could find GABHS in only 10 percent of adults with pharyngitis (*J Gen Intern Med* 1986; 1:1). Generally about half of all patients have no organism isolated so frequently we really don't have any idea what's causing the symptoms.

Not only can you not accurately diagnose strep with your physical examination, the standard argument that the WBC count or sedimentation rate can differentiate viral from bacterial idealogy is clearly bogus in this setting. I find it fascinating that the adenovirus produced the highest fevers and the greatest elevations in white counts. The message here is not to waste time and money on these worthless tests, although atypical "lymphs" may suggest mononucleosis.

Mycoplasma and *Chlamydia* may have some yet undefined role in acute pharyngitis. We are just beginning to document their presence, but it's not clear if these organisms are invasive, are associated with complications, or can play a role as a carrier state, as does strep. The article by Komaroff evaluates serology and not clinical disease, but the data are provocative and frequently quoted. Others have also implicated *Mycoplasma* in up to 30 percent of cases of teenagers and adults with acute tonsillopharyngitis (*JAMA* 1967;202:455). To further muddy the waters, however, Huss failed to find a single case of *Chlamydia* in 126 adults with pharyngitis and concluded that this organism is not an important cause of pharyngitis (*Clin Microbiol Rev* 1985;22:858). Using sophisticated culturing, immunoassays, and DNA testing, Charnock et al could not demonstrate a single case of either *Chlamydia* or *Mycoplasma* as a cause of chronic or recurrent tonsillitis in 40 patients — ages 2 to 28 years — undergoing tonsillectomy (*Arch Otolaryngol Head Neck Surg* 1992;118(5): 507). After reviewing the data, I don't think these organisms play much of a role in acute pharyngitis, and I would not factor them into treatment decisions.

THE ACCURACY OF EXPERIENCED PHYSICIANS' PROBABILITY ESTIMATES FOR PATIENTS WITH SORE THROATS: IMPLICATIONS FOR DECISION-MAKING

Poses RM, et al *JAMA* 1985,254(7) 925

This study evaluated whether experienced physicians could predict the incidence of streptococcal infection in patients with sore throats by clinical examination and how the predictions affected treatment decisions. There are actually little data in the literature to support the fact that clinical judgment plays a bona fide role in the evaluation of streptococcal pharyngitis. To the contrary, most of the literature has demonstrated that it is impossible to forecast etiology with significant accuracy, unless you find a 20-40 percent error rate acceptable (*Am J Dis Child* 1977; 131:514).

In this study 10 board certified or board eligible medical school faculty members — two internists, three pediatricians, and five family practitioners (no emergency physicians) — served as subjects. The study attempted to determine what clinical data would prompt the diagnosis of strep and precipitate treatment in 308 patients ages 17-36 years. All patients had throat cultures taken, and 27 signs and symptoms were recorded that might influence decision-making, including swollen glands, strep exposure, headache, fever, adenopathy, cough, fatigue, exudates, toxic appearance, concomitant medical problems, and time of year.

Only 15 of 308 patients (5%) had a positive throat culture for group A strep. As a group, the physicians significantly overestimated the probability of a positive throat culture. Specifically, 81 percent of the patients without a positive culture were thought by the clinicians to have a bacterial etiology. Of the 104 patients empirically treated before cultures were available because the doctors were sure that strep was the cause, only eight (7%) had a positive culture. Those clinical findings most often thought to indicate streptococcal pharyngitis were streptococcal exposure, temperature greater than 38°C, toxic appearance, pharyngeal inflammation, exudates, swollen tonsils, and cervical adenopathy. The clinical features that were actually associated with a positive culture were exudates, inflammation, and anterior cervical adenopathy, but these findings were also seen in a high percentage of culture negative subjects.

In addition to overestimating the incidence of strep throat, the physicians' treatments were strongly dictated by their erroneous clinical impressions; hence, they also overtreated. More than one-third of the patients were given antibiotics yet only seven percent of those treated (8/104) had a positive culture. Overtreatment was attributed to physician misunderstanding of the true low incidence of strep, assigning undue importance to noncorrelating clinical features, and their bias about their ability to make a correct diagnosis.

COMMENT: As with most clinicians, these doctors thought that their clinical acumen was better than it actually was, and they overestimated the incidence of strep throat in their study population. The physicians in this study shared common misconceptions — namely they

CLINICAL FINDINGS AND THROAT CULTURE RESULTS: SIGNIFICANT FEATURES BY UNIVARIATE ANALYSIS

Clinical Finding	Frequency in Patients	
	Culture Positive	Culture Negative
Pharyngeal/tonsillar exudates	77	36
Pharyngeal/tonsillar inflammation	100	75
Anterior cervical adenopathy	93	65

Source: *JAMA* 1985;254(7):925-9.

believed that fever, adenopathy, and pus certainly equals a strep throat — clearly not the case in this or any other study. Most studies have definitely found fever, exudate, and adenopathy to be more common in strep pharyngitis, especially if it is winter and the patient is 6-20 years old, but there is poor statistical correlation between any clinical finding and culture results (*J Fam Pract* 1985;21:302). The closest any study comes is an accuracy rate of 77 percent (*Am J Dis Child* 1977;131:514), but I find it difficult to use any scoring system that misses 23 percent of patients with a treatable disease. Most textbooks further promulgate the misinformation by describing the "classic" strep throat without qualifying statements (although most now state that exudates are not pathognomic of strep).

In a prodigious effort, Shank similarly compared the ability of family practice faculty and residents to predict accurately the cause of pharyngitis in almost 4,000 patients (*J Fam Pract* 1984;18:875). The false positive rate for faculty was 58 percent, compared with 70 percent for residents. False negative rates for both were about 15 percent. This and most other studies conclude that physicians are generally more accurate in predicting negative cultures than they are in predicting positive ones, and that clinicians tend to overestimate significantly the chance for patients with sore throats to have a positive strep culture.

Cough, rhinitis, and hoarseness suggest a viral cause, but 10-12 percent of patients with these symptoms have a positive culture. The rash of scarlet fever is a correlate to a strep throat, but many viruses also produce sore throat and a rash. It's a difficult concept for me to accept, but the positive predictive value of the "classic" findings in strep throat is probably around 50 percent, about as accurate as flipping a coin. Despite fancy scoring systems, my interpretation of the data is that you cannot tell what is causing a sore throat with any certainty without a number of expensive and clearly impractical laboratory tests.

Because you can't diagnose a strep throat by examination, let alone *Chlamydia* or *Mycoplasma,* how then should one make the diagnosis? More importantly, does it matter whether you make the diagnosis or is it more logical just to treat everyone with symptoms? Next month's column will attempt to tackle this difficult clinical problem. At this juncture I am personally totally re-educated on the clinical features of acute pharyngitis and expect to be similarly baffled when I try to unravel the significance of laboratory tests or to come to a conclusion about therapy.

PHARYNGITIS: THE VALUE OF LABORATORY TESTING

Studies show the clinician cannot separate viral from streptococcal pharyngitis on clinical grounds or by ED laboratory tests

This is the second in a series of discussions that attempt to put the etiology, diagnosis, and treatment of acute pharyngitis into rational clinical perspective for the emergency physician. The last chapter concluded that heretofore accepted dogma is anything but irrefutable, and the physician can quickly become frustrated if he tries to be academic or truly scientific about even the most rudimentary clinical issues. Many studies have shown that the clinician cannot reliably separate viral from streptococcal pharyngitis on clinical grounds or by laboratory tests that are rapidly available in the ED.

Although fever, tender adenopathy, and exudate are probably statistically more likely to be caused by a streptococcal infection, specifically group A beta-hemolytic streptococcal (GABHS) strains, clearly many patients with this exact scenario have a viral etiology. Children in particular tend to have "strep-looking" throats caused by adenovirus or mononucleosis. It's difficult to believe that leukocytosis, adenopathy, and pus come from a virus, but study after study confirm these observations. Actually, children under three years of age rarely have strep throat and even up to age six a viral etiology is a much more common cause of a "classic strep throat" than is GABHS. Only about 10-20 percent of young children with exudative tonsillitis have a strep infection, although teenagers and young adults tend to approach the 50 percent range when the textbook scenario is present.

Even with sophisticated laboratory evaluation, no organism can be isolated in about half of patients with acute pharyngitis. This was previously thought to represent nontreatable self-limited viral illness, but recent evidence has implicated Chlamydia and Mycoplasma and even herpes virus as culprits in at least some cases. We are just beginning to understand the role of these organisms in symptomatic acute pharyngitis, and it's possible that treatment regimens may need to be adjusted in the future to accommodate this observation. Finally, it's clear that physicians consistently overestimate the probability of GABHS in patients with sore throats, usually basing their misdiagnosis and subsequent overtreatment on preconceived dogma or bias that have no real scientific or statistical validity.

This chapter investigates the value of throat cultures in the diagnosis and treatment of GABHS pharyngitis. Unfortunately, even state-of-the-art culture techniques and other diagnostic innovations still do not diagnose streptococcal pharyngitis 100 percent of the time.

DIAGNOSIS OF STREPTOCOCCAL PHARYNGITIS: DIFFERENTIATION OF ACTIVE INFECTION FROM THE CARRIER STATE IN THE SYMPTOMATIC CHILD

Kaplan EL, et al *J Infect Dis* 1971;123(5):490

This is a classic article that is referenced in most reviews of streptococcal pharyngitis. It's from the department of pediatrics at the University of Minnesota Medical School, and it's one of the first papers to point out the fact that culturing GABHS from patients with pharyngitis is not as straightforward as has been taught and may even be misleading as to the actual cause of the symptomatic illness. In this report, 624 children were extensively studied when they presented with a sore throat during the winter months. An initial throat culture was taken by carefully rubbing the posterior pharynx and both tonsils with a cotton swab with immediate inoculation onto culture media. In addition, blood was drawn for acute phase anti-streptococcal antibody production (ASO and anti-streptococcal DNAse B). All children were cultured again at 24 hours and at three to six weeks and convalescent phase anti-strep antibodies were again drawn. Children with a tonsilar exudate and tender cervical adenopathy on the first visit and those with a positive culture for GABHS on the second 24-hour check were treated with antibiotics (usually IM benzathine penicillin).

GABHS was isolated from 35 percent of the patients. There was a bimodal age distribution for positive cultures, peaking at the 5-7 and 12-13 year age group, a finding that has been noted in other studies. GABHS was rarely found in children younger than 3 years of age. Coryza, exudate, and tender adenopathy were observed more commonly in patients with GABHS infection. Patients with streptococcal disease did not have a higher incidence of sick siblings, infected throat, or temperature higher than 101°F.

An attempt was made to determine the reliability of a single throat culture. It was noted that only 91 percent of the first cultures were positive. However, those children who had a negative first culture but a positive second culture usually grew only a few colonies on the laboratory plates, perhaps indicating a carrier state. No child in this study developed acute rheumatic fever (ARF) or acute glomerulonephritis (AGN), and there were no significant adverse reactions to the antibiotics. Interestingly there was a 38 percent incidence of therapeutic failure (as determined by reculturing) with oral antibiotics but only an eight percent failure rate with IM benzathine penicillin. Compliance with oral antibiotics was not evaluated. More than half (57%) of the children with a positive GABHS culture did not subsequently demonstrate a significant rise in ASO or anti-DNAse B titers.

The authors make a number of conclusions from their data. They believe that if only one culture is obtained, approximately 10 percent of children with GABHS infections will be missed, although many of these could conceivably be considered a carrier state rather than true infection. The presence of adenopathy and exudate were not particularly sensitive nor specific clinical markers for strep

ANTIBIOTIC TREATMENT OF PATIENTS WITH GROUP A STREPTOCOCCI INFECTIONS

Therapy	No. of patients	No. with follow-up visit	No. without Group A streptococci at follow-up	No. with Group A streptococci at follow-up Same type	No. with Group A streptococci at follow-up Different type	No. of therapeutic failures
Oral antibiotics	18	16	10	6	0	6/16
Benzathine penicillin, IM	157	137	121	11	5	11/137
No antibiotics	43	28	15	13	0	13/28
Total	218	181	146	30	5	30/218

*Source:*J Infect Dis *1971;123(5):490*

throat. Interestingly there was no correlation to a rise in antibody titer with the presence of pus on the tonsils. If a true infection is defined as a positive culture in a presence of an antibody titer rise, less than half the patients with pharyngitis who had a positive GABHS culture actually had a strep infection. The authors discount the contention that antibiotic therapy limits the antibody titer rise, and there has been general consensus on this point in the literature.

COMMENT: This article clearly demonstrates that a positive strep culture does not prove that a patient has a bona fide strep infection and that a negative culture does not always rule it out. This is especially true in children who are frequent carriers, and even more so during the winter months when the carrier rate in asymptomatic children will reach 20 to 30 percent (*Am J Pub Health* 1957;47:995). In this study, a single culture picked up approximately 90 percent of patients who had GABHS on the surface of their pharynx and tonsils. In a study of Army recruits who were cultured each day for three days, the first culture was positive only 76 percent of the time. It's important to note that only half the patients with a positive culture had serological evidence of invasive infection, considered a prerequisite for diagnosing the disease or for developing subsequent ARF/AGN.

> EVEN STATE-OF-THE-ART CULTURE TECHNIQUES DO NOT DIAGNOSE STREP 100 PERCENT OF THE TIME

The question that has not been fully answered is whether a non-rising ASO titer unequivocally means that the culture positive patient is a carrier only, but it's generally agreed that this is the case. To make things more confusing, up to 45 percent of patients with pharyngitis and negative throat cultures will have significant rises in ASO titer (*J Infect Dis* 1971;123:490).

The exact method of obtaining a throat culture is worth examining. We have all had the experience of trying in vain to get a frightened 6-year-old, a mentally retarded teenager, or someone with an overactive gag reflex to open his mouth. Clearly there is no such thing as a carefully done throat culture on many patients. Usually we end up jabbing the cotton swab into the pharynx, often getting only saliva or merely swabbing the hard palate or tongue, greatly increasing the chance for a negative culture. Brien et al demonstrated that the optimal site for a throat culture was the tonsil itself, and there is decreasing sensitivity when the posterior pharyngeal wall or other areas of the mouth are separately cultured. Other than the

tonsils and probably the posterior pharyngeal wall, swabbing any other site in the oral cavity produces unreliable culture results (*J Pediatr* 1985;106(5):781). If you do culture, it makes sense to attack both the tonsils and the posterior pharynx with vigor, repeating the swabbing at least two times. Some clinicians break the little plastic bubble on the culturette before swabbing, but it has been suggested that keeping the cotton tip dry provides the best result.

Caplan (*J Fam Pract* 1979;8:485) makes a number of reasonable arguments against the use of throat cultures in the management of streptococcal pharyngitis by quoting the following statistics: Only 68 percent of patients with documented strep-induced scarlet fever have positive throat cultures; when surgically removed tonsils are cultured, the incidence of positive cultures is twice as high as cultures taken prior to the operation. Belli et al noted that the recovery of GABHS rose from 6-20 percent when an anaerobic culture was also performed, a procedure not consistently done in all laboratories (*Am J Dis Child* 1984;138(3):274). At least two studies demonstrate that the recovery of GABHS increases by 80-90 percent when the core of ground-up tonsil homogenate is cultured and compared to cultures taken from the surface of the tonsil. (*JAMA* 1980;244:1696, and *Am J Dis Child* 1962;103:51). Wegner et al (*JAMA* 1992;267(5):695) demonstrated disappointing data on the value of laboratory variations on the recovery of GABHS. If only aerobic cultures were plated, and the results reported out in two days, cultures were only 72 percent sensitive. Even if anaerobic cultures are added, the sensitivity only reached 94 percent. Clearly most sophisticated laboratories will miss a number of positive cultures, so you can imagine the accuracy of culturing in a doctor's office. Basing your therapy decisions on the 24-hour results will likewise be very unscientific.

It is impractical, if not impossible, to do antibody titers on all patients with positive GABHS cultures so in the ED we are limited to culturing the tonsils surface (if we can see it). Because about half of patients with ARF/AGN have no history of an antecedent pharyngitis, clearly we are underdiagnosing the incidence of clinically relevant GABHS infections if we only culture symptomatic individuals.

I would summarize the salient clinical issues from this article with the following:

l. If one assumes that a immunological response is the

gold standard for evidence of infection, only half of those patients with symptomatic pharyngitis and a positive culture actually have an acute GABHS infection. In the absence of an antibody rise, the organism is probably only along for the ride and something else is actually causing the symptoms.

2. A positive throat culture cannot differentiate active infection from a carrier state, and a carrier state occurs in up to 30 percent of children in the winter living under crowded conditions. However, quantitating the colony count may suggest carrier state status.

3. One can almost double the rate of positive cultures depending on the area of the tonsil or pharynx that is cultured and by careful attention to culturing techniques. The frustrating facts are that the standard throat culture taken in the ED will miss 10 to 20 percent of streptococcal infections and overdiagnose actual disease by up to 50 percent.

With these caveats in mind, I have a difficult time reconciling the adage that mandates all patients be cultured before they are treated, and if the culture is negative, antibiotics should be discontinued. Scientific medical care is always expensive, but I was amazed that the cost of a throat culture in our hospital lab was $120. Given all the statistics, coupled with the cost concerns and the time and effort required to contact patients with a positive or negative culture (if you can even find them after they leave the ED), it is inconceivable to me that most patients with straightforward acute pharyngitis in the ED will benefit from a culture.

CONSENSUS: DIFFICULT MANAGEMENT PROBLEMS IN CHILDREN WITH STREPTOCOCCAL PHARYNGITIS

Breese BB, et al *Pediatr Infect Dis* 1985;4(l):10

This is a consensus editorial on the treatment of GABHS pharyngitis given by four pediatricians who are considered experts in the field. Two theoretical questions were raised.

1. Should all children with pharyngitis and a positive strep culture be treated? The panel of experts emphatically stated that all patients with pharyngitis and a positive strep culture should not necessarily be treated with antibiotics. They would exclude patients with a known or probable carrier state, although they agree that it is difficult (and I would add virtually impossible in the ED) to distinguish carrier state from invasive disease. More than 10

colonies per culture or classic strep symptoms are considered grounds for treatment if the culture is positive. The physicians would be more likely to treat children ages 4-12 during the winter months. Some recommend against even culturing children with non-specific or poorly differentiated symptoms of upper respiratory infections.

2. Should patients who have been treated for GABHS pharyngitis be recultured? The consensus was that it is unnecessary to reculture asymptomatic children following completion of antibiotic therapy, but to reculture if the symptoms return and re-treat with erythromycin if cultures are again positive.

COMMENT: I cannot agree with all of the conclusions from these experts, at least as they apply to emergency medicine. Pediatricians in general tend to be more conservative and prefer to culture their reliable office patients, clearly a fantasy scenario in most EDs that treat transient or indigent patients on an episodic basic. In lieu of a complete culture, it's easier and cheaper to culture only for strep in the office. However, the practice of office culturing has come under some disrepute. In one study there was a 10-60 percent incidence of office laboratories being unable to identify accurately known strep cultures, so the quality assurance issue is significant if you rely on office cultures (*Scand J Infect Dis* 1983;39(suppl):79). As mentioned, complying with complicated gathering and incubating techniques greatly increases the rate of positive cultures, but these techniques are difficult to comply with in an office laboratory.

There is considerable variation in the clinical approach among different specialists who threat sore throats. About 25 percent of physicians always culture before they treat, about 25 percent never culture but treat everyone, and about 50 percent culture selectively, meaning they do the test on patients they think are clinically likely to have the disease. The majority of physicians start antibiotics before culture results are known, but interestingly only about 60 percent of them stop the antibiotic even if they get a negative report. (I found this fascinating and wonder why the cultures were sent in the first place!) However, when the groups are broken down by specialty, pediatricians are much more likely to culture initially, wait for culture results before prescribing antibiotics, and stop therapy if cultures are negative.

The authors of this review would not treat an infant with a positive culture who is afebrile or who has conjunctivitis and other classic signs of a viral upper respiratory infection. This is particularly true in someone younger than three years of age or during the summer months. Unless I misunderstood these articles, I wonder why one would even bother culturing these patients if they would not treat if they found a positive culture. It makes no sense to me whatsoever.

STREPTOCOCCAL PHARYNGITIS IN THE EMERGENCY DEPARTMENT: ANALYSIS OF THERAPEUTIC STRATEGIES

Hedges JR, Lowe RA *Am J Emerg Med* 1986;4(2):107

This is a rather complicated statistical approach that analyzes therapeutic strategies available for the treatment of GABHS pharyngitis in the ED. A similar study has been previously done in an office setting, but under situations where follow-up was complete. The authors investigated four theoretical strategies: treat everyone with a sore throat, without a throat culture; treat only on the basis of a positive culture; treat those with a positive screening evaluation (a clinical scoring system or gram stain) without follow-up; and treat those with a positive screening test, culture those with a negative screen, and treat those with a subsequent positive culture. The study goes through a number of statistical machinations that evaluate the reliability of screening tests, the probability of rheumatic fever, the possibility of a serious drug reaction, medical costs, and follow-up concerns. Note that the rapid streptococcal screen antigen test was not included in the clinical scoring system.

Based on a statistical analysis, the authors demonstrate that lack of follow-up increases the probability of rheumatic fever and eventually increases the cost of medical care. In addition, treating solely on the basis of available screening tests without a throat culture to confirm a negative screen likewise has an unacceptable incidence of rheumatic fever.

The authors interpret their data to support the following treatment plan: use of gram stain and/or clinical criteria to permit the immediate treatment of symptomatic patients without the use of a throat culture; culture patients who do not qualify for treatment under the screening plan to detect false negative screening; and treat all patients with a negative screen who have a positive culture.

COMMENT: The statistics in this study and a similar one (*Ann Intern Med* 1977;86(4):481) are too complicated for me, but the conclusions are echoed by others (*Ann Intern Med* 1986;105:892). Because the Gram's stain approach has not caught on, clinical criteria are inaccurate, and cultures have inherent problems, one can argue with the conclusions.

Perhaps it is instructive to review the pros and cons of treatment. Standard arguments are given for treating a strep throat. With treatment, the course of the disease is shortened, the complications (peritonsillar abscess and ARF but not AGN) are decreased, and spread of the disease is decreased. Arguments against routine treatment are

INITIAL TITERS OF ANTIBODY IN CONTROL AND IN PATIENTS WITH PHARYNGITIS, WITH AND WITHOUT SUBSEQUENT RISES IN TITERS

Group (No. of patients)	Geometric mean of initial titers	
	Antistreptolysin O	Antideoxyribonuclease B
Controls (12)	135	141
Ia. No respiratory tract infection (60)	138	151
Ib. Pharyngitis without group A strep (60)	129	133
Pharyngitis with group A strep (167)	155	170
IIa. Significant antibody response (72)	125	117
IIb. No significant antibody response (95)	177	229

Source: J Infect Dis 1971;123(5):490

the overuse of antibiotics and the possibility of an adverse drug reaction in someone who did not actually require therapy (medical-legal paranoia?).

Statistics are difficult to find, but the probability of

contracting ARF if a strep throat is untreated is estimated at 0.3 percent. With treatment, this drops to 0.003 percent, so at least the concept of treating to avoid ARF is supported. I could find little data stating that treatment decreases abscess or how it influences transmission (but both make sense). Transmission must be unusual, however, because I rarely see the whole family come down with strep. Also, most peritonsillar abscesses that I see present early and I have seen abscesses in patients treated early. An old argument that currently holds no water is that documenting strep somehow influences the ENT surgeon to operate. The incidence of serious allergies to penicillin ranges from 0.6 percent to about 2 percent, although most studies show a truly serious reaction in less than 1 percent. There is no question that a patient can die from anaphylaxis to penicillin.

SUMMARY: It's clear to me that no approach is perfect, and no amount of clinical judgment, statistical analysis, or careful culturing can truly settle all of the clinical issues. A CBC and sedimentation rate are diagnostically worthless, and it's clearly absurd to order more studies such as ASO titers or do multiple cultures or complex viral studies. It appears that the gold standard (perhaps only gold plated, however) for making a reasonable scientific diagnosis is a positive culture coupled with a compatible clinical presentation. However if a $120 culture does not even establish the diagnosis with certainty and a negative test does not always exclude it, why order the test? Bad data are worse than no data.

Initially promising alternatives to cultures were the rapid strep screens. There are antigen detection tests performed on throat swabs that give results in 30 minutes. Our hospital does not offer this test routinely because of inconsistent and unreliable results. Although rather specific (90%-98%), the rapid screens miss a significant number of throats that are positive by culture (sensitivity only 75%-85%). In one recent review analyzing six different screens, these tests had a disappointing 31-50 percent sen-

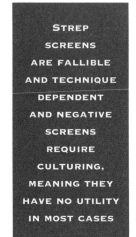

STREP SCREENS ARE FALLIBLE AND TECHNIQUE DEPENDENT AND NEGATIVE SCREENS REQUIRE CULTURING, MEANING THEY HAVE NO UTILITY IN MOST CASES

sitivity (*JAMA* 1992;267(5):695). If these data are true, I can't imagine ever doing the currently available rapid strep screens. No doubt, however, this technology will be improved in the future.

Most authors suggest a follow-up culture if screens are negative, further increasing the expense of searching for data of dubious value. Although better than clinical judgment, rapid screens have not completely solved our diagnostic problems yet (see *Ann Emerg Med* 1986;15(2):157; *Ped Infect Dis J* 1988;7(11):765).

My approach includes the following: First, I function as a realist working with an indigent population with a high incidence of strep infections, no family doctor, disconnected phones, borrowed health insurance cards, and an intolerable or nonexistent clinic system. As one committed to being practical, I am very liberal in treating sore throats in the ED and hesitant to order cultures or strep screens. If there are more than minor symptoms, I prescribe antibiotics, usually without any testing unless I suspect gonorrhea, want to diagnose mononucleosis or scarlet fever, prove to a resident the shortcomings of his clinical acumen (in this case, I demand that they do the follow-up), or if the family doctor/pediatrician is one who will ensure follow-up and is adamant about cultures.

I do not treat young infants with colds or fevers with normal-looking throats or older people with laryngitis, URI symptoms, or minimal pharyngeal complaints, but I may culture them, especially if they are immunocompromised or have confusing symptoms, but only if there is some way to ensure follow-up. If a culture is positive, I always treat. My approach will clearly overtreat, but I am willing to accept this cost-effective and practical approach unless some reader can come up with a reasonable alternative for my patient population. Because the currently available strep screens are fallible and technique dependent and negative screens require culturing, I don't think they have utility in most cases.

ACUTE PHARYNGITIS: HOW EFFECTIVE IS THERAPY?

It makes reasonable clinical sense to treat all patients with acute pharyngitis without obtaining a culture or other laboratory tests

This is the third in a series of discussions on the diagnosis and treatment of acute pharyngitis. Previous discussions concluded that despite the fact that most physicians think they can diagnose a strep throat by the clinical picture, differentiating bacterial from viral pharyngitis on physical findings is simply impossible. Specifically, fever, pus on the tonsils, leukocytosis, and tender adenopathy do not always add up to group A beta-hemolytic streptococcal (GABHS) pharyngitis.

GABHS is significantly overdiagnosed in adults with pharyngitis. With young children (under age 3) in particular, the classic textbook description of a strep throat is more often due to adenovirus. Streptococcal pharyngitis is not a disease of toddlers, but it is common in the 5-12 year age group and well into young adulthood. There is also reason to suspect that Mycoplasma and Chlamydia bacteria and the Herpes virus play some yet undefined role in pharyngitis of any age. Clearly the CBC and sedimentation rate are of no diagnostic value, and the currently available rapid strep screens have questionable value because at best they are only 80 to 90 percent sensitive, and they can't differentiate carrier state from infection. Furthermore, negative screens must be confirmed with a culture.

The clinician has previously relied upon a throat culture as the gold standard for the diagnosis of GABHS. Although a negative culture usually rules out strep, cultures are only about 90 percent sensitive, with the accuracy highly dependent on your initial swabbing and incubating technique. I had suggested swabbing both tonsils and pharynx at least twice before putting the culture swab into its container. A positive culture does not verify an active infection because the accepted proof of infection (versus carrier state) is an ASO titer rise. With a positive culture, antibody titers rise only slightly over half the time. Therefore, our so-called gold standard culture does not necessarily prove that the symptomatic patient has a strep infection if it's positive, nor does it consistently rule it out if it's negative.

My review of the literature and personal bias lead me to suggest that if follow-up is less than ideal (ideal being defined as a reliable patient and easy access to a clinic or private practice setting), and one is concerned about epidemiology and cost issues, it makes reasonable clinical sense to treat all patients with strep-like acute pharyngitis without obtaining a culture or other laboratory tests. This is an especially cost-effective approach during an epidemic (Ann Intern Med 1977;86(4): 481). This will offend the purist in the audience, and I admit *it's not an academic way to practice, but given the realities of inner city hospitals that primarily treat indigent and higher risk patients on a sporadic basis, it's the only logical way to try to control this disease. Certainly some overtreatment will occur. Surveys show that about half of physicians practice this way, but others (mostly pediatricians) still prefer to use throat cultures to guide therapy. Clearly even the experts just can't totally agree on the standard of care. In fact, I don't think there is a currently accepted standard of care.*

This chapter explores two related issues: whether treatment hastens resolution of symptoms and the effectiveness of therapy in eradicating the bacteria from the pharynx.

> ### STREPTOCOCCAL PHARYNGITIS. PLACEBO-CONTROLLED DOUBLE-BLIND EVALUATION OF CLINICAL RESPONSE TO PENICILLIN THERAPY
>
> Krober MS, et al *JAMA* 1985;253(9):1271

This article addresses the age old issue of whether treatment with penicillin hastens clinical improvement in patients with acute symptomatic streptococcal pharyngitis. The authors believe that this is the first prospective, randomized, placebo-controlled, double-blind study to evaluate this specific issue. The authors randomly assigned 44 children seen at a pediatric clinic with acute pharyngitis to either oral penicillin therapy or placebo for the first 72 hours. Treatment decisions were based on clinical criteria that have been developed to identify children likely to have GABHS (the frequently used Breeze Criteria; *Am J Dis Child* 1977;131(5):514). Therapy consisted of oral penicillin V, 250 mg TID for three days, or a similar-appearing placebo. The treating physician re-evaluated the child for fever and other signs and symptoms at 24, 48, and 72 hours. Urine samples were obtained at 48 hours to assess compliance to penicillin and to ensure that those given placebo had not received penicillin from another source. Cultures were also repeated to verify laboratory cure rates, and blood was drawn for anti-streptococcal antibodies. After three days, all patients with a positive culture were then treated with oral penicillin for 10 days.

Interestingly, only 59 percent of the patients who were entered into this study (remember these had a high clinical suspicion of having strep) had a positive throat culture. About 60 percent of those with a positive culture had a rise in antibody titers, the accepted serologic proof of a true infection. Interestingly, two patients with a negative culture also had a positive titer rise.

All penicillin-treated patients who had an initial positive culture had a negative culture at 24, 48, and 72 hours. Those receiving placebo continued to have a positive culture for three days. Urine specimens confirmed that patients given penicillin took the drug and those given placebo did not get it from another source (it's unclear if the specimens were tested for other antibiotics).

Patients in both groups were afebrile at 72 hours, however, those given penicillin had a statistically significant decrease in fever at 16 hours. Symptomatology was similar at the onset in both groups, but statistically significant clinical improvement in pain, dysphagia, headache, and abdominal pain was observed in those subjects treated with penicillin.

The authors admit that this is a small study, but they believe their statistics demonstrate a significant clinical response to penicillin. As might be expected, symptomatic patients with negative cultures did not benefit clinically from penicillin. The etiology of the pharyngitis was not confirmed in the culture-negative group, but it was presumed to be viral.

Previous clinical dogma has held that penicillin does not significantly alter the natural clinical course of strep throat. Therefore it has been suggested that one can wait to prescribe antibiotics pending culture results (*N Engl J Med* 1977;297(7):365). The authors of this study believe their data strongly refute this philosophy. Delaying treatment for three days probably does not alter the risk of rheumatic fever, but penicillin clearly makes patients feel better quicker. In addition to providing significant symptomatic improvement, penicillin produced negative throat cultures in only 24 hours, a significant issue if one is trying to decrease the spread of this disease, particularly to siblings at home and in schools and day care centers.

COMMENT: I was taught in medical school that penicillin did not alter the course of strep throat and therefore one could merely wait for the results of the culture to "decrease allergic reactions and limit the use of needless antibiotics." It's generally agreed that one can wait seven to nine days after onset of symptoms and still prevent rheumatic fever, but somehow a tradition was established that the patient suffered a similar course with his sore throat regardless of therapy. My own personal experience supports this small study, and one need only personally experience strep throat to realize that within 24 to 48 hours, one is usually 100 percent improved if penicillin is administered.

TWO COURSES OF ORAL PENICILLIN V VS. AUGMENTIN IN TREATING GROUP A STREPTOCOCCI

Treatment	Total treated	No. treated with antibiotics	Treatment failures No. (%)
Initial treatment	131	Oral penicillin V	50 (38)
First treatment	45	Oral penicillin V (24)	17 (71)
Retreatment		Augmentin (21)	2 (9)
Second treatment	19	Augmentin (17)	3 (18)
Retreatment		Oral penicillin V (2)	1 (50)

Source: J Pediatr 1988;113(2):400-3.

Textbooks state the most compelling reason for treating GABHS is to prevent rheumatic fever, but any patient will argue with this. They want to feel better as soon as possible, and they probably will if given antibiotics.

Parents frequently ask when their children can return to school. This study specifically demonstrates that at 24 hours into antibiotic therapy, a throat culture is no longer positive and presumably the disease is not contagious.

The issue is very difficult to study, and the data are mixed, but overall studies suggest that antibiotics shorten the course of strep throat. Randolph and associates also evaluated the effect of antibiotic therapy on the clinical course of strep pharyngitis and drew similar conclusions. (J Pediatr 1985;106(6):870) In a double-blind study, they analyzed 206 children who were randomized to receive either penicillin V, cefadroxil (Duricef), or placebo. At 18 to 24 hours post-therapy, antibiotics significantly decreased fever, degree of lymphadenitis, pharyngeal injection, subjective throat pain, headache, and abdominal pain. In addition to objective improvement, parents and patients reported a general overall subjective clinical improvement.

To be objective, however, I must mention a contrary study by Middleton et al in which penicillin treatment produced minimal improvement in pain and minimal general overall improvement at 48 hours (J Pediatr 1988; 113(6):1089). Because penicillin produced only slight improvement compared to placebo, the authors questioned the early use of antibiotics. Others have made the argument that allowing strep to brew for a few days prompts an immune response and hence recurrence will be less (Ped Infect Dis J 1991;10:855). Data on this seemingly bizarre suggestion are controversial; I suppose you could make the same argument for any infectious disease.

Although some physicians harbor a bias that antibiotics do not have a significant impact on the clinical course of strep throat, the opposite appears to be true. Failure to find a rapid favorable response generally means that the diagnosis of strep was incorrect. In fact, antibiotics don't just "help" symptomatology, they may have a dramatic impact on the clinical course in some patients. Why it took us until 1985 to make this observation is beyond me, but it has been demonstrated clearly enough for me to accept the concept of early treatment.

It is agreed that treatment will prevent acute rheumatic fever (ARF), but it will not prevent acute glomerulonephritis (AGN). Fortunately, the latter is a more benign disease; it is usually self-limited, and rarely produces permanent sequelae. Bennicke et al (Acta Med Scand 1951; 139:253) suggest that treatment can prevent peritonsillar abscess, and in a series evaluating patients over the age of 40, abscess developed in one of 174 penicillin-treated patients compared to nine of 175 untreated patients. This issue is not well addressed in the literature, and there are no firm conclusions. My observation is that most patients with peritonsillar abscess develop it quickly and present with the process already well along, and I have seen it develop following appropriate therapy.

ERADICATION OF GROUP A STREPTOCOCCI FROM THE UPPER RESPIRATORY TRACT BY AMOXICILLIN WITH CLAVULANATE AFTER ORAL PENICILLIN V. TREATMENT FAILURE

J Pediatr 1988;113:(2) 401

This is a fascinating study that evaluates the laboratory cure of strep throat in patients treated with penicillin. The authors believe that this issue is of importance because persistent strep infection is associated with an increased risk of disease transmission and rheumatic fever. At three to five days after completion of 10 days of oral penicillin V (dose not specified), the authors re-cultured children who had an initially positive throat culture for GABHS. Of 131 patients, an amazing 50 children (38%) continued to harbor GABHS. Careful surveillance indicated that compliance with the medication regimen was excellent, and in fact, when there was a question of noncompliance, patients were eliminated from the study. Of the 45 children still deemed to have a positive throat culture after successfully completing a full course of antibiotics, 24 were re-treated with the same course of penicillin and 21 received 10 days of oral amoxicillin with clavulanate (Augmentin). A second re-treatment course of antibiotics (actually the third treatment) was administered if the culture was still positive. When re-treated for a second time, the child who had failed penicillin was given Augmentin; if there were further failures, penicillin was given.

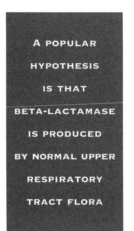

A POPULAR HYPOTHESIS IS THAT BETA-LACTAMASE IS PRODUCED BY NORMAL UPPER RESPIRATORY TRACT FLORA

In the first re-treatment course, there was a 71 percent failure rate in those given penicillin again, and a nine percent failure rate with Augmentin. Of those failing the first re-treatment (19 children), 17 were given Augmentin and two received penicillin. Even with a third course of antibiotics, four children still had a positive culture. The authors conclude that Augmentin is superior to penicillin for the eradication of GABHS from the upper respiratory tract (87% success vs. 31% with penicillin), but a 100 percent cure rate is not obtained with either regimen. In this study, no patient had complications. Diarrhea was not a problem in those given Augmentin.

The authors note that it is not earth-shattering news that patients treated with penicillin still harbor streptococci on re-culture. In the literature there is a general consensus not to re-culture patients who become asymptomatic with therapy because those with a persistent positive culture are generally considered to be carriers only. This study underscores the fact that the carrier state is probably impossible to eradicate. There are a number of theories to explain the high treatment failure rate. A popular hypothesis is that beta-lactamase is produced by normal upper respiratory tract flora, and this prevents penicillin from being totally effective. Previous studies have shown that beta-lactamase-resistant antibiotics, such as dicloxacillin, are more effective in a re-treatment regimen than is another course of oral penicillin V. Resistance to penicillin does not seem to be an issue.

The authors were concerned that the treatment failure rate with penicillin was almost 30 percent in their area. They note that this is up from eight percent in the mid-1960s. Although compliance is always an issue, as is the possibility of an inadequate potency of penicillin (the efficacy of generic drugs has sporadically been called into question), the reason for failure to eradicate strep is far from clear. The authors in this study did not look for beta-lactamase-producing organisms nor did they conduct sensitivity studies on streptococcal isolates. In addition, streptococcal antibodies were not determined and therefore it is unclear whether these were carrier states to begin with or treatment failures in established infection. Interestingly, most of the subjects whose cultures remained positive were asymptomatic children identified through surveillance techniques during outbreaks in schools, suggesting that the authors were largely treating a carrier state to begin with. However, the authors do note that two-thirds of cases of rheumatic fever occur without any symptoms of pharyngitis or after only a mild sore throat.

The data in this study were frustrating and confusing to the authors. On one hand, organism eradication has been considered the *sine qua non* in the assessment of efficacy of antibiotic therapy. On the other hand, many authors minimize or discount the importance of a persistent GABHS culture after antibiotic therapy has eradicated symptoms and associate it with a benign carrier state. The authors are unwilling to suggest that the previous gold standard, penicillin, has been tarnished, and still view initial therapy with penicillin as appropriate. The authors ask for additional studies before optimal therapy can be determined. They do, however, suggest that if a positive culture persists with therapy, Augmentin is an effective choice for re-treatment.

COMMENT: This is an extremely confusing article that does not leave one with a good clinical sense of how to proceed. Many authors have reported the concept of clinical cure in the face of a continued positive culture, but it is disturbing that 20-30 percent of patients re-cultured following compliant penicillin therapy will still have a positive culture. Try explaining that concept to a worried patient! Traditional teaching has been that if a patient is clinically cured they need not be re-cultured unless there is a sibling at home with previous ARF (because the carrier state may transmit the disease to siblings). The exact cause of the carrier state is not known, and no particular clinical characteristics or serologic subtypes have been related to its development.

The issue of invasive disease vs. carrier state is probably moot when it comes to rheumatic fever because the attack rate of ARF in patients whose cultures remain positive in spite of antibiotic therapy has been found to be identical to that observed in untreated patients. (*N Engl J Med* 1958;259:5; *Circulation* 1984;70(6):1118A). The asymptomatic carrier state probably explains why ARF is often seen without a firm history of a prior strep throat. Some authors, however, discount the significance of the asymptomatic carrier state in initiating ARF. In short, there is no real consensus on how to approach patients with positive strep cultures who are clinically cured with penicillin.

In general, the patient with the carrier state is not highly contagious, and does not develop infectious sequelae. I assume because ARF is so uncommon, many experts have decided to live with an asymptomatic carrier state even if theoretically it could predispose to ARF. ARF has not disappeared altogether, but it's clearly on the decline, attributed primarily to aggressive antibiotic treatment. Epidemiologic studies suggest that the risk of developing ARF is at most 0.5 percent for individuals in the general population who have positive GABHS cultures and are not treated. Personally I have not seen a case in many years. The attack rate may be higher for those with an untreated positive culture during epidemic outbreaks.

The disturbing issue here is that penicillin results in such a disappointing negative culture rate. The beta-lactamase theory is an interesting one, but the exact reason for treatment failures is unknown. Turner and associates were able to culture beta-lactamase producing organisms, including Staph aureus, bacteroides, and fusobacteria, in 73 percent of their patients with recurrent tonsillitis (*Scand J Infect Dis* 1983;39:83). Like other reports, in this series, penicillin could not always eradicate strep, and clindamycin was usually successful in producing a negative culture but only in 80-90 percent of cases.

In our laboratory, sensitivities are not done on positive strep throat cultures, and it's just automatically assumed that the bug is sensitive to penicillin. When Coonan et al (*Ped Infect Dis J* 1994;13:630) recently studied in vitro sensitivity to 282 pharyngeal streptococcal isolates gathered from 31 different states, all were susceptible to even low concentrations of penicillin. Also, all isolates were sensitive to clindosporins. Interestingly 3.5 percent were resistant to erythromycin, azithromycin, and clarithromycin, and 10 percent were resistant to tetracycline. It is known that up to five percent of strains of GABHS are resistant to erythromycin so if one is choosing an alternative to penicillin for treatment failures, Augmentin, a cephalosporin, or clindamycin seem to be more logical choices, clearly better than erythromycin or repeating penicillin.

Finally, a word about patient compliance to oral antibiotics is in

STREPTOCOCCAL PHARYNGITIS: DEVELOPMENT OF ANTIBODIES IN CHILDREN

Study Group	No. Patients	No. Tested	Titer Rise for ASO, AH or Anti-DNase B Antibodies No (%) with > 4X Titer Rise
Culture positive			
Received penicillin	11	11	7 (64)
Received placebo	15	13*	8 (62)
Total	26	24*	15 (63)
Culture negative			
Received penicillin	10	7*	1 (14)
Received placebo	8	5*	1 (20)
Total	18	12*	2 (17)

*Note: ASO is antistreptolysin O; AH is antihyaluronidase; anti-DNase B is antideoxyribonuclease B. * indicates patients who did not return to provide convalescent serum samples.*

Source: JAMA 1985;253:1271-4.

order. It don't matter if you are an author of an infectious disease textbook or the unemployed parent of a 6-year-old, you probably will not finish a prescribed 10-day course of almost anything. When Bergman (*N Engl J Med* 1955;252:787) assayed for penicillin in the urine of inner city children being treated for strep throat, he found that fewer than 18 percent completed a 10-day course. Frequent dosing schedules and long courses when clinical cures occur quickly were the common reasons cited for such poor compliance rates. In one study, simply going from a TID pill regimen to QID increased noncompliance by 72 percent (*Br Med J* 1987;295:814). Even though the authors of this study believed that compliance was good, they did only spot testing and the omnipresent poor compliance may have accounted for such poor culture cures. It's difficult for anyone to take a pill QID for 10 days; however, it's clear from other studies that a number of patients still harbor the streptococcal organism in the upper respiratory tract, even when symptoms are absent and compliance to antibiotics is demonstrated.

TREATMENT OF STREP THROAT: PENICILLIN

Although some speculate about its effectiveness, penicillin is still the best initial choice for acute pharyngitis

This chapter begins a discussion on the treatment of acute pharyngitis. I will focus on antibiotic therapy, beginning with penicillin, and wrap up the topic with a review of alternative antimicrobials and symptomatic adjuncts. Previous columns have emphasized that it is impossible to separate bacterial from viral etiologies of acute pharyngitis on clinical criteria alone, and I particularly emphasized that fever, tender adenopathy, and pus on the tonsils do not always equal strep. Children under the age of four years rarely have streptococcal pharyngitis — it's almost always viral even with a so-called text book presentation — and Mycoplasma, Chlamydia, *and herpes may be culprits in acute adult pharyngitis. Although the throat culture is the accepted gold standard for the diagnosis of group A beta-hemolytic streptococcal (GABHS) pharyngitis, this laboratory test is clearly not infallible. Specifically, 10-15 percent of patients with strep will not be identified by routine single culturing and about half of those who have a positive culture do not have an antibody titer rise and are probably only strep carriers with viral infections. In addition, numerous authors have demonstrated that even with compliance to antibiotic therapy, and in the setting of an initial clinical and laboratory cure, 10-30 percent of patients will again harbor the same strain of strep in the pharynx if they are recultured a few months later. This has prompted some authors to speculate on the effectiveness of penicillin and the possible value of penicillinase-resistant antibiotics.*

It's generally accepted that antibiotics shorten the duration of the disease, decrease complications, and reduce the incidence of rheumatic fever. Although penicillin has long been the standard initial therapy, it's clear that this drug can be used successfully in a number of ways.

BENZATHINE PENICILLIN G FOR TREATMENT OF GROUP A STREPTOCOCCAL PHARYNGITIS: A REAPPRAISAL IN 1985

Kaplan EL *Pediatr Infect Dis* 1985;4(5):592

This informative article is a review of the effectiveness of intramuscular benzathine penicillin G (Bicillin L-A) for the treatment of GABHS pharyngitis. The author notes that benzathine penicillin G (BPG) has long been the classic treatment (gold standard) for strep throat because of prolonged and adequate serum penicillin levels after a single injection. However, the introduction of new antibiotics and data suggesting increasing failure rates with all forms of penicillin have led many physicians to ignore the old standby or opt for more modern antibiotics.

A number of studies from the 1950s demonstrated that benzathine penicillin G is superior to oral penicillin in the treatment of streptococcal disease in children. The term "superior" means fewer laboratory failures. A laboratory failure, defined as a positive culture at the completion of therapy, is much more common than a clinical failure because almost all patients are quickly asymptomatic after either BPG or oral penicillin treatment. When studied 40 years ago, the laboratory failure rate for BPG ranged from six to 19 percent, compared to the failure rate for oral penicillin V or erythromycin, which was in the 32 percent range. If one considers a treatment failure to occur only if the same serotype is recultured, failure rates with BPG are rather negligible, about seven percent. Although the question of compliance is always present with a prolonged oral regimen, authors generally agreed that failure to take the antibiotic did not account for a large number of treatment failures. It is noted that the American Heart Association quickly endorsed the advantages of BPG over oral prophylaxis for prevention of rheumatic fever.

A number of recent studies have demonstrated a peculiar statistic: The failure rate following any form of penicillin therapy, including BPG, has risen and is currently in the 25 percent range as compared with the eight percent range 30 years ago. There are a number of possible explanations. The first explanation, and probably the most correct one, is that the statistics are bad. Most authors discount the compliance issue or a change in the manufacturing process of the penicillins, and more recently it is the trend to question whether beta-lactamase production by bacteria normally present in the upper respiratory tract is responsible for penicillin treatment failures. Symptoms may go away initially, but the bacteria are protected enough by beta-lactamase that they are only suppressed and regroup to recolonize in a few weeks. This has been supported by studies demonstrating that treatment with dicloxacillin or amoxicillin/clavulanate (Augmentin) produces higher laboratory eradication rates than a full course of penicillin. Although numerous studies have shown uniform sensitivity of Group A strep to penicillin, some form of antibiotic tolerance may be developing. Finally the issue is always raised that failure to eradicate GABHS from the upper respiratory tract is related to a carrier state, a noto-

riously difficult situation to correct.

The author concludes that there is a bona fide change in the effectiveness of penicillin in eradicating Group A strep from the pharynx. Importantly, however, the clinical significance of this laboratory observation is currently unknown. In 1985 and at present, there is no mandate to recommend alternatives to penicillin for routine strep throat, but further developments warrant close monitoring.

AN EVALUATION OF THE LITERATURE STILL SUPPORTS THE INITIAL USE OF PENICILLIN FOR ACUTE PHARYNGITIS

COMMENT: Markowitz et al (*J Pediatr* 1993;123(5):679) tried to settle the issue of the perceived recent increased failure rate of penicillin to cure strep throat. They concluded that reports of penicillin's demise for this indication are statistically premature. To support this statement, the authors conducted a meta-analysis of 32 published studies of oral penicillin treatment in children with GABHS pharyngitis that were conducted between 1953 and 1993 (about 2700 patients). When the frequency of bacteriologic treatment failure rates from 1953 to 1979 were compared to the failure rates between 1980 to 1993, there was no statistical difference. During the first 26-year period, 10.5 percent of patients recultured within 14 days of treatment again harbored the same strep strain. During the subsequent 13 years, the failure rate was 12 percent. This analysis would indicate that there has been no substantial change in cure rates for penicillin in treating strep throat.

BPG is available alone (Bicillin L-A) or in combination with procaine penicillin G (Bicillin C-R). BPG is slowly released from a deep intramuscular injection, resulting in therapeutic blood levels for approximately 14 days following the administration of 1.2 million units in adults. When used for rheumatic fever prophylaxis, the injection is used monthly. Aside from a slightly better initial cure rate, the major advantage of BPG is that only a single injection is required, a significant benefit if compliance is an issue. There are no prescriptions to fill and no pills to remember to take. I personally think that it's almost impossible for anyone to take any pill four times a day for 10 days, particularly if symptoms go away after a few days of treatment. Therefore, if one is truly realistic about the prevention of rheumatic fever, it make utmost sense to me to prescribe only BPG.

Bicillin CR combines a rapid and a depot form of penicillin. I see no particular advantage of combining the BPG with the more rapidly acting procaine (Novocaine) penicillin G, but in patients with significant symptoms I often include an oral loading dose of 1g penicillin VK with the injection of BPG. Although the textbooks would tell you that a single injection of BPG is sufficient and I could find no study supporting my bias, it's difficult for me to ignore the loading dose concept in very symptomatic patients, particularly in the easily administered oral form.

Procaine will supposedly decrease the pain of injection, but it's an ester and is more likely to cause a true allergic reaction than amides (lidocaine and others). My nurses tell me that procaine does little to reduce pain during injection. Those who are old enough to remember the use of large doses of procaine penicillin G for gonorrhea (4.8 million units IM) may have seen the peculiar nonallergic toxic "procaine reaction." It was impressive and probably due to rapid procaine absorption. About 0.1-0.3 percent of patients treated developed a bizarre but temporary state of agitation, paranoia, hallucinations, and often ran around the room in a psychotic-like state following their massive procaine load. By the way, procaine bears the trade name Novocaine, and many

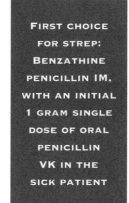

FIRST CHOICE
FOR STREP:
BENZATHINE
PENICILLIN IM,
WITH AN INITIAL
1 GRAM SINGLE
DOSE OF ORAL
PENICILLIN
VK IN THE
SICK PATIENT

patients claim an allergy to it, but this anesthetic is not used anymore by dentists.

The obvious disadvantages of the benzathine penicillin G injection are the pain, the higher incidence of anaphylaxis compared to pills, and the contention that an allergy may persist for a prolonged period. I have personally never seen an immediate or prolonged allergic reaction from benzathine penicillin G in 25 years of practice, and I use the drug frequently. Just to be on the safe side, I hesitate to use any parenteral penicillin (especially long-acting BPG) in patients with asthma, eczema, hay fever, or other obvious allergic conditions; these are known to increase the chance of a reaction to penicillin. Markowitz *(Clin Ther* 1980;3(1):49) states that allergic reactions to BPG are usually transient even though penicillin is still present, due to the rapid formation of blocking antibodies that prevent residual penicillin from combining with sensitizing antibodies. Prolonged allergy to benzathine penicillin G is probably a myth. When I posed this quandary to the drug company that makes benzathine penicillin G, I was told that the perceived prolonged reactions to benzathine penicillin G are not supported by many years of clinical

STUDIES OF THE EFFICACY OF BENZATHINE PENICILLIN G (BPG) FOR STREPTOCOCCAL PHARYNGITIS

		No. Patients	Antibiotic	Success No. (%)	Failure No. (%)
Study 1:	*1952-1954*	*1021*	*BPG*	*No. (%)*	*No. (%)*
	IM		*(600,000 units)*	*960 (94)*	*61 (6)*
Study 2:	*1954-1955*				
	Oral	*281*	*BPG*	*191 (68)*	*90 (32)*
	IM	*182*	*BPG (600,000 units)*	*148 (81)*	*34 (19)*
Study 3:	*1955-1956*				
	Oral	*489*	*Penicillin (5 regimens)*	*333 (68)*	*156 (32)*
	IM	*122*	*BPG (600,000 units)*	*103 (84)*	*19 (16)*

Source: Ped Infect Dis 1985;4(5): 592-596.

use. In fact, allergic reactions from long-acting benzathine penicillin G appear to be no different in rate, severity, or duration from those observed with short-acting penicillins (personal contact with Wyeth-Ayerst Laboratories and *N Engl J Med* 1955;252:787).

The compliance issue with oral antibiotics is of more than theoretical concern, and I don't know how the authors of the earlier studies could have realistically discounted it. Multiple studies have suggested that the overall noncompliance rate to any medication is around 30 percent. Saunders investigated patient compliance merely to filling a prescription after discharge from the emergency department (*Am J Emerg Med* 1987;5(4):283) and found that 22 percent of patients failed to even obtain a prescribed drug, let alone take it. Noncompliance was not related to gender or ability to pay, and there was no reliable method to identify patients prospectively who were unlikely to fill their prescriptions. If one of five patients fails to get his prescription filled, the number who fail to take it as prescribed has to be much higher.

In an interesting report, Cockburn et al (*Br Med J [Clin Res Ed]* 1987;295)6602):814) studied non-compliance with short-term antibiotic regimens. They demonstrated the following: There is increasing likelihood of noncompliance as the number of doses to be taken in one day increases (increasing by only one time per day increased probability of noncompliance by an amazing 72 percent); the patient's perception of his/her own current health status is important (those that thought they weren't very sick were likely to be noncompliant); and compliance goes down as the complexity of the instructions increases (such as with meals, double dose).

In my mind, BPG is the ideal treatment regimen for acute pharyngitis. It is my drug of choice for nonallergic patients if they will accept the injection (I always give them the choice but strongly recommend BPG). I especially like it for the indigent patient who is most likely to contract acute rheumatic fever and other complications of strep throat, and for the patient who is least likely to fill or take a prescription properly (a difficult judgment call).

No drug has been consistently proven superior to penicillin, and the vast majority of patients are clinically cured with penicillin. The significance of a positive reculture is unclear, but most agree that these patients are at low risk for acute rheumatic fever, and that obtaining a long-term laboratory eradication of a carrier state is nearly impossible. Because no one recommends routine reculture in clinically cured patients, the issue may be mostly academic.

Some colleagues prescribe amoxicillin/ampicillin in lieu of penicillin for strep throat. They are both effective, and the cost is comparable, but I can see no reason to use the broader spectrum drug. Ampicillin seems to be more commonly prescribed for children, perhaps a subconscious attempt to treat *Hemophilus influenzae,* a common ear pathogen. Importantly, many patients treated with ampicillin develop a rash that is incorrectly diagnosed as a "penicillin allergy," and they are branded as penicillin-allergic for the rest of their lives.

PENICILLIN V FOR STREPTOCOCCAL PHARYNGITIS

	1000 mg BID	Treatment 250 mg QID
Patients with negative streptococci A test		
At first control (Day 4)	51 (88%)	39 (64%)
At second control (Day 10)	56 (96%)	57 (94%)
Patients without pharyngeal infection		
At first control (Day 4)	26 (45%)	12 (20%)
At second control (day 10)	58 (100%)	61 (100%)
Time to clinical response, days	3.5 ±0.8	4.6±1.2
Patient with side effects	5 (9%)	10 (16%)
Nausea	1	-
Diarrhea	1	3
Diarrhea and nausea	2	3
Rash	1	1
Loose stools	-	3

Source: Curr Therapeu Res *1978;43(3): 374.*

PULSE DOSING WITH PENICILLIN VK IN STREPTOCOCCAL PHARYNGITIS: 1000 MG BID VS. 250 MG QID

Helleman K *Curr Ther Res Clin* 1978;43(3):374

This largely ignored Austrian study examines the benefit of high-dose, low-frequency administration of antibiotics vs. continuous administration of lower doses. The study was designed to determine the bacteriological and clinical response of patients with GABHS pharyngitis to treatment with two doses of oral penicillin: 1 g BID or 250 mg QID, given in a standard 10-day course. All patients had clinical signs of acute pharyngitis and a positive rapid strep antigen screen. Followup occurred at four days, 10 days, and four weeks following presentation, at which time a repeat throat swab was obtained and urine was analyzed for penicillin compliance.

Of 119 patients who received either the 1 g BID dose or the standard 250 mg QID dose, the bacteriological (laboratory) cure rates were equal: 96 percent and 94 percent, respectively. The clinical cure rate was 100 percent in both groups at 10 days. However, the pulse schedule shortened the course of the illness by approximately one day and theoretically reduced the risk of cross infection. Importantly, at four days, 88 percent in the pulse group but only 64 percent in the QID group had a negative antigen detection test. The time to clinical response was likewise significant. On day four, more than twice as many patients (45% vs. 20%) lacked pharyngeal infection if they took the high-pulse dose. When both groups were examined at four weeks, all but one subject had continued resolution of the symptoms and a negative strep screen. The authors believe that their data indicate that high-dose, low-frequency penicillin shortened the duration of illness and reduced the period of infectiousness, and that this patient-friendly protocol should be used instead of the traditional QID regimen.

COMMENT: Although largely ignored by clinicians, this is a great study! The authors note that the bacteriological and clinical recurrence rate for GABHS pharyngitis has historically been related to the length of treatment rather than the specific penicillin regimen. Currently a full 10-day course is still favored although a number of specific dosing regimens are probably equally effective. So called "pulse dosing" has been described previously (*Rev Infect Dis* 1981;3(1):1).

It is interesting to note that the more patient-friendly 1 g BID dose seemed to be more clinically effective than the traditional 250 mg QID dose. The authors do not address the fact that the recurrence rate in their population was unusually low compared to other studies; perhaps if the patients were cultured instead of screened for the antigen, the results would have been different.

Although compliance to penicillin was not specifically tested, it seems perfectly logical that patients are more likely to take a drug that is prescribed less often and at con-

PATIENT COMPLIANCE FOR TREATMENT OF STREPTOCOCCAL PHARYNGOTONSILLITIS

| | No. of Patients | | |
	Penicillin V 5 days n=70	*Penicillin V 10 days n=70*	*Cefadroxil 10 days n=69*
Complete compliance	55	55	52
1-2 doses omitted	8	13	16
3-4 doses omitted	6	2	1
5 doses omitted	1	0	0

Source: Scand J Infect Dis *1988;20:37.*

venient times (such as morning and evening). However, missing a few doses may be more significant in a BID schedule than in a QID format. The pulse dose concept may be extrapolated to the use of antibiotics for many soft tissue infections or for wound prophylaxis (not yet studied to my knowledge but quite logical), and this theory has been used for years with single daily dose phenytoin and prednisone therapy. Even the histamine blockers (cimetidine, ranitidine) are used in larger, less frequent doses than originally advocated. Note that the total daily dose of penicillin was 2 g in one group and only 1 g in the other.

At least two other studies have addressed the same issue. Krober et al (*Clin Pediatr* 1990;29(11):646) compared 1 g penicillin V given either as a single gram per day, 500 mg

BID, or 250 mg QID, to 142 children with documented streptococcal pharyngitis. There was no statistically significant difference in the prevalence of positive culture at 28 days among the regimens. Curiously the once-a-day protocol had a slightly poorer culture negative response early in the treatment course. Fyllingen et al (*Scand J Infect Dis* 1991;23(5):553) also demonstrated the effectiveness of a BID dosing regimen for oral penicillin. All things considered, it makes no sense to me whatsoever to prescribe oral penicillin for strep throat in a QID protocol.

FIVE VERSUS TEN DAYS TREATMENT OF GROUP A STREPTOCOCCAL PHARYNGOTONSILLITIS: A RANDOMIZED CONTROLLED CLINICAL TRIAL WITH PHENOXYMETHYL PENICILLIN AND CEFADROXIL

Stromberg A, et al *Scand J Infect Dis* 1988;20(1):37

The purpose of this Swedish study was to investigate the bacteriological and clinical outcome of a five-day vs. a 10-day course of oral penicillin for strep throat. In addition the effect of a 10-day treatment with the oral cephalosporin cefadroxil was evaluated. The authors note that there has been a recent tendency in Sweden to shorten the antibiotic treatment time for a number of infections, including pharyngitis.

All patients were at least 7 years old and had clinical pharyngitis and a positive culture or direct antigen test for strep. Patients were randomly assigned to one of the three following treatment groups: penicillin VK for five days followed by placebo for five days, penicillin for 10 days, or cefadroxil for 10 days. Interestingly, all antibiotics were given only twice a day. Children received penicillin 400 mg BID and adults received 800 mg BID. The cefadroxil dose was 500 mg BID for children and 1 g BID for adults. Patients were recultured approximately one week following completion of the antibiotic treatment and were re-evaluated and recultured again at two months.

Most patients experienced significant relief of their symptoms within 24 hours regardless of therapy. ASO titer conversion occurred in approximately 39 percent. During follow-up, 35 percent had a recurrence of a positive strep test and about two-thirds of these had clinical symptoms. Most recurrences occurred within the first week and were in those given the five-day course of penicillin.

The occurrence rate with a same serotype as the initial infecting strain was 27 percent in those given five days of penicillin, in six percent of those given 10 days of penicillin, and in three percent of those given 10 days of cefadroxil. At two months a total of 55 percent were recolonized in the group treated for only five days compared with 24 percent and 19 percent of those receiving a longer course of penicillin and cefadroxil respectively. The authors believe that the standard 10 days of penicillin should be maintained because it is significantly more effective in reducing the number of recurrences than a five-day course. Because most recurrences were caused by a bacterial strain identical to the original isolate, the authors believe that the initial strain was not completely eradicated by the shorter course of antibiotics. There were not enough data to make a firm statement regarding the efficacy of cefadroxil vs. penicillin, but the cephalosporin performed well. The authors conclude that the current recommendations for a 10-day course of penicillin for the treatment of strep throat is supported.

COMMENT: Although there have been some scattered reports suggesting the use of a shorter course of therapy for GABHS pharyngitis, numerous authors have found a sig-

RECURRENCES WITHIN ONE WEEK AND TWO MONTHS AFTER COMPLETION OF ANTIBIOTIC TREATMENT

	One Week	Two Months
No. patients	203	201
Recurrence with same T-type	24	46
With symptoms	18	31
Without symptoms	6	15
Recurrence with different T-type	1	9
Recurrence with T-type unknown	3	10
Total recurrences	28	65

Source: Scand J Infect Dis *1988;20:37.*

nificant difference in the recurrence rate when a seven-day course of penicillin is used instead of the standard 10-day regimen. Schwartz found recurrence rates of 31 percent vs. 18 percent in a seven- vs. 10-day course respectively (*JAMA* 1981;246:1790). Shortening the course to five days is currently an unproven regimen, and I don't recommend it. As noted in other studies, even after 10 days of oral therapy, the failure rate is high. The fact that reinfection was with the same serotype could indicate either ineffective initial treatment or reinfection from the environment (family member, school, etc.). There was a surprisingly high rate of positive cultures (50%) in family members in this group.

I found it fascinating that this is another study recommending twice-a-day therapy with penicillin VK. The dose is similar to the previous study, and the authors note that the current recommendation for adult pharyngitis in their country is penicillin 0.8 to 1.0 gram BID.

SUMMARY: A number of unresolved issues still remain to complicate the problem of the diagnosis and management of streptococcal pharyngitis. Despite the fact that there is a significant reinfection rate regardless of therapy, my evaluation of the literature still supports the initial use of penicillin. Interestingly no author in my review has suggested an alternative for initial therapy in the uncomplicated patient. For those patients with recurring infections it is logical to treat with either Augmentin, Duricef, or another cephalosporin, but I have not been convinced that such alternative initial therapy is either cost-effective or warranted. However, the use of these drugs has been reported more frequently in recent years, so stay tuned for updates. Given the compliance issue and the fact that a full 10 days of therapy is strongly recommended, my first choice would be benzathine penicillin IM, adding an initial 1 gram single dose of oral penicillin VK in the sick patient. An option would be 1 gram of oral penicillin VK given twice a day for 10 days, a reasonable alternative that addresses both efficacy and the realities of patient compliance. Next month's column will discuss other alternatives, especially erythromycin, and focus on symptomatic therapy.

STREP THROAT: ALTERNATE THERAPIES AND SYMPTOMATIC RELIEF

Although most patients with strep are clinically cured with penicillin, up to 20 percent harbor the strain weeks later and need alternate antibiotics

Studies indicate that although most patients are clinically cured with penicillin, a large number (10%-20% range) will harbor the same streptococcal strain in their throat if they are recultured a few weeks or months later. The majority are asymptomatic, and it's assumed that one is dealing with a benign carrier state. It's almost impossible to rid these carriers of the strep organism, even with multiple repeat courses of penicillin. A number of studies have demonstrated that penicillinase-resistant antibiotics are more effective than simple penicillin in producing a laboratory cure rate over both the short and long haul. An attractive theory is that normal upper respiratory flora produce penicillinase to render penicillin partly inactive. This chapter explores the value of alternative antibiotics.

ONCE-DAILY CEFADROXIL VERSUS ORAL PENICILLIN IN THE PEDIATRIC TREATMENT OF STREPTOCOCCAL PHARYNGITIS

Goldfarb J, et al *Clin Ther* 1988;10(2):178

This is a relatively small study of 32 children with acute pharyngitis who were randomly assigned to receive either cefadroxil 30 mg/kg (maximum 1 g) once a day, or oral penicillin VK in a dose of 15 mg/kg BID (maximum 750 mg/day). Both regimens were maintained for 10 days. Patients had a throat culture at the beginning of therapy, after antibiotics, and again at one month. All were also evaluated for ASO titer rise. In the subgroup of patients who had both a positive throat culture and a significant rise in antibody titers, cultures were negative immediately following treatment in 75 percent in the penicillin group and 92 percent in the cefadroxil group. One patient had a persistent positive culture, and one became recolonized. Eleven of 12 in the cefadroxil group had an initial cure, and one became recolonized. The authors conclude that once-daily treatment of strep throat with cefadroxil is as efficacious as BID treatment with oral penicillin.

A COMPARISON OF CEFADROXIL AND PENICILLIN V IN THE TREATMENT OF STREPTOCOCCAL PHARYNGITIS IN CHILDREN

Gerber MA *Drugs* 1986;32(suppl 3):29

This is a study that is similar is design to the previous Goldfarb study although it included 555 patients ages 1 to 25 years. Treatment consisted of a 10-day course of cefadroxil (15 mg/kg BID or 30 mg/kg daily), penicillin VK (250 mg BID), erythromycin estolate (15 mg/kg BID), or a single dose of benzathine penicillin G (900,000 U) plus procaine penicillin G (3000,000 U). All treatment regimens were well tolerated and produced a good clinical response in 24 hours. At an 18-to 24-hour reculture check, all the patients treated with cefadroxil and 98 percent of those treated with penicillin were negative. At the 11-month follow-up, the following bacteriologic failure rates (or continued positive culture) were noted: cefadroxil, 4 percent; penicillin V, 12 percent; benzathine penicillin G, 12 percent; and erythromycin 2 percent. Compliance was better with the cefadroxil group when compared to the penicillin group (96% vs. 88%). The authors conclude that cefadroxil is as effective as penicillin and that the once-daily cephalosporin may improve patient compliance.

> MOST PATIENTS ARE CLINICALLY CURED WITH PENICILLIN, BUT 10-20% HARBOR THE STRAIN A FEW WEEKS OR MONTHS LATER

COMMENT: These two articles are representative of a large body of literature comparing alternatives to penicillin for the initial treatment of strep throat. Although the statistics vary somewhat, they all have a common theme: Many drugs are as effective as penicillin for initial therapy, and penicillinase-resistant antibiotics tend to have a higher initial bacteriologic cure rate and less recurrence on distant follow-up. There is no question that most patients rapidly experience a clinical cure with a variety of antibiotics. In the simple cases, it is impossible to demonstrate that the more expensive newly developed drugs work any faster or are clinically any better than penicillin. However, there is a clear message in the literature that the recolonization rate is less when a non-penicillin drug is used, and penicillin is not the drug of choice for frequently recurrent tonsillitis. The critical issue is to determine the real significance of a persistent or recurrent positive culture in the asymptomatic patient. The consensus in the literature is

that clinically cured patients should not be routinely recultured and those with a persistent asymptomatic positive culture need not be treated since they are at no increased risk for suppurative or non-suppurative complications (*J Pediatr* 1980;97(3):337). The only exception is that the carrier state should be identified and treated if a family member has rheumatic fever or there is an inordinate (quantified?) number of symptomatic recurrences of pharyngitis in the patient or family members. Rifampin has been advocated as an effective way to obliterate the carrier state, but this drug is not used to treat acute tonsillitis.

Interestingly many authors now advocate the pulse-dosing concept that was discussed in the last chapter. Specifically, penicillin can be given as 1 g BID rather than 250 mg QID. Likewise, erythromycin or even the cephalosporins can be used in this much more patient-friendly routine. A common theme in all references, however, is that treatment should be maintained for a full 10 days. There are scattered reports suggesting that five or seven days of therapy may be sufficient, but these newer short-term regimens cannot be recommended at the current time, especially if penicillin is used.

Cefadroxil is a widely prescribed semisynthetic cephalosporin that is well tolerated, rapidly absorbed from the GI tract, very effective against strep, and is marketed heavily for its once- or twice-a-day dosing scheme. It is a reasonable choice for the treatment of penicillin failures or recurrent tonsillitis, but it will also be effective for initial therapy.

COMPARISON OF ORAL CEPHALOSPORINS WITH PENICILLIN THERAPY FOR GROUP A STREPTOCOCCAL PHARYNGITIS

Stillerman M *Pediatr Infect Dis* 1986;5(6):649

This is a review of the literature on cephalosporin therapy for strep throat as well as a prospective study of 104 children with proven streptococcal pharyngitis who were randomly assigned to receive either oral cefaclor or penicillin VK for 10 days. The bacteriological failure rate for the cephalosporin was 14 percent, compared with 30 percent for penicillin. The clinical response to both drugs was satisfactory and similar, and neither had unacceptable side effects. The author reviewed four earlier studies on the initial use of cephalosporins for streptococcal pharyngitis and concluded that in all studies these drugs were consistently more effective than penicillin, but the small number of patients did not allow a statistical significance to be calculated. When the author combined the data of previous studies, a 11 percent failure rate was noted for cephalosporins and a 23 percent failure rate for penicillin, a highly significant difference when this meta-analysis was performed (P<0.001). Based on the combined data, the author concludes that all cephalosporins are more effective than penicillin for the treatment of strep throat.

COMMENT: This author is from the department of pediatric infectious diseases at the State University of New York at Stony Brook, and in his opinion the failure rate with penicillin is unacceptable. An oral cephalosporin is favored as a first-line drug. Despite good results with cefaclor, the author prefers cephalexin (Keflex) because of a cost analysis and a slightly better safety profile. This is one of a few articles that takes a strong stand in favor of cephalosporins as initial therapy, but the majority of papers I reviewed disagree with using cephalosporins as initial therapy in uncomplicated cases. I have no particular argument with this opinion, and the statistics make a good case if the end point is a bacteriological cure rate. Cefadroxil as once-a-day therapy is the most logical route if one is choosing a cephalosporin.

Brook (*Clin Pediatr* 1985;24(6):331) was able to demonstrate beta latamase production in an amazing 96 percent of patients with a history of recurrent tonsillitis (not first time, easily cured infection) with GABHS. His study demonstrated the superiority of clindamycin (Cleocin) over penicillin or erythromycin in lowering the recurrence rate of tonsillitis. The recurrence rate over 18 months was quite high (higher than most studies) and consisted of the following: penicillin, 86 percent; erythromycin, 57 percent, and only seven percent of those receiving clindamycin. This author suggests clindamycin is superior to penicillin in those with severe recurrent tonsillitis in whom beta-lactamase production is demonstrated. (Of course, no one would routinely assay for penicillinase.)

The cost of new antibiotics is always of some concern. Private pharmacy prices are all over the map, and you should always urge patients to shop around. Generics are not available for many of the most expensive drugs, but

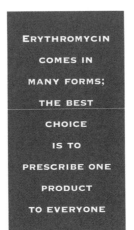

ERYTHROMYCIN COMES IN MANY FORMS; THE BEST CHOICE IS TO PRESCRIBE ONE PRODUCT TO EVERYONE

many cephalosporins are now off patent; as of this writing, there is no generic for cefadroxil. On a practical basis, it seems silly to argue the difference between $40 for a prescription vs. $10 if the cheaper drug doesn't work, requires a repeat ED visit within six months, or even if a repeat throat culture is necessary to check for cure rates. In the long run, the more expensive antibiotic may actually be cheaper. It seems clear that patients who come to the ED with recurrent strep throat (defined loosely as two or more episodes per year) should not be treated with multiple courses of penicillin, and you should probably forgo even an initial try with penicillin. I would currently choose cefadroxil in this situation.

There is little doubt that numerous cephalosporins adequately treat a strep throat, and every drug rep has an article touting his brand. A recent meta-analysis (*Pediatr Infect Dis J* 1991;10:276) supported cephalosporins as initial therapy, but a criticism of the work is that many of the included studies had methodological flaws. The price issue is no longer a major concern with many generics available. I have no problem with cephalosporins as initial therapy, but they are often overkill from a microbiological view. So far, there is no evidence that penicillin has lost its therapeutic edge against strep.

IN VITRO SUSCEPTIBILITY OF RECENT NORTH AMERICAN GROUP A STREPTOCOCCAL ISOLATES TO ELEVEN ORAL ANTIBIOTICS

Coonan KM, Kaplan EL
Pediatr Infect Dis J 1994;13(7):630

The authors of this study attempted to investigate possible antibiotic resistance of strep to commonly prescribed antibiotics. They determined the minimum inhibitory concentration of 11 antibiotics to 282 pharyngeal isolates from patients with strep throat from 31 states, with specimens collected over a three-year period (1989-92). The study was prompted by a resurgence of serious GABHS infections and their sequelae. The susceptibility of 43 isolates from severe invasive strep infections ("flesh-eating bacteria") was also studied.

All the isolates were exquisitely sensitive to low doses of penicillin, but a few strains (4%) were resistant to erythromycin and the newer marcrolides, azithromycin and clarithromycin. Cephalosporins exhibited varying potencies, but all strains were sensitive to cephalothin, cefixime, cefaclor, cefpodoxime, and clindamycin. Clindamycin probably performed best. Interestingly, there was no difference in susceptibility between the simple pharyngeal pathogens and the strains associated with severe infections. Resistance was common to tetracyclines and ciprofloxacin, making these drugs ineffective. The authors conclude that streptococci are not developing resistance to penicillin, and there is no need to alter the standard penicillin/erythromycin approach to a simple strep throat.

COMMENT: This study would indicate that penicillin, even in very modest oral doses, will cure a strep throat as well as the broader spectrum antibiotics. Interestingly, a few strains were resistant to all of the macrolides, so prescribing clarithromycin (Biaxin) or azithromycin (Zithromax) over erythromycin won't cure more patients, but may make them a bit poorer, albeit less ill from the therapy. Clindamycin is a good cephalosporin in vitro, but it has more significant side effects than caphalexin or cefadroxil. These data would lend credence to the theory that failure to eradicate strep from the throat is due to

ANTIBIOTIC ALTERNATIVES FOR STREPTOCOCCAL PHARYNGITIS

Drug	Dose*	Comments
Penicillin	• 1.2 mu Benzathine - single dose • 1 gm Pen VK (oral BID) • 250 mg Pen VK (oral QID) rash common	• Still drug of choice for uncomplicated infections • No rationale for amoxicillin or ampicillin;
Erythromycin	• Erythromycin base 250-333 mg TID • Erythromycin estolate 20-30 mg/kg/day • Erythromycin ethylsuccinate/stearate 40 mg/kg/day • May use BID regimen (about 1 gm/day)	• Drug of choice in penicillin anaphylaxis • As effective as penicillin • Resistance an issue outside U.S. • GI side effects common • No single preparation consistently better tolerated • Careful of drug-drug interaction, especially theophylline
Azithromycin/ Clarithromycin	• Standard doses • Efficacy similar to erythromycin and may be better tolerated	• Not first-line • Not well studied
Cephalosporins	• Cephalexin 1 gm BID or 500 mg QID • Cefadroxil 1 gm/day or 500 mg BID • Cefaclor, cefuroxime, cefpodoxime, and cefixime have been successful • Ceftriaxone not recommended	• All types have equal or slightly better laboratory cure rates compared to penicillin; clinical cure rate similar • Recommended for recurrent infections • Cefaclor has higher incidence of skin rashes and GI side effects • Single daily dose of cefadoroxil attractive
Quinolones	Not recommended	• Poor activity against strep
Tetracycline	Not recommended	• Resistance common
Sulfa/Trimethoprim	Not recommended	

*10-day course recommended for all oral antibiotics.

Source: James R. Roberts, MD.

coexisting penicillinase-producing bacteria in the respiratory tract. I don't think cefaclor is a good alternative; it's the cephalosporin most commonly associated with side effects, especially allergic reactions and serum sickness.

In a recent study of antibiotic sensitivity, Kelley et al (*Clin Pediatr* 1993;32:744) found that of 187 strep isolates, all were sensitive to penicillin. None were fully resistant to erythromycin, but five percent had intermediate susceptibility.

Significant erythromycin resistance has been documented in Finland and Japan (20%-60%), enough to render the drug useless in that country (*Am J Dis Child* 1979; 133(11):1143 and *N Engl J Med* 1991;326:292). Resistance to erythromycin does not seem to be a significant problem in this country; it's still only about five percent. The concern over erythromycin resistance should not limit its use for those who like the drug.

ORAL ERYTHROMYCIN

Med Let Drugs Ther 1985;27(678):1

This is a review of all the available oral erythromycins as of 1985. I am unaware of any significant additions to the list since then, so I believe this is still an impartial and important review. With regard to bioavailability, many advertisers claim superior serum concentration from their products. Such claims are difficult to prove because of study methodology problems and conflicting and even contradicting results, but the entire issue of bioavailability is probably moot. Most pathogens susceptible to oral erythromycin are killed in relatively low concentrations and all preparations are absorbed well enough to reach serum concentrations high enough to be effective. In fact, the authors were unable to find a single study that demonstrated a clinical failure with erythromycin due to inadequate bioavailability. However, erythromycin estolate may be more bioavailable and thus require a lower dose than erythromycin ethylsuccinate or stearate.

The major problems with oral erythromycin are gastrointestinal intolerance and drug-drug interactions. GI distress is quite common, and it often causes patients to discontinue the drug; it can make them quite ill. In the authors' opinion, there are no data indicating that any type of erythromycin or any particular brand causes less GI toxicity than another. All can cause abdominal cramps, vomiting, and diarrhea, and even pseudomembranous colitis has been reported. Other adverse side effects include cholestatic hepatitis, a condition related to the estolate (Ilosone) formulation. Hepatitis can occur with the ethylsuccinate and transient deafness has also been reported.

Of specific importance is the effect of erythromycin on the hepatic metabolism of commonly used drugs, including theophylline, warfarin, digoxin, and carbamazepine. For example, patients with asthma who take theophylline may become theophylline toxic when given erythromycin for bronchitis, due to inhibition of the theophylline clearance. The authors conclude there is no evidence that any erythromycin formulation is more effective or better tolerated in adults than another. They suggest the use of estolate for children but advise that this formulation not be used for adults because of the risk of hepatitis.

COMMENT: Erythromycin is available in a number of tablet and suspension forms: erythromycin base and enteric coated (E-mycin, ERYC, Ery-tabs); erythromycin stearate (Erythrocin), estolate (Ilosone), and ethylsuccinate (E.E.S., Pediazole); and a parenteral form. It's almost impossible to keep these drugs straight in your mind, so the best thing to do is to choose one erythromycin product that you can prescribe to everyone. My choice is to write for erythromycin base, and let the pharmacist decide which preparation to use. Interestingly, I came across two studies that suggested that the enteric-coated form produces the most GI side effects. The advertising for better GI tolerance of some products is probably hype, but it's clear that many patients cannot tolerate this drug. To decrease GI side effects, use a smaller dose and give it after meals. Almost 75 percent of patients on higher doses will have bothersome side effects. One study reported an amazing 28 percent dropout rate due to side effects with 1.5 g/day but only nine percent discontinuance with 1 g/day.

To sidestep problems with erythromycin, my first alternative to penicillin is usually a cephalosporin. I don't usually prescribe erythromycin for the initial treatment of strep throat unless the patient has a convincing hisotiry of a severe allergy to penicillin. With true allergy, it's the drug of choice. Those little red bumps many people get with amoxicillin/ampicillin are not an allergy, but it's often difficult to be sure because patients are convinced that they are allergic and rarely know the details. I have never seen a patient with a penicillin allergy have a reaction to a cephalosporin, and this concern is likely overdone. Although there is some allergic crossover, most physicians believe cephalosporins are safe unless penicillin anaphylaxis has occurred.

One argument for the use of erythromycin for acute pharyngitis (without a culture) is that it will cover *Mycoplasma* and *Chlamydia,* but this clinical dilemma is far from solved. McDonald found no great advantage of treating adults with nonspecific (non-strep) pharyngitis with erythromycin (*J Infect Dis* 1985;152(6):1093).

Hovi (*Scand J Infect Dis* 1987;19(6):651) demonstrated that erythromycin was effective for the treatment of acute strep throat, with a 90 percent cure rate. It was equally effective when given as 500 mg BID or 250 mg QID, but side effects occurred more commonly with the higher dose so don't prescribe more than 1 g/day.

SECTION VIII

TENDON DISORDERS

DIAGNOSING ACHILLES TENDON RUPTURE

The Thompson test is the only definitive method for diagnosing ruptures of the Achilles tendon

Although rupture of the Achilles tendon is a somewhat rare entity, the practicing emergency physician will surely see (or miss) an occasional case during a busy year. A very disabling injury, Achilles tendon rupture (ATR) requires prompt diagnosis and treatment. A major pitfall in emergency medicine is that this injury is often not appreciated on the first visit. Patients with ATR rarely complain of a specific problem with the function of this tendon but simply present with pain and a limp, telling the triage nurse that they have a sprained ankle. The unwary physician can easily be lulled into agreeing with the patient's misdiagnosis, and can treat a major injury like a minor sprain. This chapter discusses the clinical features of Achilles tendon rupture and review diagnostic considerations and therapeutic modalities.

COMPLETE ACHILLES TENDON RUPTURES

Landvater ST, Renstrom PA
Clin Sports Med 1992;11(4):741

This is a recent and extensive review of the problem of Achilles tendon rupture. Although it was probably written for orthopedics surgeons, it certainly puts the problem into perspective for emergency physicians. ATR has been recognized since the 1500s. Although there are no epidemiologic studies on its incidence, it appears to be an increasing problem, although this may reflect more accurate diagnosis or better reporting techniques. Interestingly, this is a disease of seemingly healthy, relatively young patients, occurring at a mean age of 35 years. This age group is significantly lower than the age for other types of tendon rupture. The injury usually occurs during recreational sports where sudden acceleration or jumping is required. Basketball and racquet sports seem to be the most common ways to obtain this injury. Curiously, ATR is uncommon in well-trained athletes and usually occurs in sporadically active, nonprofessional athletes who intermittently participate in vigorous sports activities ("weekend athletes"). The authors note the increased incidence is in professionals and white collar workers who have a sedentary occupation. ATR is clearly more common in men, with the ratio being about 4:1 to 10:1, males: females.

Many authors have noted the tendency for ATR to occur following steroid use (injection or oral) or in those with degenerative diseases. However, most injuries occur *de novo*, without known preexisting medical problems or symptoms of tendinitis.

The pathogenesis of ATR is unclear. Because the tensile strength of a tendon is normally significantly greater than that of a muscle belly, it is presumed that the Achilles tendon ruptures before the calf muscles tear because the tendon is weakened. Achilles tendons classically rupture 2-6 centimeters proximal to their insertion to the calcaneus, rather than at the expected site of rupture, the weaker insertion site. This observation is further evidence for pre-existing tendon pathology. From a pathologic standpoint, many tendons demonstrate degenerative changes, termed tendinosis. Importantly, tendinosis is asymptomatic, usually only demonstrating itself by rupture. Tendinosis is often calcific, lipoid, or mucoid in nature, and is probably the result of chronic hypoxic changes. The blood supply to the tendon is poorest in the area that most commonly ruptures. It's postulated that a sedentary lifestyle and the aging process decreases blood supply, creates hypoxia, and results in degenerative changes that predispose to rupture. The observation that the majority of patients have no symptoms of tendinitis or dysfunction

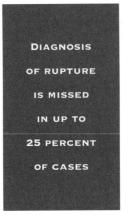

DIAGNOSIS OF RUPTURE IS MISSED IN UP TO 25 PERCENT OF CASES

prior to rupture supports this theory. (In a report of 292 cases of ATR by Jozsa (*Am J Sports Med* 1989;17(3):338), all of the tendons studied histologically demonstrated degenerative changes.)

Most patients who experience ATR report a sudden pop or snap in the foot that is accompanied by pain. The pain may resolve spontaneously or be minimal after the initial event. A common complaint is a feeling of being kicked from behind. A defect in the tendon may be palpated in the acute stages, but edema or hemorrhage quickly obscure the gap. The Thompson test (discussed later) is a particularly useful diagnostic test, but it is unknown to

many physicians.

The diagnosis of ATR is missed in up to 25 percent of patients by the initial examiner. The authors emphasize that a completely ruptured Achilles tendon may have one very misleading feature on physical exam. Specifically, the patient is able to actively plantar flex the foot if no resistance is applied because numerous other muscles (toe flexors, peroneus) also perform this function. Standard radiographs are useful to rule out fracture but cannot be used to diagnose ATR. Ultrasound and MRI will demonstrate disruption of soft tissue planes. There are occasional false positive and false negative tests with ultrasound, but MRI is diagnostic. These expensive tests are usually not required because the clinical diagnosis is easily confirmed by the examiner once the condition is considered.

The objectives in treating ATR are to restore normal length and function. Both surgical and nonsurgical approaches have been advocated. There is controversy in the literature as to the preferred modality, and options include immediate surgical repair or long-term casting. A re-rupture is a known complication of unsuccessful therapy. The re-rupture rate is highest (up to 30%) with non-surgical treatment. Other complications include skin and tissue necrosis, nerve damage, infection, venous thrombosis, and rarely pulmonary embolism. Some

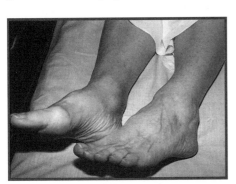

This elderly woman came to the ED complaining of pain in the ankle after stepping up to a curb. The triage note stated sprained ankle. She was able to walk with a limp and had minimal pain. Note the soft tissue swelling about the ankle. X-rays were negative, and she was able to weakly plantar flex the foot. Such an injury could be mistaken for a simple sprain. See color plate in center well.

authors prefer nonoperative therapy, consisting of casting the foot in equinus, but surgery seems to get the therapeutic nod by most specialists. Significant functional disability can occur if the tendon is lengthened by therapy. Casting is generally restricted to the non-athletic patient or the weekend athlete, particularly if he is more than 50 years of age.

COMMENT: Fortunately, emergency physicians need not become embroiled in the treatment controversies of ATR, but they should be expert in suspecting the injury, making the diagnosis, and instituting proper and timely referral. As with any soft injury where surgery is an option, a delay of even a few days can result in complications and poor results, so this is not a condition that can be allowed to declare itself days to weeks later by producing continued pain and dysfunction. It is imperative that the emergency physician make this diagnosis in the ED on the first visit and obtain immediate referral, allowing the orthopedic surgeons to hash out the details of the most efficacious treatment. An Achilles tendon rupture is an injury with major morbidity, even in the best of hands, and the average time lost from work is two to four months. The reader is referred to Wills et al for a detailed discourse on therapy (*Clin Orthop* 1986;207:156).

It is important to note that ATR is an injury that occurs predominantly in healthy young to middle-aged males who usually present with signs and symptoms of a sprained foot or ankle. Only 10 to 20 percent have any symptoms in the Achilles area prior to complete rupture, so a major tendon injury may not be suspected by the inexperienced clinician. Often a pop or snap is heard or felt, but this sensation also occurs with lateral ankle sprains and a number of other non-important ligamentous injuries. Although the patient usually has pain and swelling in the posterior ankle, a superficial examination will localize the pain in areas commonly injured by less serious inversion or eversion injuries.

In my experience, the defect in the tendon can only be felt about half the time, so this is an unreliable clinical finding. One might intuitively think that patients with a complete Achilles tendon rupture would be unable to stand on the toes, but this is also not a totally reliable finding. While only a few patients can actually stand on the toes, all can certainly plantar flex the foot when asked to do so in the ED, especially while sitting in a chair or lying on a stretcher where gravity can help. Plantar flexion may be weak, but it is always possible because structures other than the Achilles tendon will still be intact. Radiographs are useful to rule out fractures and other injuries, but the diagnosis cannot be supported or ruled out with plain films.

Although many patients will give a history of onset of pain during a sports activity that includes lunging, jumping, or acceleration (soccer, basketball, tennis, gymnastics, and handball), the injury can occur from simply walking briskly, stepping off the curb, or pushing a car. The association of Achilles tendon rupture and steroid use is interesting, and it should be a well-known axiom that weight-bearing tendons — such as the Achilles and patellar ten-

don — are rarely injected with steroids because this may weaken the tendons. Although steroid injections work wonders for tendinitis about the shoulder or elbow, such injections to tendons around the knee and ankle should not be part of the ED routine.

Some authors go to great lengths to distinguish other causes of pain in the Achilles area. Generally, distinguishing rupture from inflammatory disorders is all that is required (or possible) in the ED. Clearly there are other causes of pain in this area besides tendon rupture. (See the excellent review by Plattner, *Postgrad Med* 1989;86(3): 155.) Achilles tendinitis can cause pain in the posterior ankle. There is some debate whether this common symptom seen in runners is an actual inflammatory process or microtears. So-called tendinitis is actually a peritendinitis because the Achilles has no true synovial sheath. There is also a superficial and deep bursa around the insertion of the Achilles tendon that can be inflamed from mechanical processes, especially from wearing high heels, and a painful condition termed "pump bumps" has been described. Regardless of the exact pathophysiology, once tendon rupture is ruled out, pain in the Achilles tendon area is treated conservatively with rest, local heat, and NSAIDs. Steroids

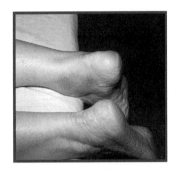

In addition to swelling about the malleoli, there is ecchymosis and swelling posteriorly, but this was not appreciated until the patient got out of the wheelchair and onto the stretcher. A palpable defect in the Achilles tendon could not be appreciated due to swelling. See color plate in center well.

should not be given routinely because they may weaken the tendon and predispose to subsequent rupture.

From a diagnostic standpoint, once the condition is considered, one should be able to confirm ATR in the ED from the history and by clinical examination. Authors have commented on the ability of ultrasound (*AJR Am J Roentgenol* 1988;151:127) and MRI (*Am J Sports Med* 1989;17:333) to diagnose Achilles tendon rupture, but the astute emergency physician should be able to spot this one from across the room; it's a bona fide "doorway diagnosis."

From an ED treatment standpoint, all patients should

be referred to a specialist. Because casting is a viable option, outpatient follow-up is reasonable, but a proper splint must be applied. For a soft tissue injury of the foot or ankle, the ankle is usually placed in a posterior splint at 90 degrees, but for an Achilles rupture, the foot should be plantar flexed. Plantar flexion limits tendon lengthening while healing, a complication that results in significant dysfunction. I prefer to use a bivalve plaster splint consisting of a short leg anterior and posterior splint, with crutches to prohibit touchdown. Importantly, patients cannot be given an Ace bandage or sugar tong splint and told to arrange their own follow-up; it's best if the EP personally arranges specific follow-up.

BILATERAL ACHILLES TENDON RUPTURE: AN UNUSUAL OCCURRENCE

Hanlon DP *J Emerg Med* 1992;10(5):559

This is a case report that discusses spontaneous bilateral Achilles tendon rupture, an unusual but previously reported injury. The patient was a healthy 33-year-old man who complained of pain in the lower legs following a hard landing on his forefeet in a skydiving exhibition. He experienced a sharp pull in the heel area upon landing, with palpable defects in the Achilles tendon and a diagnostic Thompson test bilaterally. Importantly and characteristically, the patient was able to plantar flex both feet. Radiographs were normal, and at operation bilateral Achilles tendon ruptures, occurring in the classic area 4-6 centimeters proximal to the calcaneal insertion, were documented. The authors note that this patient had not received previous steroid injections, was not on chronic oral steroid therapy, and had no underlying systemic diseases that would predispose to tendon weakness (rheumatoid arthritis, lupus, gout, renal failure, or metabolic abnormalities).

COMMENT: Other authors have reported bilateral ATR (*BMJ* 1961;1:1657; *Clin Orthop* 1986;213:249), but the condition has usually been associated with predisposing systemic diseases or chronic steroid use. This case is classic for ATR: the patient was a healthy male, age 30-40 years, who experienced a sudden force to the tendon. He

was able to plantar flex the feet, and the rupture occurred 4-6 cm proximal to the Achilles tendon insertion.

SPONTANEOUS RUPTURE OF TENDON OF ACHILLES: A NEW CLINICAL DIAGNOSTIC TEST

Thompson T, Doherty J *J Trauma* 1962;2:126

In this original article, Thompson and Doherty describe the now well-known Thompson test for diagnosing ATR. The authors note that the gastrocnemius muscle arises from two heads on the posterior femur and extends distally to form approximately one half of the Achilles tendon. The soleus muscle, originating from the posterior aspect of the tibia, blends with the gastrocnemius in the distal calf to complete the Achilles tendon. The test consists of squeezing the calf of the affected leg and noting if the foot will passively plantar flex. If the foot does not plantar flex, the test is positive and the Achilles tendon is ruptured.

Following an initial clinical observation, the authors tested their technique on freshly amputated limbs and found a similar result: the foot would plantar flex if only

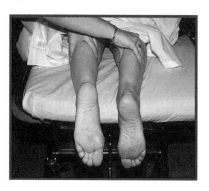

To perform the Thompson test, the patient is prone on the stretcher with the legs overhanging. The calf is squeezed briskly and motion of the foot is noted. In this case, one foot does not plantar flex. At operation, she had complete rupture of the Achilles tendon in the non-flexing foot. See color plate in center well.

a small portion of the tendon was intact, and the foot remained in neutral position with the squeeze maneuver when the tendon was completely cut.

To perform the test properly, the patient should be placed prone on a table with the feet extending over the end. The calf muscles are squeezed just distal to their widest girth and movement of the foot is observed. The unaffected foot serves as control. Thompson states that a positive test is the absence of plantar movement of the foot, indicating a rupture of the heel cord. In this original report, the squeeze test was accurate in 19 of 19 cases.

The authors also describe their experience with 47 cases

of spontaneous rupture of the Achilles tendon. They note that their patients' ages ranged from 20-72 years, but the majority were between 20-40. Most patients were male (42 males, five females). Most patients were white collar workers, and there were only three conditioned athletes in the group. No patient did heavy manual labor. The mechanism of injury was a sudden push-off in 29 cases, sudden dorsiflexion in 10, fall from a height in six, and struck from behind on the heel in one.

Importantly, 22 cases were initially misdiagnosed by the first physician, who believed the patients had a partial tear or simple sprain. The injury was not detected for up to four months in some patients. The clinical findings included calf swelling, palpable depression of the tendon, loss of plantar flexion, and loss of push-off. X-rays of the foot and ankle were of no diagnostic help. The most common site of rupture was a few inches proximal to the insertion to the Achilles tendon on the calcaneus. At operation, it was found that the basis for the squeeze test was rupture of the soleus portion alone. If the soleus was completely ruptured and a portion of the gastrocnemius remained intact, the test was still diagnostic.

The authors conclude that injuries to the Achilles tendon occur primarily in middle-aged white collar workers engaging in part-time athletics, but the diagnosis is often initially missed by physicians. The authors believe that rupture is almost always complete and that partial tears do not occur. The squeeze test, heretofore termed the Thompson test, is a valuable diagnostic sign of complete rupture, which is present in almost every case.

COMMENT: It has also been my experience that many physicians do not appreciate that partial tears of the Achilles tendon are uncommon events, and that such injuries are usually complete ruptures. Partial tears can theoretically occur, but I don't know how they can be diagnosed because operative repair is usually not considered. The Thompson test will be negative in partial injuries. Most review articles do not mention or discuss the concept of a partial tear. Perhaps a partial tear is what some term tendinitis.

Performing the Thompson test should be part of the evaluation of every patient with a sprained ankle or foot, and the clinician should approach this test in the manner specifically described by the author. If one attempts to evaluate Achilles tendon function by merely asking the patient to plantar flex the foot, the injury will invariably be missed.

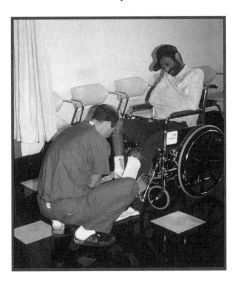

The best way to miss an Achilles tendon rupture is to examine a patient in the hallway in a wheelchair. This patient had a complete rupture, could plantar flex the foot while sitting, and was sent home with the diagnosis of a sprained ankle. See color plate in center well.

The Achilles tendon function is only isolated with the calf squeeze test. Importantly, one cannot adequately perform the Thompson test with a patient sitting in a chair or on the edge of the stretcher. Patients should be placed on their stomachs on a stretcher with the feet extended over the end of the stretcher. The mattress should go no further distally than the middle third of the lower leg to allow for free motion of the foot. Patients are told to relax and not to use any active motion. The examiner than briskly squeezes the calf with lateral and medial compression, and notes the presence or absence of passive plantar flexion of the foot. The intact tendon briskly plantar flexes the foot while the ruptured tendon allows no motion whatsoever. This is not a subtle test; when performed properly, the diagnosis is obvious to even the most inexperienced operator. The good foot can serve as a control, assuming, of course, that the pathology is not bilateral.

Although it may be possible to feel the defect in the tendon, this is not an accurate test. The patient may have complete ATR and not exhibit a palpable defect, especially if there is soft tissue swelling or hemorrhage. Finally, I have noted that ecchymosis around the posterior calcaneus is usually present, but I have not seen this described the literature. It may take a number of hours for the hemorrhage to be evident.

QUADRICEPS TENDON RUPTURE

QTR is relatively uncommon, but it should be suspected in all patients with knee trauma

Avoiding a potentially embarrassing misdiagnosis of Achilles tendon rupture, as I outlined in the last chapter, is as simple as checking for Achilles tendon function with the Thompson test in all patients who present with ankle and foot trauma. This chapter focuses on a similarly deceptive process in the knee, specifically quadriceps tendon rupture (QTR). It is a relatively uncommon injury, yet it is one that should be suspected and investigated in all patients who present with trauma to the knee. It's quite easy to mistake QTR for a simple knee sprain or minor hemarthrosis and to delay needed surgical repair of this significant tendon injury.

QUADRICEPS TENDON RUPTURE: A DIAGNOSTIC TRAP

Ramsey RH, Muller GE *Clin Orthop* 1970;70:161

Although this article is more than 20 years old, it is worth reading and one of the few I could find in the literature that specifically addresses QTR. The authors report their experience with 17 cases gathered over a 10-year period. They note that only 10 of the 17 patients were properly diagnosed and treated within the first week of injury. Treatment was delayed because the condition was not recognized by the initial examining physician. The authors emphasize the two clinically diagnostic criteria necessary to identify QTR: loss of ability to maintain the knee in full extension against gravity and a palpable soft tissue defect proximal to the superior pole of the patella. The condition is usually one of total rupture, but partial tears can occur. The disability noticed by the patient is buckling of the knees and inability to climb stairs or walk up an incline.

The authors stress that this frequently missed injury may not present in a dramatic fashion. Importantly, the knee may not be excessively painful or swollen, and plain x-rays are not diagnostic, usually being interpreted as normal. Most physicians readily examine for lateral stability and other ligamentous injuries and, finding none, diagnose this condition as a simple sprain. The problems associated with a delay in diagnosis are compounded because consultation is not routinely sought and follow-up is not rigorous.

The average age of the patients in this series was 56 years, reflecting the opinion that age-related degenerative change is a necessary predisposition for tendon rupture. Some type of degeneration of the tendon apparatus is usually noted when pathologic sections are taken. (This is similar to the degenerative condition tendonosis that was discussed in reference to Achilles tendon rupture in the last chapter.) The mechanism of injury is a forced flexion of the knee against quadriceps contraction. As may be expected, this condition occurs more commonly in obese individuals, but any body habitus is at risk. Often the patient forcibly contracts the quadriceps to prevent a fall or slip, resulting in a complete rupture even in the absence of an actual fall or direct trauma. Any portion of the tendon may be involved, and the injury usually extends to the medial and lateral fascial expansions. QTR usually affects one knee, but the process can be bilateral, as was described in three cases in this series.

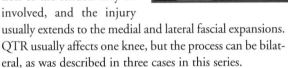

Treatment for QTR is surgical, and it is indicated as soon as the diagnosis is made. Surgery is followed by cast immobilization for about six weeks. When diagnosed and treated expeditiously, the final result is usually quite acceptable, and most patients have a normally functioning knee after a period of physical therapy.

COMMENT: I have seen about half a dozen cases of quadriceps tendon rupture over the past 20 years, and was initially introduced to this entity when I missed my first case. The usual scenario involves an elderly patient who has a minor fall without direct trauma, often walking up or down steps. It can occur after a relatively minor stress that would not suggest a major destructive mechanism, such as stepping up to a curb or getting out of a car. Another mechanism of injury that can occur in younger patients would be sporting activities involving jumping, like basketball or track, or as noted in one case in the series presented, jumping off a diving board.

QTR can be a subtle injury. Patients may not readily describe their dysfunction, knowing only that they cannot stand up. Pain is usually deceptively mild. During its initial stages, swelling may not be excessive or is confined to the suprapatellar area. In my experience, it is often difficult to appreciate a definite rent in the tendon. The same difficulty with trying to feel for a tendon disruption was noted for Achilles tendon rupture. Palpating the defect can

This elderly man tripped on a sidewalk but caught himself before he hit the ground. When he tried to walk, the leg consistently gave way. In the ED, the diagnosis was knee strain and hemarthrosis (note prep for arthrocentesis). The x-ray was normal except for soft tissue swelling. If one looks for it, the classic soft tissue defect superior to the patella is obvious, but in this case it was not initially appreciated. He could not lift his heel off the stretcher, but when put in a knee immobilizer and given crutches, he could walk quite well. See color plate in center well.

be especially deceptive if there is some associated swelling. The injury appears to many physicians as a strained knee with a hemarthrosis, and knees often are drained by arthrocentesis. If some blood is withdrawn, it confirms the missed diagnosis, but some taps are dry, and this may be a tip-off to the diagnosis. Although it may seem like a simple diagnostic maneuver, many physicians do not begin their examinations by asking patients to straight leg raise. If one examines the patient on a stretcher with only various lateral and anterior stress maneuvers and palpation for bony tenderness, the knee examination seems rather benign. If the nurse then puts on a knee immobilizer, the patient will be able to walk just fine because the brace takes the place of the quadriceps tendon. Occasionally an avulsion chip from the patella is noted, but x-rays usually look normal. If one compares both sides, there are possible subtle changes in patellar positioning and tissue planes, but this is usually impossible to appreciate if only one knee is x-rayed. The easiest ways to look for QTR are to have the supine patient raise the heel from the stretcher with the knee kept straight, assessing for ability to move the patella with quadriceps tightening, and to have the patient dangle the legs over the stretcher and extend them against gravity. However, pain from a number of injuries prohibits

A PROBLEM WITH QTR IN THE ELDERLY IS THAT THEY POORLY TOLERATE CASTING; PROLONGED IMMOBILIZATION CAN PREDISPOSE TO THROMBOSIS

patients from fully extending the knee in this position.

If the injury is suspected clinically, it is relatively simple to confirm the diagnosis with ultrasound. QTR would also be noted on an MRI scan, but it's easiest to obtain a study from the experienced ultrasonographer. However, unless the operator has experience, a lot of equivocal readings of the ultrasound will occur. It would be difficult to

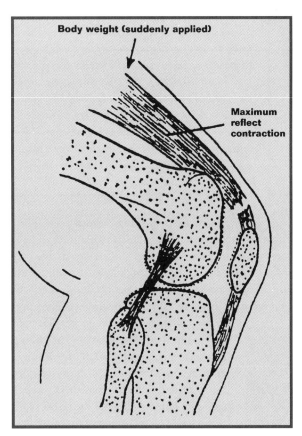

Body weight (suddenly applied)

Maximum reflect contraction

Site of quadriceps disruption in the adult with indirect force. Source: Clinical Orthopedics and Related Research, J.B. Lippincott Co., May-June 1970, No. 70, p. 163.

diagnose the less common partial rupture because function would remain intact. However, complete rupture is more common than a partial tear, and one should be careful about diagnosing "quadriceps strain," especially in an elderly patient who can't walk.

It is interesting that about half of the cases were initially misdiagnosed in this series. Similar data are found in other series. Hopefully, trained emergency physicians are clued in to this diagnosis and look for it routinely. It was disheartening, however, to review a number of emergency

medicine textbooks only to find QTR not mentioned or only briefly described. Although this is a relatively uncommon injury, it is certainly an embarrassing one to miss. All EPs should routinely consider QTR when examining injured knees.

BILATERAL SIMULTANEOUS RUPTURE OF THE QUADRICEPS TENDONS: A REPORT OF FOUR CASES AND REVIEW OF THE LITERATURE

Keogh P, et al *Clin Orthop* 1988;Sep (234):139-141

This article discusses the case histories of four patients with bilateral QTR. In the first case, a 70-year-old man jumped from a ladder and was unable to stand. He was admitted to the hospital and treated with physical therapy and was amazingly discharged without a definitive diagnosis. A month later, the diagnosis was finally made and surgical repair was performed. In the second case, a 71-year-old woman fell on the stairs and was unable to stand. She was correctly diagnosed with bilateral QTR and histology of the tendon was consistent with ischemic degeneration. In the third case, a 72-year-old man slipped on steps and experienced a tearing sensation in both knees. He could not stand, but his diagnosis was missed until 10 days later when he underwent surgery. In the last case, a 74-year-old woman experienced knee pain while walking. There was no specific severe sudden flexion injury in this case.

The authors note that a sudden collapse or weakness in both legs and the inability to stand should make one suspect bilateral QTR. They offer little in the way of a detailed description of the physical examination in their patients, but the underlying theme is that the patients could not stand. As noted by other authors, half of these cases were initially misdiagnosed. The patients in this report did not have significant degenerative diseases such as gout or rheumatoid arthritis, although these are considered predisposing conditions. Conservative therapy may result in partial function return, but when the knee is again stressed, rupture usually occurs.

COMMENT: I have seen two cases of bilateral QTR, and in my experience it is a rather obvious presentation. The majority of cases involve elderly patients with relatively minor flexion types of injuries with resulting inability to stand. Neither patient had swelling or significant pain. Elderly patients rarely strain or sprain ligaments or tendons so one should keep a high index of suspicion in this age group when there is disability and fractures are not seen. A similar orthopedic scenario is the elderly patient who falls and has hip pain. X-rays may look normal, but my rule is that any little old lady who has fallen and has hip pain has a fracture until ruled out by tomograms or CT scan. Plain x-rays are not sensitive enough to pick up subtle fractures in osteoporotic bones. I guess a general rule for QTR is that no patient should go home with bilateral knee immobilizers. Other authors (*J Bone Joint Surg [Br]* 1984;66(1):81; *Injury* 1977;8(4):315) have reported QTR as being bilateral. Most authors note that patients with this condition have an underlying metabolic disturbance, such as degenerative disease. Curiously, hyperparathyroidism is associated with QTR

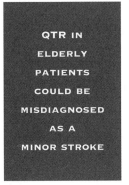

QTR IN ELDERLY PATIENTS COULD BE MISDIAGNOSED AS A MINOR STROKE

(*JAMA* 1972;221(4):406).

It may be difficult to make this diagnosis in confused, intoxicated, or aphasic patients or in those with conditions that do not allow them to explain their history or symptoms. Some authors note that because of the minimal trauma required to produce QTR in elderly patients, the inability to use the legs could be misdiagnosed as a minor stroke. Keep this in mind when you examine the next demented or post-cerebrovascular accident nursing home patient who had a minor fall and can't walk. As with most medical conditions, the diagnosis of QTR is easy when it is considered.

A problem with this condition in the elderly is that they poorly tolerate six weeks of casting. Prolonged immobilization leads to stiffness and can predispose to deep vein thrombosis.

DEFINITIVE TREATMENT FOR OLECRANON BURSITIS

Physicians often opt for a conservative approach while a more aggressive one of drainage and steroid injection should be routine

Although not a life-threatening or limb-threatening situation, patients with olecranon bursitis commonly visit the emergency department expecting accurate diagnosis and definitive treatment. One may simply refer them to the local orthopedic surgeon or rheumatologist, but there is no reason why this condition cannot be handled definitively in the ED.

Physicians who are familiar with the entity often opt for a conservative approach; however, once the diagnosis is made, I believe the EP should be more aggressive with olecranon bursitis and consider drainage and steroid injection as routine therapy. The only way to get in trouble with olecranon bursitis is to miss a case of septic bursitis, a condition that is usually quite evident on examination. Septic bursitis is, however, a potentially serious infection that requires more aggressive therapy and occasionally hospitalization. Olecranon bursitis is bread-and-butter clinical medicine, but it was difficult to find articles that specifically addressed this problem while emergency medicine textbooks often provided only a superficial discussion.

IDIOPATHIC OR TRAUMATIC OLECRANON BURSITIS. CLINICAL FEATURES AND BURSAL FLUID ANALYSIS

Canoso JJ *Arthritis Rheum* 1977;20(6):1213

This is a concise (but difficult to find) review of the clinical presentation of 30 consecutive cases of idiopathic olecranon bursitis (OB) and an analysis of the fluid that was withdrawn from the Bursal sac. All patients were treated at a veterans hospital so only male subjects were included. All patients underwent radiograph study (with comparison views) and Bursal fluid aspiration with subsequent fluid analysis and culture. Subjects were excluded if they had gout, rheumatoid arthritis or other systemic rheumatic diseases, or suspected infections. The average time for Bursal swelling to accumulate and prompt evaluation was 17 days, although some patients noted it for as long as six months. Repetitive trauma, such as leaning on the elbows or a minor blow to the olecranon area preceded the soft tissue swelling in the majority of cases, but some developed spontaneously and were termed idiopathic. The fluid collection was unilateral in all cases and was virtually painless and not tender. Minor pitting edema on the posterior aspect of the forearm was present in about half of the cases. X-rays demonstrated bony spurs in a third of the cases, but such defects were frequently seen in the unaffected arm. Non-specific calorific deposits were found in about a quarter of the patients.

Bursal fluid was drained by needle aspiration (specific technique not explained). In all cases the aspirated fluid was pink or bloody, and when spun down, the supernatant was xanthochromic. The WBC count in the fluid averaged 878/mm3 (range 50-4700 mm3). Mononuclear cells predominated, but erythrocytes, macrophages, lymphocytes, and polymorphonuclear cells were also noted. Fluid analysis demonstrated a glucose and protein level approximately 60-80 percent of corresponding serum values. Bilirubin and lactate dehydrogenase (LDH)levels were higher than serum, probably reflecting destroyed red cells. The characteristics of the bursal fluid did not correlate with the duration of the bursitis. The mucin clot test was rated poor or fair in all cases.

The authors speculate that trauma or recurrent intrabursal hemorrhage are somehow involved in the pathogenesis of olecranon bursitis, but the exact etiology has not been established. Most patients relate a history of minor trauma although the process can appear spontaneously in many cases.

COMMENT: Bursae are small fluid-filled sacs that are lined with a synovial membrane. They reduce friction between tendons and muscles, and there are about 150 throughout the body. Many are nameless, but the ones to come to the attention of physicians are the olecranon, prepatellar, subdeltoid, trochanteric, and anserine bursa.

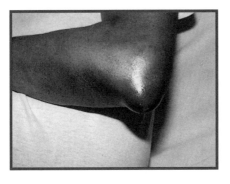

Typical presentation of nonseptic olecranon bursitis. This patient presented with a seven-day history of a soft, non-tender, non-painful swelling in the olecranon area. No specific trauma was recalled. The mass was fluctuant, and radiographs were normal.

Most of the time inflammation is sterile, but any type of bursitis can occasionally be septic. Physicians generally recognize bursitis in the shoulder or knee, but many cases of painful bursitis elsewhere are misdiagnosed as nonspecific musculoskeletal pain, tendonitis, arthritis, cellulitis, or strains/sprains.

Patients with nontender, nonpainful swellings over the olecranon occasionally present to the ED for an explanation of this rather peculiar structure and advice on treatment. Occasionally, they have a history of trauma, although in my experience, a specific traumatic event is rarely elicited. I think the majority of patients assume that they must have injured the area and erroneously indict an unrelated minor traumatic episode. I suspect that sitting at the local tavern is a common precipitating event when the elbow consistently comes in contact with the bar surface. An associated process, such as rheumatoid arthritis or gout, rarely can be identified, but the majority of patients do not have these predisposing conditions. The olecranon bursal distention can be quite impressive (golf-ball size) and there may be some surrounding edema, but the area is not hot, red, painful, or tender. The term

The preferred treatment for nonseptic olecranon bursitis is aseptic needle aspiration and instillation of long-acting steroids. To drain the bursa, hold the barrel of a 10 cc syringe parallel to the forearm and advance until fluid is aspirated via a 20 gauge needle. Note the classic serosanguinous fluid. With the needle still in the bursal sac, the syringe containing steroid is substituted for the aspirating syringe. See color plate in center well.

bursitis may actually be a misnomer because OB does not present like other painful inflammatory processes associated with the term.

I have not yet met a resident who could comfortably treat such conditions without obtaining an x-ray, but plain films are always worthless and can be deleted from routine therapy. The presence of a bony spur probably does not contribute to the etiology of fluid accumulation because the spur is often bilateral, present without the bursitis, or absent in the presence of bursitis. X-rays may be helpful if there is significant trauma involved, but obtaining one when there is little clinical evidence of olecranon fracture is certainly a waste of time and money. When significant trauma is present, the collection may actually be a hematoma and not merely synovial fluid.

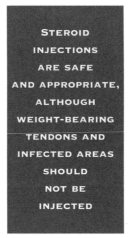

STEROID INJECTIONS ARE SAFE AND APPROPRIATE, ALTHOUGH WEIGHT-BEARING TENDONS AND INFECTED AREAS SHOULD NOT BE INJECTED

It is important to make the distinction between simple OB and septic bursitis. The olecranon bursa is the bursa most likely to become infected, but the presence of septic

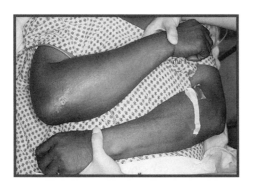

This patient has septic olecranon bursitis (cultures positive for S. aureus*). Note the skin defect from a previous trauma, the obvious diffuse cellulitic appearance, and the lack of a distinct fluctuant mass. The area was painful and tender. The patient was febrile. He failed outpatient treatment and required seven days of intravenous antibiotics for complete resolution. See color plate in center well.*

bursitis should be obvious on clinical examination. Infection mandates a completely different clinical approach. Findings that might suggest a septic process include significant bursal tenderness, an overlying abrasion or wound, redness, warmth, obvious surrounding cellulitis, and fever. Septic bursitis is usually a diffuse process that looks like other soft tissue infections, whereas OB is a localized and distinct non-painful fluid collection. Patients with septic bursitis have pain on extension and flexion of the elbow, but patients with simple nonseptic bursitis have painless full range of motion.

Although usually clinically obvious, in confusing cases one can attempt to make the distinction between septic and nonseptic bursitis by analyzing bursal fluid for cell count, Gram's stain, and culture. I emphasize that fluid analysis is helpful, but, except for cultures, not totally accurate. Infected bursae don't respond with high cell counts like infected joints. Nonseptic bursal fluid is characteristically xanthochromic, and septic fluid is often purulent, cloudy, or otherwise obviously infected. Infected bursal fluid should have a glucose less than 50 percent of serum levels, and the Gram's stain may be positive for organisms (but only in 60%-70%). Polymorphonuclear cells should be predominant.

In one review of 47 episodes of septic bursitis, Pien et al (*Orthopedics* 1991;14(9):981) noted that 72 percent of the cases occurred in the olecranon bursa. The other infections were located in the prepatellar bursa. Septic bursitis frequently had some predisposing trauma or occupational injury and/or immunocompromise, such as diabetes or long-term steroid therapy. Half of the patients had obvious surrounding cellulitis and lymphangitis, but only one-quarter were febrile. *Staphylococcus aureus* was isolated in 70 percent of the aspirates, although three patients had gram-negative infection and eight had mixed bacterial infections.

When the Gram's stain was done, almost 80 percent were negative for organisms. Only five patients had complete synovial fluid analysis, but the mean WBC count was surprisingly low, at 6110/mm3 following antibiotic therapy. All the patients had complete resolution of their infections without permanent sequelae. Half of the patients were hospitalized; the remaining were treated as outpatients with oral antibiotics. Antibiotic therapy was prolonged to about four weeks. This report emphasizes the cellulitis aspect of olecranon septic bursitis, but comments on the low WBC count in aspirated fluid, the need for fluid culture, and the need to treat for an extended period with antistaphylococcal antibiotics.

Septic bursitis is best treated with an antistaphylococcal penicillin (oxacillin, dicloxacillin). Cephalosporins may work, but penicillins are known to concentrate in bursal fluid. In the nonimmunocompromised patient who is not toxic, outpatient therapy can be considered. Treatment should continue for 12-14 days, and resistant cases should be hospitalized for intravenous antibiotics. Surgical incision or removal of the bursa may be required in selected cases.

Smith et al (*Arch Intern Med* 1989;149(7):1581) studied the surface temperature of the skin overlying the olecranon bursa as a method to differentiate septic from nonseptic cases. They demonstrated a skin temperature difference between the involved and contralateral side as being of diagnostic importance. Although this may be of some help, I believe that the distinction is usually clinically obvious. Perhaps the infrared thermometer could have application here?

TREATMENT OF NONSEPTIC OLECRANON BURSITIS. A CONTROL, BLINDED PROSPECTIVE TRIAL

Smith DL, et al *Arch Intern Med* 1989;149(11):2527

This is a prospective blinded trial comparing treatment protocols in patients with nonseptic olecranon bursitis. This is the first prospective double-blind placebo controlled trial, and it examines various anecdotal therapies prescribed in 42 cases. All patients were males (mean age 60 years) who were seen at a veterans hospital during one year. The diagnosis of nonseptic olecranon bursitis was based on surface skin temperature, analysis of bursal fluid, Gram's stain, crystal examination, and fluid cultures. Following bursal fluid aspiration with aseptic technique, patients were randomized into one of four treatment regimens:

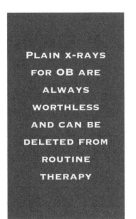

PLAIN X-RAYS FOR OB ARE ALWAYS WORTHLESS AND CAN BE DELETED FROM ROUTINE THERAPY

- Methylprednisolone acetate (20 mg) by intrabursal injection and oral naproxen (500 mg BID for 10 days).
- Methylprednisolone injection and oral placebo.
- Oral naproxen alone.
- Oral placebo.

All patients were instructed to wear a compression dressing around the elbow continuously for 10 days. Patients were examined at 1, 3, and 6 weeks and six months post-treatment.

Subjects treated with intrabursal steroid demonstrated significantly less bursal swelling than patients receiving either the oral NSAID alone or placebo. Adding naproxen to the steroid injection did not influence the clinical

course. During the six months, re-aspiration of the bursal fluid was necessary in some patients. The mean number of repeated aspirations per patient treated with intrabursal methylprednisolone (with or without naproxen) was only 0.1. Patients treated with the oral NSAID alone or placebo required 1 and 0.4 mean aspirations respectively. No patient developed adverse effects from the treatment, and there was no evidence of skin or subcutaneous atrophy or secondary infection with intrabursal steroids. The authors conclude that intrabursal injection of methylprednisolone is superior to other regimens in controlling fluid accumulation in olecranon bursitis. If the steroid is used, the addition of an oral NSAID is of no clinical benefit. Steroid injection is less expensive than prolonged treatment with NSAIDs, and it also avoids potential GI and renal complications.

COMMENT: This report indicates that following complete aspiration of the olecranon bursa, a single steroid injection with long-acting methylprednisolone acetate (such as Depo-Medrol) is superior to other treatment modalities. There is no need to include supplemental NSAID therapy. Concerns over steroid injections, such as predisposing to infection or causing skin atrophy, were not seen in this study. Other authors have, however, noted these complications with steroid instillation (*Ann Rheum Dis* 1984;43(1):44).

In my limited noncontrolled experience, patients treated with any method other than steroid injection were likely to experience recurrent fluid accumulation. Emergency physicians are generally reluctant to use steroid injections in patients with tendonitis or bursitis, despite the fact that such therapies are safe, easy, and often associated with a miraculous recovery. I think this reticence is largely due to insecurity about the diagnosis and lack of familiarity with soft tissue injection techniques. Injecting tendonitis/bursitis is actually a rather simple straightforward technique. When mixed with lidocaine or saline to increase volume, the steroid can be infiltrated into the general area of pain and need not be as anatomically exact as the neophyte might expect. Certainly, any orthopedic surgeon would not hesitate to consider steroid injections under such circumstances and emergency physicians should offer the same chance for a cure to their patients.

As long as one uses common sense, steroid injections

are very safe and very appropriate. A few caveats should be mentioned. First, one should never inject major weight-bearing tendons, such as patellar or Achilles tendon, injection should be limited to a single time, and one should make sure one is not injecting an infected area. When it comes to olecranon bursitis, the approach is technically easy. One can easily differentiate infection from non-infection, this is not a weight-bearing structure, and generally a single injection is curative.

Prior to steroid injection, the olecranon bursa should be completely drained of fluid. This is best accomplished by using 20 gauge needle and 10 cc syringe. Be sure to maintain sterile technique. I usually anesthetize the skin with lidocaine, but it's not a very painful process. The barrel of the syringe is held parallel to the forearm and advanced to the center of the fluid collection. Fluid is withdrawn until the bursa completely collapses. This fluid is classically serosanguinous and clear. With the needle tip left in the bursal sac to ensure intrabursal injection of the steroid, the aspirating syringe is disconnected and the steroid-containing syringe is attached to the needle nub.

Methylprednisolone acetate in a dose of 20-40 mg is a standard regimen. I prefer to add a few milliliters of saline or lidocaine to increase the volume. This re-expands the bursa and can be disconcerting to both patient and physician, but this swelling will subside over the next day. An Ace bandage is then applied to administer continuous pressure. I personally do not add oral NSAIDs to my therapy, and do not make a routine referral or follow-up visit. Patients are referred to their primary care physicians or given the name of an orthopedic surgeon for follow-up if the fluid should recur.

For the majority of cases, there is no need to order routine x-rays or to send the aspirated fluid for analysis. Fluid analysis is not an accurate way to rule in infection, and it is certainly a waste of time and money to order glucose, protein and cell counts, and Gram's stains on fluids drained from an asymptomatic site. If done, cell counts greater than 5,000/mm3 suggest infection, but the cell count varies considerably and is not diagnostic. Some physicians routinely send fluid for culture only and those seem reasonable data to have if the patient returns.

ZEROING IN ON DE QUERVAIN'S TENOSYNOVITIS

Definitive treatment is long-acting steroid injection, which has virtually no disadvantages

Although there are many reasons why patients present to the emergency department with pain in the wrist, de Quervain's tenosynovitis (or de Quervain's disease) is one entity whose diagnosis and treatment should be familiar to all emergency physicians. de Quervain's disease is an inflammatory tendonitis, and the diagnosis is made entirely by clinical examination. Once recognized, it is relatively easy to treat if one chooses to take the definitive step: steroid injection. With other inflammatory conditions, such as olecranon bursitis, many emergency physicians are unfamiliar with the techniques of steroid injection and shy away from using them even though this therapy is quite simple and can be remarkably effective. I strongly believe that all emergency physicians should become skilled in the diagnosis and treatment of tendonitis and bursitis, and this means becoming familiar with the use of injectable steroids.

de Quervain's disease is commonly misdiagnosed as a wrist sprain or arthritis, and the literature is relatively sparse on the subject. I could find only a few references in the emergency medicine literature. This entity is bound to show up in your emergency department a few times each year, but the findings are not impressive and are easily dismissed as a nonspecific minor non-emergency. I'm sure the diagnosis of de Quervain's disease is commonly missed, usually because it's not considered.

DE QUERVAIN'S DISEASE

Field JH *Am Fam Physician* 1979;20(1):103

This general overview of de Quervain's tenosynovitis was written for family practitioners, but it has relevance to emergency physicians who are also likely to see this pathology. de Quervain's disease is named after the Swiss physician who first described the disease in 1895. The process is a tenosynovitis of the abductor pollicis longus and extensor pollicis brevis tendons of the wrist. In the distal radius, a tunnel is formed in the bone through which these tendons pass. The tendons are enclosed by sheaths, and they are surrounded by the radius bone and covered by fascia, so the tendons run in an osseofiborus tunnel. Either tendon or both are subject to inflammation as a result of the repeated use of the thumb. The key symptom of de Quervain's disease is pain with use of the thumb. Patients also describe an aching pain at rest that is referred to the radial side of wrist and occasionally up

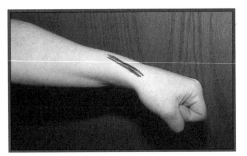

de Quervain's tenosynovitis produces pain in the radial aspect of the wrist due to inflammation of the abductor pollicis longus and extensor pollicis brevis tendons. Pain may radiate up the forearm or into the thumb, but it is maximal at the radial styloid (area marked). See color plate in center well.

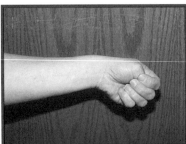

Finkelstein's test involves grasping the thumb in the palm and ulnar deviation of the wrist. When the pain is reproduced, this test is sensitive for de Quervain's disease, but it's probably not very specific. See color plate in center well.

near the radial styloid. The pain is often quite striking, and the patient may resist doing this test a second time. One may also reproduce the pain by passively flexing the thumb. Because of its location, de Quervain's disease is confused with arthritis of the carpal-metacarpal joint of the thumb, an occult fracture, cellulitis, or other types of tendon inflammation, such as gonococcal, tenosynovitis, or soft tissue contusion. The author of this report states that an osteoarthritic joint — the most common misdiag-

the arm or into the distal thumb. (Figure 1.)

The diagnosis is confirmed clinically by performing Finkelstein's test. (Figure 2.) To perform this test, the patient's thumb is held in the palm by the fingers and the wrist is ulnar deviated. This produces a diagnostic pain

nosis — will demonstrate pain if the physician pulls the thumb with longitudinal traction combined with gentle back and forth rotation, whereas this will not produce pain in patients with de Quervain's disease. Also, patients with significant arthritis will often have changes on radiographs.

INJECTABLE CORTICOSTEROIDS

Intrasynovial Preparations	Trade Name	Strength per ml	Range of Usual Dosage
Hydrocortisone tebutate	Hydrocortisone TBA	50 mg	12.5-75 mg
Prednisolone tebutate	Hydeltra TBA	20 mg	5.0-30 m
Methylprednisolone acetate	Depo-Medrol	20 mg	4.0-30 mg
Triamcinolone acetonide	Kenalog-40	40 mg	4.0-40 mg
Triamcinolone diacetate	Aristocort Forte	40 mg	4.0-40 mg
Triamcinolone hexacetonide	Aristospan	20 mg	4.0-25 mg
Betamethasone acetate and disodium phosphatate	Celestone Soluspan	6 mg	1.5- 6 mg
Dexamethasone acetate	Decadron-La	8 mg	0.8- 4 mg

A number of long-acting steroids are available for injection therapy of tendonitis. Patients should be warned that occasionally pain is made worse for a few days by the injection, and it takes three or four days for the steroids to work their magic.

Source: Clinical Procedures in Emergency Medicine, Roberts JR and Hedges JR, editors, W.B. Saunders Co., Philadelphia, PA 1991.

X-rays will be normal in patients with tendonitis.

Treatment consists of resting the involved area, occasionally with a thumb spica/wrist splint, and local injection of a long-acting corticosteroid. The physician should attempt to place the steroid directly in the osseofiborus tunnel and tendon sheaths. The author of this article prefers dexamethasone suspension (Decadron-LA) and notes that this preparation does not produce the post-injection pain flare that is occasionally experienced with some other steroid formulations. Steroid injection may fail if both tendon sheaths are not injected. The extensor pollicis brevis may be rather narrow and somewhat inaccessible to the injection.

In some cases surgery is required. Surgical therapy includes incision of the tendon sheaths so tendons can glide freely over the distal radius. From an anatomical standpoint, there may be more than one tendon for the abductor pollicis longus; failure to inject this tendon, or to free it during surgical therapy, can lead to recurrences.

COMMENT: de Quervain's tenosynovitis generally develops because of overuse of specific tendons whose function is somewhat hampered or subject to trauma by one's intrinsic anatomy. Workmen, especially individuals who use their thumb or wrist repeatedly, are at risk for developing the process. In my experience, however, a good percentage of patients seem to develop it spontaneously without any predisposing factors. It's not a process that should prompt a work-up for a collagen vascular disease or degenerative arthritis. Many patients will offer a history of antecedent trauma to the wrists to the triage nurse, but when one carefully questions the relationship between a specific traumatic episode and the development of de Quervain's disease, it is often tenuous at best. As with most cases of tendinitis/bursitis, patients (and occasionally their doctors) assume that the pain must be due to some sort of injury and diligently search for some past minor accident or injury to confirm the spurious etiology. Physicians almost always order an x-ray because of lingering concerns about trauma or an occult fracture. I have seen this process in all age groups, but it seems to be more common in women aged 40-50. Some texts mention the fact that it is common in mothers who repeatedly lift their infants (but I don't know of any mother who doesn't).

If one can get the patient to relax, the physical exami-

nation is diagnostic. On the physician's first attempt, patients often tend to jump or withdraw no matter where you touch them on the wrist, so it may require three or four gentle attempts to localize the area of tenderness accurately. Physical examination should reveal pain over the radial styloid only. It may be associated soft tissue swelling, redness, or warmth, and when the process has been present for a long period of time, one may actually appreciate crepitus by placing the fingers over the radial styloid and moving the tendons back and forth. Finkelstein's test is quite sensitive and is generally well correlated with the process, although false positives can certainly occur. I haven't seen the specificity of this test studied prospectively, and I intuit that it's not high. If one examines the thumb with compression and longitudinal stress, it should be simple to differentiate de Quervain's disease from the most common misdiagnosis, carpal-metacarpal arthritis.

Conservative treatment would be to apply a thumb spica splint and prescribe an oral NSAID, but this probably is only worthwhile for patients with minor symptoms. The disadvantage is that patients usually require the splint for a week to 10 days, and resolution is slow or absent. I occasionally see patients who have failed such conservative therapy. Although there are no well-controlled prospective studies, the majority of physicians familiar with this disease claim that steroid injection provides prompt and effective relief. Oral steroids are usually not prescribed. Certainly any orthopedic surgeon who is confronted with this diagnosis will first opt for the long-acting steroid injection, and there's no reason why the EP should hold off on definitive therapy. Because there is virtually no disadvantage to a single steroid injection in this disease, I think it ought to be done routinely in the emergency department. One problem of slow resolution and ineffective therapy is that this inflammatory condition can produce stenosing tenosynovitis, which then requires surgery. It's easy to blow off nonspecific wrist pain, prescribe an NSAID, and refer to a consultant, but I believe that a diagnosis and cure are possible in the ED.

Although I believe that emergency physicians should be liberal with the use of steroid injections for inflammatory conditions, a few caveats bear repeating. Before steroids are injected, you must be certain that you are not dealing with an infectious process. It would be difficult to confuse de

> SURGERY IS SOMETIMES REQUIRED AND INVOLVES INCISION OF THE TENDON SHEATHS SO TENDONS CAN GLIDE FREELY OVER THE DISTAL RADIUS

Quervain's disease with an infection, although cellulitis and possibly gonococcal tenosynovitis could be impostors. Gonococcal infections can present with a tenosynovitis picture, but usually a differentiation between this and de Quervain's is rather easy. One should routinely inquire about the presence of urethritis or a vaginal discharge, sore throat, exposure to gonococcus, and carefully look for the petechial hemorrhagic rash associated with gonococcemia. de Quervain's disease does not cause a fever or an elevated sedimentation rate. Also, it is more common in the older age group, which is less likely to get gonorrheal infections. One must, however, maintain vigilance.

Another caveat concerning the use of steroid injections is that one should avoid injecting tendons multiple times, and one should never inject major weight-bearing tendons, such as the Achilles or patellar tendons. Steroids can weaken these structures and predispose to rupture. I personally would not inject a wrist that has been previously injected. Recalcitrant cases should probably be referred to a hand surgeon; many of them come to surgery if they fail steroid injections. Finally, the choice of steroid is probably one of personal preference, but I routinely use the long-acting methylprednisolone acetate (Depo-Medrol). Physicians have had equal success with other long-acting preparations, and I believe there is no major advantage of one over the other. A number of authors have commented on the fact that patients can experience a poststeroid injection painful flare, which actually increases symptoms. This is a real phenomenon, and patients should be warned about it.

The actual steroid injection is rather simple and straightforward. You need not be as anatomically correct as some authors stress. Mix one to two milliliters of a long-acting steroid with a few milliliters of lidocaine. The injection should be done with sterile technique using a relatively painless 25 or 27 gauge needle. (See figure.) I prefer to use an inch and a half needle as opposed to the shorter ones so you can disburse the steroid over a wider area with a single stick. The best place to inject liberally is the area that the patient localizes as being the source of his problem. I have patients define the painful area two or three times by putting a single finger on the most painful spot, and then mark this with a pen. If one uses lidocaine with the steroid, the immediate relief of pain signifies that your steroid has been placed in the right spot. One should be generous with the injection and inject enough volume to cause moderate soft tissue swelling. Although theoretically one should inject the tendon sheaths individually, I

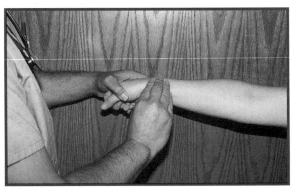

When inflammation is severe, crepitus may be felt under the skin by the examiner's fingers when the inflamed tendons are moved. See color plate in center well.

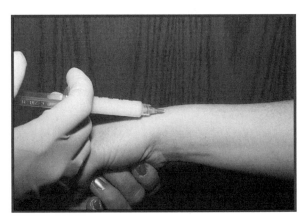

The definitive therapy for de Quervain's disease is injection of the tendon sheaths and peritendinous area with a long-acting corticosteroid. If the steroid is mixed with lidocaine, the accuracy of the injection is immediately known. The lidocaine also gives additional volume so injections do not have to be so anatomically precise. Although it's difficult to appreciate clinically, the steroid should be placed in the tendon sheath (but not the tendon itself) for best results. See color plate in center well.

believe that this is difficult to do or confirm, and one can compensate by just putting more medicine in a wider area. The injection should be free-flowing and if you have to push hard on the syringe, the procedure should be terminated and the needle moved slightly. Failure to obtain a free-flowing injection probably means that the needle is in the tendon itself, a condition that is not sought. One wants to inject the tendon sheaths or peritendon area only.

It's probably not a bad idea to prescribe two or three days of splinting post injection and also prescribe aspirin or another analgesic for additional relief when the local anesthetic wears off. It is important to instruct the patient that it takes three or four days for the steroid injection to be curative, and that the original pain will return when the lidocaine wears off. It's also important to advise them of the possibility of a postinjection painful flare phenomenon that may temporarily increase their pain. I could find no studies on the value of oral NSAIDs following steroid injection, and I don't routinely prescribe them. The local steroid injection should be curative, and adding an expensive NSAID with possible side effects appears to have no added benefit.

Because recurrence is not uncommon, patients should be given proper referral and not be given unrealistic expectations. Those who fail their first steroid injection are probably good candidates for referral.

MYTHS AND MISCONCEPTIONS IN EMERGENCY MEDICINE

MYTHS AND MISCONCEPTIONS IN EMERGENCY MEDICINE

Many practices regularly used in the ED are based only on anecdote and tradition, and many are downright worthless

Physicians tend to be stubborn and inflexible when it comes to adopting new or different medical strategies, especially when they go against the dogma they learned in medical school or residency. The old timers know that yesterday's heresy is tomorrow's tradition, and vice versa. Even so, it's difficult to accept change when it goes against the teachings of your gray-haired professors, your senior resident role model, or commonly accepted textbooks. Over the years, I have noticed many dogmatic approaches fall by the wayside, yet physicians, even when confronted with hard, indisputable facts, are reluctant to change what's familiar. Unfortunately, many of our strongly held rules and prejudices have no basis in fact. Often they are based only on anecdote, tradition, animal studies, or 50-year-old case reports. Many are expensive and clinically worthless, while some even subject patients to needless discomfort or inconvenience.

With this in mind, and in effort to teach old dogs new tricks, this section focuses on some of the medical myths and misconceptions I have come across in the medical literature. This chapter discusses some orthopedic examples. These articles debunk many of the age-old axioms that have long guided the ED management of some common orthopedic problems.

TREATMENT OF CLAVICULAR FRACTURES. FIGURE-OF-EIGHT BANDAGE VERSUS A SIMPLE SLING

Andersen KP, et al *Acta Ortho Scand* 1987;58(1):71

The authors of this prospective Scandinavian study compared the outcome of two treatment modalities prescribed to 61 patients with simple, closed, mid-clavicular fractures. All patients were older than age 13 years. There were no associated neurovascular symptoms, and the only injury was the clavicle fracture. Thirty-four were treated with the standard figure-of-eight bandage, and 27 were given a simple sling. Those given the figure-of-eight were told to wear it for three weeks and have it adjusted weekly by their doctor. Those given a sling wore it as needed and had no scheduled physician visits. All patients were encouraged to perform early shoulder mobility exercises when it was comfortable to do so.

Patients were followed for 10 to 17 weeks and were questioned about the discomfort of the dressing, number of outpatient visits, use of analgesics, duration of immobilization, and satisfaction with treatment. Functional and cosmetic results were assessed upon completion of the study.

Using a numerical rating score, patients with figure-of-eight bandages had twice as much discomfort and impairment to normal activity (sleep, bathing) than those given a sling. The mean duration of immobilization was three weeks with a figure-of-eight while most patients given the sling discarded it within one week. Patients with the traditional figure-of-eight were much more dissatisfied with the treatment (26%) than those treated with the sling (7%).

There was no significant difference in final clinical outcome parameters, such as deformity, skin problems, neurovascular dysfunction, impairment of shoulder motion, pain, tenderness, weakness of the shoulder muscles, or x-ray findings. In the final evaluation, the alignment of the fracture was essentially not reduced by either treatment, but all demonstrated satisfactory radiographic healing. Early in the treatment the figure-of-eight was refused by 10 patients because of excessive pain from the device or edema and paresthesias of the arm. One patient developed deep vein thrombosis. The device was discontinued by the physician in two patients because the strapping displaced a primarily non-displaced fracture. Other changes in alignment secondary to treatment are listed in the table.

For the treatment of uncomplicated mid-clavicular fractures, the authors conclude that the figure-of-eight bandage is unnecessary. It is associated with complications, commonly causes needless discomfort and inconvenience, and provides no better functional or cosmetic result than a sling. Patients clearly preferred a simple sling to the cumbersome and annoying figure-of-eight bandage. The use of a sling is recommended as first-line treatment.

COMMENT: We have all been taught that a figure-of-eight dressing should be routinely applied to patients with clavicular fractures. This misconception is reiterated by many textbooks. The uncomfortable hunched shoulder position is theoretically used to align or reduce the fracture fragments, relieve pain, and promote healing, yet these claims have never been proven and are probably untrue. Having put these dressings on patients, I can attest to the fact that they are uncomfortable and initially usually increase pain. To use a figure-of-eight as suggested, one has to adjust or tighten the straps on a recurrent basis, a major inconvenience to physician and patient. This article makes the case that we are not enhancing the healing process with this cumbersome and expensive device. We are, in fact, making patients more uncomfort-

FIGURE-OF-EIGHT DRESSINGS: MYTHS AND MISCONCEPTIONS

Clinical Dogma:	*A figure-of-eight dressing should be used to align fractured clavicles and promote healing.*
Fact:	*The figure-of-eight does not reduce fractures, may worsen alignment, and is associated with annoying and harmful side effects. (Final cosmetic and functional results with a simple sling are comparable, and the sling is much more patient friendly.)*
Clinical Dogma:	*After a fall on the outstretched hand, tenderness of the scaphoid often suggests an occult (x-ray negative) fracture. All patients with snuff-box tenderness and normal x-rays should be immobilized for 10-14 days, and the x-ray repeated. Delay in immediate casting immobilization of the thumb are associated with a high incidence of nonunion.*
Fact:	*Scaphoid fractures are rarely occult, and the vast majority of such injuries are evident on initial plain films when the study includes special navicular views. The scaphoid compression test is much more sensitive than snuff-box tenderness. In those few that are initially occult, long-term prognosis is little affected by an initial conservative approval and close follow-up. Short-term immobilization with follow-up is much more appropriate.*
Clinical Dogma:	*To evaluate suspected acromioclavicular injuries, obtain normal and weighted radiograph. Adding stress to the AC joint will unmask injuries not apparent on unweighted x-rays. Weights should be tied to the wrist as opposed to having patients hold them.*
Fact:	*Weighted x-rays add no usable clinical information to unweighted films, and may, in fact, mask injuries. There is no difference in how the weight is applied.*

Source: James R. Roberts, MD

able with our misguided attempts to reduce or immobilize simple clavicle fractures.

Despite a number of similar studies, I still see the figure-of-eight applied routinely, even to children with greenstick type fractures that are not displaced. Stanley et al (*Injury* 1988;19(3):162) similarly studied the healing of clavicle fractures treated with a conservative broad arm sling versus the traditional figure-of-eight dressing. In their study, 140 patients without associated skin tenting or neurovascular problems were treated in a random fashion; 108 received a sling and 40 received a figure-of-eight. All patients experienced eventual complete recovery. Although previous authors have reported nonunion when the figure-of-eight dressing was used, there were no cases of nonunion in this series.

There were no significant differences between the groups in any outcome parameter or the time required to achieve full recovery. The authors likewise failed to find an advantage of a figure-of-eight bandage in patients with uncomplicated clavicular fractures and suggest conservative treatment with a sling.

McCandless et al (*Practitioner* 1979;233 (1334):266) conducted a similar study. Forty patients with displaced fractures of the clavicle were alternately treated with either a sling or a figure-of-eight. Those given a figure-of-eight returned every other day for adjustments. As in the other studies, the final outcomes were similar, although these authors also found significant disadvantages for the figure-of-eight. In their study, two patients experienced increased angulation of the fracture fragments with the strapping, and deformity was increased in four subjects due to depression of the outer fragment. Four patients developed a swollen blue arm on the side of the fracture, thought to be secondary to the figure-of-eight. The condition resolved when a sling was substituted, but the authors raised the possibility that axillary vein thrombosis may have supervened had the axillary compression not been removed. It was concluded that attempts to correct deformities of clavicular fracture using a figure-of-eight bandage are ineffective and may be harmful. A simple triangular sling results in similar healing and cosmetic results with less discomfort and hassle to the patient.

It's important to note that candidates for a sling have simple closed fractures of the clavicle without neurovascular compromise or significant skin tenting. Immediate orthopedic referral is suggested if either of these complications are present. As one old orthopedic surgeon once told me, the only requirement for a clavicle fracture to heal properly is that both pieces be in the same hemothorax. Clearly, minimally displaced fractures do not require reduction for satisfactory healing. Studies indicate that all our efforts and fancy dressings intended to provide stabilization and reduction are to no avail. Moreover, the figure-of-eight dressing is uncomfortable, inconvenient, pro-

CLASSIFICATION OF AC JOINT INJURIES

Grade 1: <3 mm (or <50%) increase of the injured vs. the uninjured AC joint width with a normal CC distance (defined as <5 mm or <50% difference between injured and uninjured sides).

Grade 2: ≥3 mm (or ≥50%) increase of the injured vs. the uninjured AC joint width with a normal CC distance.

Grade 3: ≥5 mm (or ≥50%) increase of the injured vs. the uninjured CC distance with or without AC widening and with or without clavicular elevation.

Source: Ann Emerg Med *1988;17:20-24.*

hibits showering, causes skin irritation to the axilla, can predispose to neurologic injury or axillary vein thromboses, and is much more expensive than a sling. All these downsides are in addition to making your patients generally dissatisfied with their treatment.

It's time to throw away the figure-of-eight dressings for simple clavicular fractures and adopt the more rational therapy consisting of a simple sling and early motion. For those of you who are cost-conscious, a figure-of-eight costs $25 in our hospital, compared with $1.75 for a sling. One final important caveat. Many patients and primary care physicians are conditioned to seeing a clavicle fracture treated with a figure-of-eight strap. Unless you want to look like a dilettante, be sure to explain to the patient why you are prescribing a simple sling. Otherwise, when the family doctor sees the patient at follow-up, both may suspect your orthopedic prowess. (I have even received angry notes about my lack of knowledge in treating clavicle fractures that said, "Everybody knows a clavicle strap is standard of care.")

SCAPHOID FRACTURES AND WRIST PAIN— TIME FOR NEW THINKING

Staniforth P *Injury* 1991;22(6):436

This editorial review challenges the axiom that patients who fall on an outstretched hand who have snuff-box tenderness without evidence of fracture on x-ray have a high incidence of occult scaphoid (navicular) fractures and therefore should be routinely immobilized in plaster and x-rayed again in two weeks. This contention is in addition to the widely held belief that failure to immobilize such fractures immediately and properly guarantees subsequent nonunion, chronic pain, and a lawsuit. The author contends that much of this dogma has been created from fear of litigation, yet the actual compensation or malpractice proven for missing scaphoid fractures, at least in England, is extremely small. The downside of the traditional approach is that too many patients are immobilized and disabled for two weeks without any good reason.

In a review of the recent literature, the author notes that in reality only about seven percent of scaphoid fractures are actually occult and therefore 93 percent of patients with minor wrist injuries are overtreated. In addition, evidence indicates that a short-term delay in casting a scaphoid fracture makes little or no difference in long-term prognosis. Finally, with the availability of the bone scan, no scaphoid fracture should remain occult for long.

The author concludes that patients with normal x-rays who complain of wrist pain following trauma should be treated initially in a conservative manner with a simple bandage or splint. This approach assumes a reliable patient and access to follow-up in four to five days. The author contends that it is not negligent to leave the painful wrist — with a normal x-ray — out of plaster when the patient leaves the ED.

COMMENT: This author, like many others, questions the knee-jerk response of long-term (10-14 days) immobilization of every x-ray negative patient with a painful wrist, a common procedure in EDs across the country. He also refutes the contention that scaphoid fractures are clinically and radiologically difficult to diagnose. A bone scan is admittedly the gold standard that may be used in selected cases, but the study is by no means a routine test. Finally the point is made that there really is no difference in long-term outcome when conservative treatment is compared to immediate casting or full immobilization.

The occultness of scaphoid fractures and their propensity to cause long-term problems if nonunion occurs did not, however, get into the literature by accident. The sprained wrist deserves your respect and careful attention. Statistics vary, but up to 12 percent of scaphoid fractures may not be seen on routine wrist films. It is prudent, therefore, to recognize the problem but to tailor your treatment to individual cases and not blindly immobilize everyone for two weeks.

In a study by Dias et al (*J Bone Joint Surg [Br]* 1990; 72(1):98), the diagnostic accuracy of plain radiographs was not enhanced by performing repeat studies two to three weeks following injury in patients with wrist pain. They note that scaphoid fractures are often overdiagnosed in the presence of snuff-box tenderness, and 20 percent of the x-rays in their series were interpreted as positive when they were actually negative controls shown to a blinded radiologist. It's easy to miss a subtle scaphoid fracture, and one should always be leery of making the

ALIGNMENT OF HEALED FRACTURES

Displacement	Figure-of-Eight	Simple Sling
Diminished	1	2
Unchanged	30	21
Increased	3	4
Number	34	27

Source: Acta Orthop Scand *1988;57:71-74.*

diagnosis of wrist sprain. Likewise, it's certainly easy to call a minor blip on the wrist film or be faked out by a vascular channel. It does not take much to talk yourself into a probable fracture, especially if that's where the patient hurts.

In suspicious cases, the EP should not be satisfied with the standard wrist series of x-rays. In a study by Mehta (*Ann Emerg Med* 1990;19(3):255), adding a supination and pronation x-ray — the so-called six-view study — on 36 patients with a negative four-view study identified 11 additional fractures. In the 25 patients with an initial negative six-view survey, repeat x-rays in two weeks failed to identify a single new fracture. These authors suggest additional x-rays initially to evaluate further the scaphoid bone in patients with snuff-box tenderness after a fall on an outstretched hand. If this extended series is negative, they also suggest that minimal immobilization is a reasonable approach. It is certainly reasonable to always order additional scaphoid views in high-risk patients.

A number of authors have emphasized the value of the physical examination to pick up occult scaphoid fractures. Longitudinal compression of the thumb has been found by Waeckerle (*Ann Emerg Med* 1987;16(4):733) to be a sensitive and specific physical finding for scaphoid injury. This so-called scaphoid compression test is much more sensitive than snuff-box tenderness. With this maneuver, inward longitudinal stress is applied along the axis of the thumb's metacarpal, and pain in the wrist strongly suggests scaphoid injury (*J Hand Surg* [BR] 1989;14(3):323). The scaphoid compression test is a useful adjunct in decision-making for the management of selected cases. A positive test in the setting of a negative x-ray should alert you to a possible occult fracture.

It is obvious that the occult carpal scaphoid fracture is often an illusionary diagnosis. In my experience, most so-called occult fractures were actually misread on the initial ED x-ray, stressing the need for good attention to the mechanism of injury, being liberal with ordering special scaphoid views, and tight quality control on x-ray interpretation. The old axiom of mandating full immobilization for two weeks, followed by another x-ray in all patients, is clearly overkill. The most reasonable approach is to immobilize patients who are x-ray negative and who present with the proper mechanism for a scaphoid fracture. If there is a positive compression test, specific orthopedic follow-up is arranged in four to five days, when the patient is more comfortable and the physical examination more reliable. It is certainly common for patients to hurt all over during their first evaluation in the ED, and you can get almost anyone with a painful wrist injury to jump when you apply pressure directly over the scaphoid. If there is general diffuse pain and a negative thumb compression test, I have the patient take off the splint in four to five days and seek follow-up only if the pain persists.

In many cases, however, a final decision cannot be made in the ED so it's prudent to be conservative and care-

ful. I always specifically tell patients about the possibility of occult fracture. It makes no sense, however, to keep someone out of work for two weeks when the vast majority have no significant injuries.

Finally, if one chooses to immobilize a scaphoid fracture, one probably only need apply a volar wrist splint from the forearm to the head of the metacarpals.

MID-CLAVICULAR FRACTURES

Fracture Types/ Dislocations	Figure-of Eight Bandage	Simple Sling
Two-fragment fracture	25	20
One intermediary fracture	7	5
Two or more intermediary fractures	2	2
Undisplaced	3	3
Minor displacement	15	12
Major displacement	16	12
Number	34	27

Source: Acta Orthop Scand *1988;57:71-74.*

Traditionally, it has been recommended that scaphoid fractures also require immobilization of the thumb, although the necessity for this is unclear. Yanni (*J Bone Joint Surg* [BR] 1991;73(4):600) states that only the wrist should be immobilized, ideally in a neutral position or slight palmar flexion, avoiding wrist dorsiflexion and without ulnar or radial deviation. It is instinctive to put the wrist in some degree of dorsiflexion when immobilizing it, but in a cadaver study the fracture gap was actually increased with wrist dorsiflexion and closed with palmar flexion. In essence, splinting the wrist in dorsiflexion reproduces the injuring force, and is intuitively illogical. Thumb movement had no effect on fragment motion unless the wrist was in ulnar deviation. From the ED standpoint, there is no downside of including the thumb in the splint for a few days so I suggest that it still be done. Proper splinting requires that the physician carefully mold the splint and hold it until it becomes hard because patients reflexively dorsiflex their wrist when you leave the room. Removable velcro wrist splints are acceptable for the first three or four days of immobilization for x-ray negative patients.

LACK OF EFFICACY OF 'WEIGHTED' RADIOGRAPHS IN DIAGNOSING ACUTE ACROMIOCLAVICULAR SEPARATION

Bossart PJ, et al *Ann Emerg Med* 1988;17(1):20

This study prospectively examines the value of the weighted x-ray in identifying acromioclavicular (AC) strains in 83 patients with shoulder injuries. The authors claim that this is the only study that systematically investigates this universally accepted technique, but the widely subscribed maneuver is anecdotal at best. Plain x-rays to include both shoulders were first ordered, followed by radiographs with the patient stressed with 10-pound weights, either held or suspended from the wrist. Films were given to a radiologist who blindly read the films in a random order. The injuries were classified as grade 1, 2, or 3 separation by evaluating AC and coracoclavicular (CC) measurements.

In only three of 70 cases with grade 1 or 2 sprains did the addition of the weights result in enough of an increase in CC distance to make the diagnosis of a grade 3 separation. Interestingly, in seven cases the addition of weights produced a less severe radiographic picture than was demonstrated on the plain films without weights. Apparently weights can decrease or increase the CC distance in a normal shoulder. There was no difference when the patient either held the weights or the weights were tied to the wrist.

The authors conclude that adding weights did not produce predictable or reliable distraction of the AC joint in patients with an acute injury to the shoulder; the procedure had virtually no diagnostic significance. Because current trends are to treat all AC strains conservatively — even grade 3 separations — the routine performance of weighted x-rays is discouraged. The increased cost, radiation exposure, and associated discomfort do not warrant routine weighted x-rays.

COMMENT: It is common practice to obtain unweighted and weighted views of both shoulders and measure the AC joint space and the CC distance in order to evaluate the extent of injury to the AC joint. Theoretically, the integrity of the AC and CC ligaments is reflected in the relationship of the clavicle with the acromion and coracoid process. It has long been taught that splinting or muscle spasm during an acute injury may mask third-degree injuries so stress films are routinely ordered. Most agree that weights should be hung from the wrist rather than having the patient hold them to minimize muscle contraction that may mask the degree of injury. This apparently is another myth.

It's difficult to talk patients out of routine x-rays following trauma, and it's certainly reasonable to obtain a radiograph to rule out a clavicle or humerus fracture. Many patients actually have an AC injury with normal x-rays. Unless there is an obvious deformity, the diagnosis of AC strain can be substantiated by physical examination alone by eliciting pain, tenderness, and swelling at that AC junction. Patients with these findings have a clinical AC separation, regardless of x-ray findings.

Although it is of academic interest to grade AC strains, it makes little practical difference. AC separations are rarely repaired surgically, and surgery is not guided by the x-ray findings; even third-degree strains are usually managed conservatively. It is clearly impossible to justify the expense and radiation exposure of routine weighted films, and the tradition should be stopped. If one insists on using weighted films, it makes ultimate sense to use these views initially and abandon the unweighted radiographs altogether. This article nicely demonstrates that weighted films are not only useless, but they may on occasion do just the opposite of their intent.

MYTHS AND MISCONCEPTIONS ABOUT NSAID GASTROPATHY

The problem with long-term NSAIDs is that the family doctor frequently follows the EP's advice by renewing the NSAID many times

Because medicine is not an exact science and because of the super-strong egos of many physicians, it's a relatively easy task to find true scientific data that invalidate commonly held myths and misconceptions in emergency medicine. Numerous procedures and protocols are established and religiously adhered to that are based purely on tradition, anecdotal reports, personal belief, or seemingly logical parameters, but when studied rigorously, the dogma is found to be bogus. Yet these myths and misconceptions are continually handed down from housestaff to housestaff (or attending to attending) with such zeal and charismatic adherence that they quickly become ingrained as absolute truth. Even respected textbooks promulgate erroneous concepts, often to the delight of malpractice lawyers.

Although I won't go into detail here, there is a benefit to the use of H2 blockers for the treatment of an acute GI bleed and for the prevention of an immediate recurrence of the hemorrhage. But this chapter will touch on some commonly held misconceptions of NSAID therapy. H2 blockers are a wonderful addition to chronic ulcer therapy; however, they are also used almost universally while patients are actively bleeding. Multiple studies have demonstrated their lack of effectiveness in either stanching the hemorrhage or decreasing the rate of recurrence during the initial hospitalization. In short, H2 blockers are of no value in the therapy of an acute GI bleed. This chapter is an evaluation of some other GI mythology, specifically various methods commonly used to quell NSAID-induced gastropathy.

CIMETIDINE THERAPY IN NONSTEROIDAL ANTI-INFLAMMATORY DRUG GASTROPATHY: DOUBLE-BLIND LONG-TERM EVALUATION

Roth SH, et al *Arch Intern Med* 1987;147(10):1798

The purpose of this study was to address the efficacy of cimetidine in treating or preventing gastric ulcers in patients taking maintenance nonsteroidal anti-inflammatory drugs (NSAIDs). Because cimetidine is a useful agent for the treatment of traditional peptic ulcer disease, it has been postulated that it would have some beneficial effect in preventing NSAID gastropathy. Patients with rheumatoid arthritis who were taking long-term NSAIDs underwent baseline endoscopy and were assigned a grading of their gastrointestinal mucosa with regard to irritation or ulceration. The NSAIDs included piroxicam, indomethacin, ibuprofen, naproxen, and meclofenamate. Subjects were randomly assigned in a double-blind fashion to receive cimetidine or placebo for up to 12 months. The dose of cimetidine was either 400 mg at bedtime or 300 mg QID. After eight weeks of therapy, patients underwent repeat gastroscopy. If improvement were noted on endoscopy findings, patients were continued in a maintenance phase on either cimetidine or placebo. If the condition had worsened, subjects were termed treatment failures. Patients who had been taking placebo during the time their endoscopic lesions worsened were then switched to open label cimetidine and re-endoscoped within another two months.

Overall, 48 patients initially entered the cimetidine therapy group, and 46 patients were assigned to the placebo group. At eight weeks, about half of the patients in both groups improved, but progression of the endoscopic lesions was noted in 56 percent of those taking cimetidine and 52 percent of those randomized to placebo. Of those who improved and were placed on maintenance therapy for 10 months, worsening of the lesions occurred in 50 percent of the placebo group and 42 percent of the cimetidine-treated group (no statistically significant difference). Cimeditine also failed to be better than placebo when the active drug was substituted for the failed placebo in the second phase of the study. Interestingly, 27 patients were dropped from the study initially because they had asymptomatic severe ulcer changes prior to randomization. This study demonstrated that more than half of the NSAID-induced ulcers don't get better on their own, nor do they improve with cimetidine therapy.

The authors comment on the high incidence of gastropathy with chronic NSAID use, noting that up to 20-30 percent of patients in previous studies have demonstrated ulcer disease. Most importantly, there was a poor overall correlation between peptic symptomatology and endoscopy findings, a commonly reported phenomenon. The failure of cimeditine to offer protection against NSAID gastropathy was discouraging. The results of this study paralleled those found in many others (*Br J Rheumatol* 1986;25(1):54; *Dig Dis Sci* 1982;27(11):976; *Am J Gastroenterol* 1981;75:104; *Gastroenterology* 1980; 78:1230; and *Arch Intern Med* 1987;147(10): 1798).

CHARACTERISTICS OF NSAID GASTROPATHY

- *Etiology: Likely due to inhibition of prostaglandin production*
- *Incidence: Three- to fivefold increase over controls*
- *Ulcers tend to be gastric rather than duodenal*
- *Injury is diffuse: Hemorrhages, petechiae, erosions, ulcers*
- *Symptoms do not reflect extent of mucosal damage*
- *Symptoms occur without demonstrated mucosal injury*
- *Ulcers tend to be "silent" until bleeding/perforation*
- *Lesions occur within weeks of therapy*
- *Not prevented with H2 blockers/sucralfate/antacids*
- *Possible prevention with misoprostol and omeprazole*
- *Lesions heal quickly when drugs are withdrawn*
- *Healing can take place while therapy continues*
- *Possible risk factors: Advanced age, rheumatoid arthritis?, previous ulcers, concomitant smoking, alcohol or steroid use*
- *All NSAIDs have been implicated; safest not yet determined (possibly increased risk with NSAIDs of long half-life or those with greatest anti-inflammatory effect?)*

Source: James R. Roberts, MD

The authors speculate that the failure of cimetidine to provide benefit probably reflects a fundamental difference between NSAID gastropathy and classic peptic ulcer disease. This is probably related to the fact that prostaglandins provide a protective mechanism in the GI tract, and NSAIDs interfere with this physiologic protection due to their potent anti-prostaglandin effect.

COMMENT: NSAIDs are great drugs for certain pathologies, and they have been a godsend to patients with inflammatory conditions. Their use is not without risk, and for this reason, they should be used for the proper indications. Although designed to fight inflammation, NSAIDs are probably the most commonly prescribed analgesic for all types of pain, and they are effective analgesics. It is almost unheard of for any patients to leave our

ED with any painful condition — from back pain, ankle sprain, soft tissue contusion to headache — without a mandatory prescription for some nonsteroidal. These drugs are basically forced upon many patients when either no therapy, acetaminophen, or less potent forms of over-the-counter NSAIDs clearly would be more appropriate.

The incidence of GI side effects from NSAIDs is probably underestimated by the majority of emergency physicians; we just don't see complications (or recognize them) on a regular basis. Because many patients don't take our prescribed drugs for long periods of time, the problems with NSAIDs seldom surface for the run-of-the-mill sprained ankle or contusion. The problem with long-term NSAID maintenance therapy is that many patients are unaware of serious side effects until they experience anemia, perforation, or an acute GI bleed. Pain is the body's way of telling the patient to stop taking the offending agent that is tearing up their intestinal tract, but NSAIDs are such good analgesics that they mask this important warning symptom. Many authors have found that even healthy patients without a history of ulcers will develop endoscopic evidence of mucosal injury following only a few weeks of NSAID use. Importantly, no NSAID is immune to this problem.

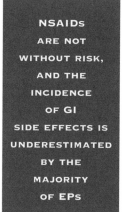

NSAIDs ARE NOT WITHOUT RISK, AND THE INCIDENCE OF GI SIDE EFFECTS IS UNDERESTIMATED BY THE MAJORITY OF EPs

Because all clinicians are now aware of the association between gastropathy and NSAIDs, numerous strategies have been developed to prevent such side effects. It never ceases to amaze me that while the best way to prevent side effects is obviously to prescribe an alternative to NSAIDs, clinicians instead often opt for another expensive drug in an effort to further mess with the body's physiology. H2 blockers are probably ineffective against NSAID ulcers or gastritis because this gastropathy is not the same pathophysiology that is seen with classic peptic ulcers: excess acid, *Helicobacter pylori,* excess alcohol, or a stress-induced etiology. In short, methods developed to combat conventional peptic ulcers cannot be extrapolated to NSAID gastropathy because the two entities are fundamentally two distinctly different processes.

It's routine to suggest taking NSAIDs after eating, and this seems to make sense. Patients probably experience fewer GI side effects with this advice. I have, however, never seen a study that demonstrates that this advice offers any cytologic protection whatsoever. I would intuit that taking NSAIDs with food does not prevent mucosal injury

in the long run. I don't know of anyone who would tell a patient to take a NSAID on a empty stomach, but we may be fooling ourselves.

It seems absurd to prescribe $50-$60 of the newest NSAID (and they commonly cost that much for a 7- to 10-day course) when acetaminophen would suffice. But on top of this, one prescribes another $50 worth of cimetidine (Tagamet), ranitidine (Zantac), famotidine (Pepcid), or whatever your favorite H2 blocker is. You have now changed a $3 analgesic regimen into a $100 one, and put at least 20-30 percent of your patients at risk for possible side effects. This mistake is most egregious for soft tissue injuries, where the common mistaken belief is that trauma produces an inflammation similar to the inflammation produced by rheumatoid arthritis. In short, NSAIDs do not help injured, strained, or contused tissue heal faster by quelling some mythical "trauma-induced" inflammation.

Taking NSAIDs for five to seven days is relatively innocuous for otherwise healthy patients, and these are good drugs when used properly. Despite many attempts to prove otherwise, no one specific NSAID is consistently any better than another in respect to side effects. Importantly, prescriptions tend to have a half-life much longer than the emergency physician may intend. The family doctor frequently will follow the EP's advice by renewing that ED-prescribed NSAID many times over . Giving NSAIDs needlessly is sort of like prescribing antibiotics for a upper respiratory infection. Generally no harm is done, but occasionally significant side effects are seen, and probably more importantly, patients get used to taking prescription drugs when they are not needed. I have seen many patients prescribed more than one NSAID when a second physician is involved after the patient leaves the ED (or the patient was already on one NSAID, but forgot to tell the EP). I still remember one elderly lady who had four NSAID prescriptions in her purse (all from different doctors) when she arrived in the ED in hypovolemic shock from her silent GI bleed.

Other authors have demonstrated the inability of conventional ulcer therapy to benefit NSAID gastropathy. Ehsanullah et al noted that although ranitidine did initially, but not over the long-term, reduced the incidence of duodenal ulcerations, it had no significant effect on gastric lesions when NSAIDs and this H2 blocker were concurrently prescribed (*BMJ* 1988;297(6655):1017). The prevalence and severity of gastrointestinal symptoms, such as epigastric pain, heartburn, nausea, and vomiting were unaffected by the concomitant use of ranitidine. Although there was some protection of duodenal ulceration with ranitidine, ulcerations still occurred. Taha et al (*N Engl J Med* 1996;334:1455) believe that high-dose famotidine significantly reduces the cumulative effects of long-term NSAID therapy with regard to gastric and duodenal ulcers, but this merely lowers and does not eliminate ulcer formation.

In summary, numerous double-blind placebo-controlled studies have demonstrated that H_2 receptor antagonists are no better than placebo in the treatment or long-term prevention of NSAID-induced gastric ulcers. The message here is straightforward for the emergency physician: prescribe NSAIDs for short periods of time for predominantly inflammatory conditions or self-limited painful conditions and choose an alternative non-NSAID whenever possible. NSAIDs are great analgesics and are safe for short-term use, but they have no special ability to hasten healing in painful traumatic soft tissue injuries. An obligatory NSAID prescription should not be routine for minor musculoskeletal conditions. Advise patients to take NSAIDs with food, but avoid the temptation to increase side effects, increase costs, and lull both patient and clinician into a false sense of security by concomitantly writing an H_2 blocker prescription. Although the purest may argue that there is some statistical benefit for patients with duodenal ulcerations with H_2 blockers, the benefit of routinely combining H_2 blockers and short-term NSAIDs makes no physiologic, medical, or financial sense.

> **THE PROBLEM WITH LONG-TERM NSAID THERAPY IS THAT PATIENTS ARE UNAWARE OF SIDE EFFECTS UNTIL THEY EXPERIENCE ANEMIA, PERFORATION, OR GI BLEED**

SUCRALFATE TREATMENT OF NONSTEROIDAL ANTI-INFLAMMATORY DRUG-INDUCED GASTROINTESTINAL SYMPTOMS AND MUCOSAL DAMAGE

Caldwell JR, et al *Am J Med* 1987;83(3B):74

The authors of this study evaluated the effect of sucralfate (Carafate) vs. placebo in 143 patients with established NSAID gastropathy. This was a randomized double-blind trial comparing placebo with 1 g sucralfate QID. One aim of the study was to address the dilemma of what to do other than discontinue the drug when patients who really require NSAIDs develop gastropathy.

Patients were entered in the study if they experienced GI side effects while receiving their daily dose of a variety of NSAIDs for a number of rheumatologic disorders. Patients were first given placebo for two weeks while their intensity, frequency, and pattern of GI symptoms (heartburn, epigastric pain/burning, belching, nausea, vomiting, diarrhea) was established. If they became asymptomatic while taking placebo, they were excluded. At baseline prior to randomization, the symptomatic patients received endoscopy to grade the extent of the lesions. Amazingly, 42 percent had mucosal lesions at baseline. Subjects were then randomly assigned to receive sucralfate or placebo for four weeks. Following the four-week period, subjects were again endoscoped and given open label sucralfate for up to six months and then reinvestigated. Antacids were allowed as needed, and gastrointestinal symptoms were recorded on a weekly basis.

Interestingly, 30 percent of patients had their symptoms abate with placebo. In one subgroup, sucralfate did reduce (but not eliminate) the frequency and intensity of peptic symptoms and improved mucosal lesion compared to placebo. However, only patients taking NSAIDs with a long half-life demonstrated a benefit, and there was no difference in favor of sucralfate or placebo in symptom frequency or intensity in patients receiving salicylates or short half-life NSAIDs. Long half-life drugs were piroxicam (Feldene), naproxen (Naprosyn), sulindac (Clinoril) and diflunisal (Dolobid). The most common short half-life NSAID was ibuprofen.

Overall, however, gastric mucosal healing was not statistically different between the two groups. The authors conclude that sucralfate is partially effective in relieving symptoms and in reducing mucosal damage in some patients receiving concomitant long-term NSAID therapy but only if the NSAID has a long half-life. Although the mean endoscopy scores and symptoms were better in this subgroup of patients, sucralfate did not cure or eliminate the pathology. It is postulated that sucralfate may be beneficial in situations where H_2 blockers have not been helpful because sucralfate is cytoprotective. Cytoprotection is a physiological and pharmacological activity that is independent of acid secretion, and because NSAID-induced ulcers are not secondary to excessive acid, this approach is reasonable. The authors conclude that their data demonstrated that sucralfate, used as an adjunct to NSAID therapy, can partially relieve both GI symptoms and gastric mucosal damage in some patients who develop these symptoms and must be maintained on long-term NSAID therapy.

COMMENT: Sucralfate is an aluminum salt of a sulfate disaccharide that forms a protective barrier on the gastric

mucosa. The drug appears to have comparable healing rates for conventional ulcers when going head-to-head with H_2 blockers, but it must be given four times a day. Pharmacologically, sucralfate is not an antacid, but it exerts its anti-ulcer effect by bonding to proteinaceous exudate in ulcer craters and therefore forms a protective barrier against food, acid, and other insults. It appears magically to seek out injured tissue to form an ulcer-adherent complex and does not distribute to normal gastric surfaces. It has some mild pepsin-inhibiting activity and can have a slight effect on the GI absorption of some drugs. Sucralfate is minimally absorbed, has no significant renal, hepatic or hematologic toxicity, and rarely produces systemic symptoms. It's a rather interesting drug, one that I use frequently for the treatment of ill-defined dyspepsia or gastritis, and it's a mainstay in my GI cocktail.

One should be careful in analyzing the conclusion of this article because it deals with the treatment of endoscopic lesions and symptoms of gastropathy once they have developed. It does not address the prevention of these symptoms and therefore the data have limited applicability to the emergency physician who prescribes NSAIDs for a short period of time. Although sucralfate may be partially helpful once symptoms are established, I could find no literature that addressed its ability to prevent NSAID gastropathy. The benefit was found only in patients taking NSAIDs with a long half-life, and while it may be helpful for the patient with rheumatoid arthritis who is taking piroxicam, sulindac, diflunisal, or naproxen, it appears to be of no value to patients on ibuprofen. EPs will not prescribe most of the very long-acting NSAIDs, but may be tempted to use naproxen, and this is now available over-the-counter. As a side point, many of

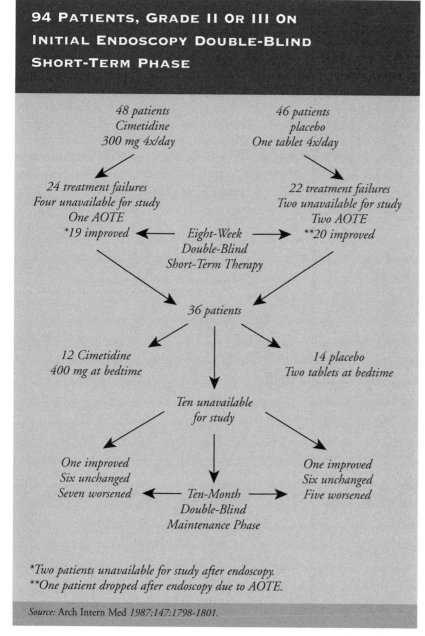

94 PATIENTS, GRADE II OR III ON INITIAL ENDOSCOPY DOUBLE-BLIND SHORT-TERM PHASE

48 patients
Cimetidine
300 mg 4x/day

46 patients
placebo
One tablet 4x/day

24 treatment failures
Four unavailable for study
One AOTE
*19 improved ← Eight-Week → **20 improved
Double-Blind
Short-Term Therapy

22 treatment failures
Two unavailable for study
Two AOTE

36 patients

12 Cimetidine
400 mg at bedtime

14 placebo
Two tablets at bedtime

Ten unavailable
for study

One improved
Six unchanged
Seven worsened ← Ten-Month →
Double-Blind
Maintenance Phase

One improved
Six unchanged
Five worsened

*Two patients unavailable for study after endoscopy.
**One patient dropped after endoscopy due to AOTE.

Source: Arch Intern Med 1987;147:1798-1801.

my residents prescribe diflunisal (Dolobid), and make the brand name sound suspiciously like Dilaudid in an effort to get rid of drug-seeking patients.

Although this article contains some data which are statistically significant, I thought it interesting that 30 percent of patients treated with the baseline placebo had their symptoms disappear. Most importantly, side effects and endoscopic lesions were lessened not eliminated with therapy. If I saw a patient in the ED who had GI symptoms while on arthritis medicine, I would personally advise discontinuing the offending drug rather than try to fix the problem by adding sucralfate. Other authors have been unable to find a benefit of sucralfate over placebo for this condition (*Am J Gastroenterol* 1988;83(2):143). Another interesting bit of data from this study is a very impressive 42 percent incidence of gastric mucosal lesions in symptomatic patients. Also of note is the fact that 58 percent of patients with symptoms had a normal endoscopy. Although this article may tempt you to prescribe sucralfate in patients who are taking NSAIDs and develop symptomatology of gastric irritation, it does not support the concomitant use of the two medications initially. If the patient does not have severe arthritic problems mandating the continued use of NSAIDs, the most prudent strategy is merely to stop the offending drug rather than to try to treat the side effects with another medication. If the NSAID is mandatory, this patient should be carefully followed by a consultant.

One side effect of NSAIDs that may not be well known and may have short-term therapy consequences is that NSAIDs negate the antihypertensive effect of many blood pressure medicines. Beta blockers, diuretics, and ACE-inhibitors can lose their effectiveness if NSAIDs are used concomitantly. This reduction in hypotensive effect can be important in some patients.

Although many clinicians erroneously believe that H_2 blockers and sucralfate can protect patients from NSAID-induced gastropathy or prescribe them "just to be safe," there are actually no scientific data to support this practice. The bottom line is that conventional ulcer therapy is no better than placebo in reducing the frequency or severity of gastric mucosal injury from short-term NSAIDs. The manufacturers of these medications do not claim an indication for this purpose nor has the medical literature suggested significant benefit. Although both drugs have minimal downsides, they are expensive, can provide a false sense of security, and can occasionally produce side effects.

MORE MYTHS AND MISCONCEPTIONS ABOUT NSAID GASTROPATHY

One study showed that gastropathy worsened with the antacids, a totally unexpected finding that was contrary to intuition

The last chapter began a discussion of strategies to decrease the incidence and severity of NSAID-induced gastropathy and methods to treat mucosal lesions and symptoms once they develop. The bottom line of that discussion was that the almost universally prescribed H2 blockers and sucralfate (Carafate) were no better than placebo in preventing or treating NSAID gastropathy and routinely prescribing these conventional ulcer medications was needless and basically worthless concomitant therapy. Although neither of these anti-ulcer drugs have a significant downside — and both are great therapies for peptic ulcers — they work no special magic on NSAID-induced GI pathology. The suspected physiological reason for the failure of these otherwise useful medications is that NSAID-induced gastropathy is not the same pathophysiology as the run-of-the-mill peptic ulcer. NSAIDs wreak their GI havoc through an inhibition of prostaglandin activity. H2 blockers merely decrease acid production while Carafate forms a protective barrier around an already established ulcer crater. The etiology of an NSAID ulcer is not simply excessive acid production. While many physicians still continue to prescribe conventional anti-ulcer regimens, neither the Food and Drug Administration, the *Physicians' Desk Reference*, nor the drug companies claim an indication for H2 blockers or sucralfate when it comes to NSAID-induced gastropathy.

My suggestion is that physicians limit the use of NSAIDs to patients who have truly inflammatory conditions or when using them as analgesics, prescribe them for only short periods of time. Obviously many alternative analgesics can be used, although NSAIDs are rather effective at providing pain relief caused by a variety of noninflammatory conditions. I also mentioned the common misconception that soft tissue trauma (sprains, strains, and contusions) has an arthritis-like inflammatory component that is somehow quelled by NSAIDs. I know of no data that show that NSAIDs help heal sprained ankles or muscular back pain any faster than acetaminophen.

This chapter is a critical look at commonly co-prescribed oral antacids and an analysis of a relatively new approach that specifically attacks the etiology of NSAID gastropathy.

LOW DOSE ANTACIDS AND NONSTEROIDAL ANTI-INFLAMMATORY DRUG-INDUCED GASTROPATHY IN HUMANS

Sievert W, et al

J Clin Gastroent 1991;13(Suppl 1):S145

This randomized double-blind crossover study evaluated the effect of low-dose antacid therapy on 40 healthy volunteers who were taking a three-week course of the NSAID naproxen (500 mg BID). After initial baseline endoscopy, all subjects were begun on the NSAID regimen and randomly assigned to receive either placebo or four Maalox TC tablets (aluminum hydroxide) daily. The Maalox therapy was considered low-dose and had an acid neutralizing capacity of 104 mEq/day. The low-dose regimen was chosen because higher doses are associated with annoying diarrhea. After the first three-week phase, subjects were again gastroscoped to grade the condition of the gastric and duodenal mucosa, noting the severity and number of the lesions. This was followed by a 21-day washout period that culminated in a third endoscopy to ensure healing of any lesions. The subjects were then crossed over into the alternative therapy and again underwent endoscopy after an additional three-week period.

The low-dose antacid failed to prevent abdominal discomfort, heartburn, and nausea any better than placebo. There was basically no difference in symptom scores with Maalox or placebo. Curiously, endoscopic findings in both the stomach and duodenum were more prominent in patients who had taken the antacid than in those who were treated with placebo. This apparent worsening of gastropathy with the antacids was totally unexpected and contrary to intuition. Other authors have demonstrated that Maalox increases prostaglandin synthesis and is cytoprotective, so the findings were provocative (*Gut* 1989; 30(2):148).

The authors conclude that low-dose aluminum hydroxide antacids offer no protection against mucosal ulceration and do not diminish GI symptoms in patients taking therapeutic doses of NSAIDs. The possible detrimental effect of the antacids suggested by this study could not be explained, but it could be due to the unopposed action of the aluminum component of the antacid on the gastric mucosa.

COMMENT: Yet another way for physicians to attempt to short-circuit gastropathy in patients taking NSAIDs is to suggest the concomitant use of oral antacids. Large doses of antacids, enough to create total neutralization of gastric pH, often result in diarrhea, and such regimens are usually discontinued by the patient. Giving a low-dose tablet of Maalox TC may be more patient-friendly, but this study failed to show a protective effect, either on symptoms or endoscopy findings. I could find no corroborating studies on this topic, but the data question the value of a common strategy prescribed to combat the GI effect of relatively short-term NSAID therapy. There are two findings in this study that bear emphasis. The first is that mucosal erosions were evident within three weeks of a modest dose of a popular NSAID. Secondly, it's rather amazing that 40 individuals subjected themselves to four endoscopic procedures (thinking about that alone may be enough to give anyone gastric upset, if not a true ulcer).

Because NSAID gastropathy is not acid-mediated, it makes physiologic sense that merely buffering gastric acid is not a logical defense. It doesn't hurt — and seems to help

ENDOSCOPIC GRADING SYSTEM AND RESULTS OF PLACEBO VS. MAALOX

Grade	Description
0	Normal mucosa
1	1 erosion
2	2-4 erosions
3	5-10 erosions
4	>10 erosions or ulcer
Gastric	**Lesion Grade**
Placebo	1.40±0.18
Maalox	1.91±0.17
Duodenal	
Placebo	1.22±0.35
Maalox	1.61±0.33*

*Not significant

Source: Clin Gastroenterol *1991;13(Suppl 1):S145-8.*

— to take NSAIDs with food, but adding an obligatory oral antacid is probably an unnecessary expense and evidently a waste of time. If your patient on short-term NSAID therapy develops gastric distress from the drug, the only reasonable approach is to stop the offending agent. It makes so much intuitive sense that antacids should help, it's not surprising that the regimen was never studied previously, and that it is simply accepted as routine. In fact, I frequently have given antacids with NSAIDs when the first dose is started in the ED and the patient has not eaten recently.

Maalox usually contains both magnesium hydroxide and aluminum hydroxide, but the contents of the preparation used in this study were not specified. Apparently only aluminum hydroxide was given. The aluminum component of most antacid products is often constipating, and the magnesium component can cause diarrhea, so both are often used in combination to offset the adverse GI effects.

I think the observed worsening of gastric lesions with Maalox in this study is interesting, but it may be merely a statistical glitch that does not have clinical significance. Finally, a few shortcomings of this study should be mentioned. The pH of the gastric secretions was not measured, and the actual clinical significance of the mucosal lesions was not investigated. No patient experienced perforation or GI bleeding, and the real significance of short-term changes in gastric mucosa from NSAIDs is not known. It is possible that the pathology found in this study had endoscopic, but not clinical significance. It's important to note, however, that NSAID-induced gastric ulcers are not self-limited changes that heal spontaneously while NSAID therapy continues.

> MISOPROSTOL CAN PREVENT GASTRIC ULCERS, BUT IT CAN CAUSE SPONTANEOUS ABORTION IN PREGNANT WOMEN AND DIARRHEA IN MOST PATIENTS

DUODENAL AND GASTRIC ULCER PREVENTION WITH MISOPROSTOL IN ARTHRITIS PATIENTS TAKING NSAIDs

Graham DY, et al *Ann Intern Med* 1993;119(4):257

The purpose of this study was to determine the efficacy of misoprostol (Cytotec) in preventing duodenal or gastric ulcers in arthritis patients who were receiving maintenance NSAID therapy. It was a randomized double-blind multicentered placebo-controlled trial of 638 patients. Previous studies have demonstrated that misoprostol, a synthetic prostaglandin E₁ analog, decreases the incidence of gastric ulcers in patients on chronic NSAID therapy without interfering with the systemic anti-inflammatory effect of the arthritis drugs.

All subjects were patients at a Veterans Affairs clinic, but the number of men and women was approximately equal. Patients were eligible for the study if they had any type of arthritis requiring at least three months of NSAID therapy with either ibuprofen, piroxicam, naproxen, sulindac, tolmetin, indomethacin, or diclofenac. All women were required to be post-menopausal or otherwise incapable of becoming pregnant. Patients were also excluded if they were taking anticoagulants, other ulcer therapy, or prednisone. The outcome parameter that was used to determine treatment failure was the development of gastric or duodenal ulcers (defined as a circumscribed mucosal defect of 0.5 cm or greater in diameter).

Following an initial baseline endoscopy, patients received either misoprostol (200 μg) or placebo four times a day for 12 weeks while they were maintained on their NSAID in anti-arthritic doses. The endoscopy was repeated at 4-, 8-, and 12-week intervals, and the condition of the gastric mucosa was evaluated each time. Approximately 320 patients in each group had a negative endoscopy on initial screening and participated in the study. About 70 percent (455) of the patients completed the trial.

At the 12-week endoscopy evaluation, a duodenal ulcer had developed in 0.6 percent of patients (2/320) taking misoprostol and in 4.6 percent (15/ 323) of those receiving placebo. The incidence of gastric ulcer was 1.9 percent (6/320) in those taking misoprostol vs. 7.7 percent (25/ 323) of those on placebo. There was no difference between the two groups in the presence or absence of gastrointestinal symptoms. Adverse effects were few, although 3.8 percent of patients taking misoprostol (vs. 0.9% for placebo) developed diarrhea.

This study confirms other reports that have demonstrated that both gastric and duodenal ulcers commonly develop in outpatients taking long-term NSAIDs. The authors conclude that misoprostol significantly lowers the frequency of both duodenal and gastric ulcers in such patients. They state that misoprostol is the only drug shown capable of preventing ulcers in chronic NSAID users. Because it is impossible prospectively to identify all patients at risk for NSAID gastropathy, the authors could not promulgate conclusive recommendations about whom should routinely be given concomitant misoprostol therapy; however, prophylaxis with misoprostol can be a prudent clinical decision in selected cases.

COMMENT: Released in 1989, misoprostol (Cytotec) is the only drug to have received FDA approval for the prevention of gastric ulcers in high-risk patients taking NSAIDs. It is generally accepted that this drug will prevent gastric ulcerations caused by NSAIDs (*Med Lett Drugs Ther* 1989;31:808, *Lancet* 1988;2(8623):1277, and *Ann Intern Med* 1991;115(3):195). There are data suggesting a prophylactic effect against duodenal ulcers, but the final vote on duodenal lesions is not yet in. Importantly, the drug does not interfere with the systemic anti-inflammatory activity of NSAIDs. Misoprostol is a synthetic analog of prostaglandin E_1, a protective substance normally secreted by the gastrointestinal mucosa in response to injury. Because NSAIDs inhibit the synthesis of prostaglandins, adding prostaglandins locally theoretically short-circuits the NSAID-induced gastropathy yet does not interfere with the systemic effect of the arthritis drug. Misoprostol is not absorbed and has no systemic effects. Misoprostol is also about as effective H_2 blockers in healing ulcers of non-NSAID etiology, but it is not commonly used for this indication.

Two side effects of misoprostol must be understood. Importantly, the drug is contraindicated during pregnancy because it can cause (and has been used to induce) spontaneous abortion. Secondly, many patients will develop a troublesome diarrhea that is generally dose related, and it occurs in about a quarter of those patients taking 100 μg QID. The recommended dose is 200 μg QID, and 100 tablets cost about $50 wholesale. The 100 μg QID regimen is statistically less effective than the 200 μg QID protocol, but the lower dose is still better than placebo and has fewer side effects.

Misoprostol's prostaglandin enhancement is believed to augment mucosal defenses that have been disrupted by NSAIDs. Therefore, in order to understand the physiology of the drug, one must understand the pathophysiology of NSAID-induced ulcers. NSAID ulcers are thought to be due to a mechanism different from classic gastric or duodenal ulcers. The E series of prostaglandins (PGE) are synthesized from fatty acids in the GI tract where they provide a natural protection to the gastric mucosa. PGEs enhance mucus production, which acts as a protective barrier from mechanical abrasion and acid/drug insults. PGEs also stimulate gastric bicarbonate ion secretion. In addition, mucosal blood flow, an important factor in providing nutrients to the mucosa and an aid to the removal of

DEVELOPMENT OF ULCERS FOR PATIENTS WITH AND WITHOUT HISTORY OF ULCER

| | *Ulcer Type* | | | | | |
| | *Duodenal* | | *Gastric* | | *Either* | |
Group	*Placebo*	*Misoprostol*	*Placebo*	*Misoprostol*	*Placebo*	*Misoprostol*
All patients[1]	*4.6%*	*0.6%*	*7.7%*	*1.9%*	*11.5%*	*2.5%*
No ulcer history[2]	*3.8%*	*0.4%*	*6.7%*	*1.7%*	*9.6%*	*2.1%*
Ulcer history[3]	*7.2%*	*1.2%*	*10.8%*	*2.5%*	*16.9%*	*3.7%*

[1]*Placebo patients=323; misoprostol patients=320.*

[2]*Placebo patients=240; misoprostol patients=239.*

[3]*Placebo patients=83; misoprostol patients=81.*

Source: Ann Intern Med *1993;119:257-62.*

excess hydrogen ions, is prostaglandin mediated. Finally, some gastric acid secretion is under prostaglandin control. The ability of NSAIDs to inhibit local gastric prostaglandin production will therefore remove at least four protective mechanisms that the body has developed to combat the development of mucosal erosions and ulcers.

Misoprostol, acting in a manner similar to naturally occurring prostaglandin, will stimulate local mucus secretion in a dose-dependent manner, increase bicarbonate secretion, increase gastric mucosal blood flow, and will inhibit gastric acid secretion. Therefore, this drug is an almost theoretically perfect substance. Because misoprostol has little systemic activity, it does not interfere with the anti-arthritis effect of NSAIDs. It also has no effect on NSAID nephropathy. The medical literature is generally in agreement that misoprostol is an important protective therapy in patients who require long-term NSAID therapy.

The dilemma for the emergency physician is that misoprostol is expensive, not required by the vast majority of patients who receive NSAID prescriptions from the emergency physician, and indications for its use are not clear cut. It is generally accepted that misoprostol will prevent gastric ulcers from developing (it's not so clear for duodenal ulcers), but the ability of the drug in preventing GI bleeding or perforation over the long haul is not known. Diarrhea is a common and bothersome side effect, and heartburn, dyspepsia, and nausea can also occur as side effects. It's important to know that the drug is contraindicated in pregnant women. Although one may be correct in prescribing misoprostol to high-risk patients, it does not appear to be logical to me to prescribe it routinely. Perhaps it may be of value in the elderly patient with gout who requires short-term NSAIDs but who has had previous GI problems associated with NSAIDs. Adding it to a patient on long-term therapy who presents to the ED with GI complaints is also a possible strategy (although this is probably a decision best made by the primary physician). Elderly patients are also at higher risk, but I would not advocate prescribing misoprostol routinely for short-term NSAID regimens. It would likely not be prudent simply to prescribe misoprostol to symptomatic patients while continuing the NSAID; they may have serious pathology, and a shotgun approach (aimed only at relieving symptoms) can be problematic. While misoprostol is not a perfect drug, at least we have something to consider.

A relatively new edition to anti-ulcer therapy is the drug omeprazole (Prilosec). Omeprazole is the first of a new class of ulcer drugs with potent antisecretory properties. The drug binds to the proton pump of the parietal cell and inhibits the $H+/K+$-ATPase mechanism that secretes hydrogen ions into the gastric lumen. Omeprazole is the most potent acid inhibitor, being more powerful than any of the H_2 blockers (*Med Lett Drugs Ther* 1990;32 (813):19). At higher doses, acid inhibition is nearly complete, and the drug probably heals duodenal peptic ulcers faster than H_2 blockers. Some important side effects are associated with this new drug; especially of concern are many drug-drug interactions. Currently omeprazole is only approved for the short-term (not maintenance) therapy of duodenal ulcers (*N Engl J Med* 1989;320(2):69).

For now there are little data on the ability of omeprazole to prevent NSAID-induced ulcers. While omeprazole may be more effective than H_2 blockers, the etiology of NSAID ulcers would lead one to intuit that even very effective blockers of acid production won't be totally effective in preventing NSAID-induced ulcers (*N Engl J Med* 1989;320:69).

How does the gastric mucosa defend itself? When a gastric insult has occurred, the body has a repair mechanism ready to respond, but that repair mechanism is largely dependent on an intact ability to produce prostaglandins at the site of injury. NSAIDs are weak acids that inhibit prostaglandin production, both systemically and locally in the gastric mucosa. Being acids, NSAIDs cause direct topical damage to the gastric mucosa. Hence, NSAIDs have a dual mechanism by which they cause gastric ulcers: they are both the initial insult and the antagonist to the body's normal defenses.

The stomach's natural defense mechanism is a complex interaction between mucus, bicarbonate, mucosal blood flow, and other factors. The production of protective substances and the physiology of cellular regeneration following mucosal injury is largely under the influence of prostaglandins. Following disruption of cell membranes, prostaglandins are produced. Prostaglandins will stimulate secretion of bicarbonate and the synthesis of mucus, and will thereby augment local defense mechanisms. In addition, prostaglandins will enhance mucosal blood flow that is required to maintain the integrity of the mucosa and eliminate excess hydrogen ions.

FACT AND FICTION: KIDNEY STONES

Flat plate x-rays are essentially useless for diagnosing kidney stones, and there is no support for forced diuresis or fluid restriction as therapies

Emergency physicians frequently evaluate patients who have signs and symptoms of ureterolithiasis. Most of us have our routine work-up, and all of us have our particular bias and dogma that we expound to anyone who will listen. As with any medical entity, there are a number of myths and misconceptions that have been promulgated concerning the diagnosis and treatment of ureteral calculi. Some approaches are adhered to religiously despite the presence of data that are questionable, non-existent, nonsupportive, or downright contrary.

In this chapter, I review some of the commonly held clinical beliefs and practices concerning kidney stones in an attempt to evaluate which are truly axioms and which are merely unsubstantiated rumors.

USEFULNESS OF ABDOMINAL FLAT PLATE RADIOGRAPHS IN PATIENTS WITH SUSPECTED URETERAL CALCULI

Zangerle KF, et al *Ann Emerg Med* 1985;14(4):316

The authors of this study tested the ability of clinicians to detect and localize ureteral calculi on plain abdominal radiographs. The scout film of intravenous pyelograms (IVPs) of 120 patients undergoing this study for various reasons were presented, without a medical history or laboratory data, to a staff radiologist and a staff emergency physician. These plain films were blindly read by the two specialists who were instructed to make an interpretation of the presence or absence of a ureteral stone, localize the calculus, and then grade their degree of confidence in that interpretation. To minimize the chance that the calculus had moved during the time from the flat plate and the IVP performance, the plain radiographs were actually the scout films used for the IVP. Approximately half of the IVPs (51 cases) demonstrated a ureteral calculus (40 cases) or obstruction without definite calculi (11 cases). Out of 69 calculi-negative IVPs, 23 were ordered for suspected calculi and 46 were for evaluation of hematuria, tumor, or trauma. In order for the interpretation to be considered a true positive, the reader had to assign a "likely" or better confidence level to their reading and the suspected calculus had to be in the same position as noted on the IVP.

Overall, only half of the readings were correct as to the presence or absence of a calculus, but the incidence of true positives was only 33 percent for the radiologist and 25 percent for the emergency physician. (See tables.) The incidence of true negatives was 76 percent and 71 percent for the radiologist and EP, respectively. The interpretations of the radiologist and emergency physician agreed with the IVP 51 percent and 48 percent of the time respectively. The radiologist was correct on 36 percent of the positive and 64 percent of the negative films. The corresponding percentages for the emergency physician were 33 percent and 60 percent, respectively. Both readers rarely registered a high confidence or "definite" prediction for the presence of the calculus, a criteria for being called a true positive. For example, out of 133 readings by the radiologist, a "definite" prediction was given only eight times; and for five of those, the interpretation was incorrect.

Although the study only used two physicians for x-ray interpretation and the readers were presented the films without the benefit of a history or laboratory data, the authors conclude that the plain abdominal radiograph is highly unreliable in patients with suspected ureteral calculi. This x-ray adds no useful information to the evaluation of suspected kidney stones. The false positive and false negative interpretation rates were high, making the plain film a virtually useless study. An IVP was recommended for definite diagnosis in all cases of suspected ureteral calculi.

COMMENT: Tradition is difficult to change, and many of my colleagues continue to order plain films (flat plate, KUB) for the evaluation of patients with suspected kidney stones. For some odd reason, most can quote these studies but still order the films anyway. Radiologists often request this study before agreeing to perform an IVP, even though they repeat the plain film as part of their preliminary evaluation. If an IVP is scheduled, it's absurd for the EP to also order a plain film. Urologists seem to be the most enlightened on this subject, although they will never even consider evaluating a patient without a full IVP and/or an ultrasound study. Although one can occasionally see a stone on a plain film, it is such an inaccurate study that the procedure should be abandoned. Once a radiopaque stone is confirmed by an IVP, occasionally the flat plate may be used on an outpatient basis to follow the movement of that stone, but this is the only reason that I can see for ordering such a low-yield study.

Roth et al (*Ann Emerg Med* 1985;14(4):311) conducted a similar study that appears in the same issue as the Zangerle et al article. These authors retrospectively reviewed the IVPs of 206 adult patients who underwent an emergency dye study as part of their evaluation for possible kidney stones. A staff radiologist was asked to interpret blindly a plain film, and the results were compared to the IVP reading. (See table.) It's noted that the incidence of true positives was again less than 50 percent. The sensitivity and specificity was only 62 percent and 67 percent, respectively. These authors similarly conclude that the sensitivity, specificity, accuracy, and negative predictive value of a plain film are low, and the x-ray provides no more diagnostically useful information than the history, physical examination, and urinalysis. They suggest that a plain film should never be used in place of an IVP for the diagnosis and management of patients with suspected kidney stones.

FILM READINGS: RADIOLOGIST VS. EP

	Radiologist	Emergency Physician
True positive	20/60 (33%)	13/51 (25%)
True negative	55/72 (76%)	49/69 (71%)
False positives		
Negative IVPs	17/72 (24%)	20/69 (30%)
Positive IVPs	19/61 (31%)	10/51 (20%)
All IVPs	36/133 (27%)	30/120 (25%)
False negatives	22/61 (36%)	28/51 (55%)

The radiologist made 133 readings (61 on positive films, 72 on negative) on 120 films. The EP made 120 readings (51 positive, 69 negative) on 120 films, hence the different denominator for true positive and true negative results.

Negative IVPs assume a confidence of "likely" or better (see text).

Calculus on negative IVPs was predicted but there was no evidence of a calculus on IVP. On positive IVPs, calculus was predicted, but it was in a different position than predicted.

Source: Ann Emerg Med *1985;14:316-319.*

NUMBER OF CORRECT PLAIN ABDOMINAL RADIOGRAPHS (PARs)

	Radiologist	Emergency Physician
Positive PARs	36% (22/61)	33% (17/51)
Negative PARs	64% (46/72)	60% (41/69)
All PARs	51% (68/133)	48% (58/120)

All readings taken together = 50% (156/253)

Positive PARs were taken from patients with IVP-proven ureteral calculus. Negative PARs had IVP-proven absence of ureteral calculus.

Source: Ann Emerg Med 1985; 14:316-319.

CHARACTERISTICS OF PAR IN PATIENTS WITH AND WITHOUT IVP EVIDENCE OF URETERAL STONE

	No.	%
True positives	92	45
False positives	19	9
False negatives	56	27
True negatives	39	19
Total	206	100

Source: Ann Emerg Med 1985; 14:311-315.

There are many reasons why the abdominal plain film is a useless test. Although textbooks state that 90 percent of stones are radiopaque, this is a misleading statistic. It is true that most stones will contain radiopaque calcium. Once you know that the stone is present by the IVP, it may be possible to diagnose it accurately 90 percent of the time with a retrospective review of the flat plate. In my experience, however, the incidence of radiopaque stones that can be seen on the initial plain film and localized to the genitourinary tract does not come close to 90 percent. In the studies reviewed here, less than half of the stones were prospectively called on the initial reading of the plain film; it's more accurate to flip a coin! Even if a stone contained calcium, bowel gas, GI contents, feces, and underlying bone, the myriad calcific densities (vascular, nodes, cartilage) normally seen in the pelvis and abdomen make those little white specks almost impossible to interpret with any accuracy.

One argument for the continued use of the flat plate has been that it is occasionally diagnostic and the IVP is expensive, and it may save the patient a possible allergic reaction to dye. It is impossible to predict which patients will develop anaphylactoid reactions, and there are other untoward dye reactions, so these are logical concerns. In patients with previous anaphylactoid reactions to dye, the incidence of a repeat reaction is actually quite low and very acceptable if one has the options to pretreat (over 12 hours) with antihistamines and steroids. Other osmotically related problems are minimized with the newer non-ionic dyes with low osmolality. Of course, an ultrasound can safely settle the issue, and it is the procedure of choice if the patient is pregnant or in those claiming an allergy to dye, especially if you suspect drug-seeking.

Although many patients can have the diagnosis of kidney stone made on history, physical, and urinalysis findings, I'm an advocate of the liberal use of IVP/ultrasound to document the condition. There are relatively few times in the ED that we can definitely diagnose the cause of acute, severe pain. Although a kidney stone has a rather classic presentation, I've seen appendicitis, renal infarction, ovarian torsion, ectopic pregnancy, dissecting aneurysms, hematoma from tumor, and drug-seeking behavior mimic the classic presentation. If a patient with a past history of a kidney stone presents with textbook characteristics, and states, "This one is just like my other stones," I will occasionally forego the study. One argument for routine IVP that is often made is that the dye study confirms complete obstruction. The degree of obstruction is, however, usually not the reason patients are admitted or discharged.

Most emergency medicine textbooks have acknowledged the data in these papers and recommend foregoing the routine flat plate. Some still hedge or do not address the issue squarely. It would be nice if physicians would either read the enlightened texts or believe their own experiences and the results of well-designed studies.

ACUTE URETERAL COLIC AND FLUID INTAKE

Edna TH, Hesselberg F

Scand J Urol Nephrol 1983;17(2):175

The authors of this prospective study assessed the effect of forced IV fluid administration or strict fluid restriction on the pain and stone passage rate in 60 patients with acute ureteral colic. During the first six hours after diagnosis, half of the patients were managed with total fluid restriction and the other half were treated with a generous 3 liters of IV fluids (2 liters D5W and 1 liter Ringer's lactate). All patients had an IVP prior to entering the study. The location and diameter of the stone, the sex and age of the patient, and the duration of the pain prior to evaluation were similar in both groups. The patients graded their pain after six hours of treatment. Meperidine, in less than generous doses, was given for pain control.

The authors concluded that the amount of fluid intake had no practical influence on the degree of pain or clinical outcome in patients with renal colic. (See table.) The authors note that while the pain of ureteral colic is thought to arise from distension of the renal pelvis and ureter above an obstructing stone, an increase in pressure is not the only factor producing pain. This concept of fluid-induced proximal distension resulting in increased pain has been the basis for recommending fluid restriction. In the presence of ureteral obstruction, however, the majority of administered fluid is filtered by the opposite kidney. Volume expansion does not necessarily produce additional urine flow in the obstructed side.

The authors admit that their study only evaluated a short period in the life span of a kidney stone. Of importance, the patients were treated from 11 to 13 hours after the onset of pain, and the results might have been different had the fluid manipulations occurred earlier in the course.

Most stones spontaneously passed, but the fate of the stone was not related to fluid intake. The authors conclude that fluid intake has no effect on initial pain relief or spontaneous stone passage in patients with acute ureteral colic.

COMMENT: Many physicians are under the impression that fluid infused in a peripheral vein ends up in the obstructed ureter, applying proximal pressure to flush out a stone. Other physicians are just as adamant that excess hydration increases pain by increasing distension of the proximal ureter and pelvis. Physiological studies seem to indicate that neither assumption is correct. This study is one of the few clinical trials that actually studies the subject. Textbooks continue to promulgate biases and myths,

PAIN AND OUTCOME IN ACUTE URETERAL STONE COLIC

Pain gradation after six hours of treatment*	Group A No fluid intake	Group B High fluid intake
No pain	12 (2)	11 (1)
Some pain, but less than before	9 (2)	10 (4)
Pain as before treatment	3 (1)	0
Pain worse than before, or requiring new analgesic before six hours	6 (3)	9 (3)
Total	30 (8)	30 (8)

Fate of the ureteral stone	Group A No fluid intake	Group B High fluid intake
Stone surgically removed	5	6
Stone cystoscopically manipulated	6	4
Stone spontaneously expelled	17	18
Patient did not attend check-up	2	2
Total	30	30

*Figures in parentheses denote patients with pain of less than six hours when treatment began.

Source: Scand J Urol Nephrol *1983;17:175-178.*

MYTHS AND FACTS ABOUT KIDNEY STONES

Myth: *A plain abdominal radiograph is clinically useful in the diagnosis and treatment of renal calculi. It is a cost-effective screening study.*

Fact: *Plain films have such a high incidence of false positive and false negative readings that they are virtually useless for making diagnostic and treatment decisions. An IVP or ultrasound examination is required to confirm all cases.*

Myth: *Patients with kidney stones should receive high volumes of intravenous fluids to increase urine flow and to flush out stones. Patients with kidney stones should be fluid-restricted because excess fluids will distend the proximal ureter and increase pain.*

Fact: *Neither fluid loading nor fluid restriction affects the incidence of stone passage or degree of pain. Most of the parenteral fluid is shunted to the contralateral kidney and never reaches the involved ureter.*

Myth: *Almost all patients with kidney stones will have at least microscopic hematuria. If hematuria is absent, complete ureteral obstruction is likely.*

Fact: *Up to one in four patients with documented stones will not exhibit hematuria. The magnitude of hematuria does not correlate with the degree of obstruction.*

Source: James R. Roberts, MD

and the latest edition of a standard emergency text (Schwartz et al, *Principles and Practice of Emergency Medicine,* 3rd Edition, Lea and Febiger) states that aggressive IV hydration aggravates the degree of obstruction and can increase the patient's discomfort. The author of this chapter believes that oral hydration is adequate and does not advise IV fluids. The American College of Emergency Physicians study guide (Tintinalli et al, McGraw-Hill) takes an opposite approach and advises IV saline to ensure urine volumes of up to 200 ml per hour. Neither author references his statement, probably because there are little data in the literature to back up the contentions. Although the study reviewed here is limited and has a few methodological flaws (especially the lack of consistent evaluation of urine flow, volumes, and a dynamic pain score), it is one of the few studies of its kind in the literature. I would

agree that 3 liters of fluid over six hours is aggressive fluid management, and such a fluid load should have provided an obvious benefit if it were to make a difference.

Most patients with kidney stones are vomiting. They come to the hospital very quickly because of the severity of renal colic, and significant dehydration is usually not an issue. Certainly, dehydrated patients should be fluid-loaded prior to receiving an IVP because dehydration is a risk factor for the development of dye-induced nephropathy. A possible downside of over-hydration is that the IVP dye is diluted and the study may be inadequate. Excess fluid is also detrimental to patients with limited cardiac reserve.

We have all seen patients who miraculously become pain-free after their IVP. This is attributed to the fact that IVP dyes are highly osmotic. The high osmotic load into the ureter may be somewhat therapeutic, although this is also speculation and has not been well studied. Because 90 percent of calculi pass spontaneously, usually in the first few hours, such clinical observations are difficult to interpret.

Finally, the use of glucagon and other anticholinergic or antispasmodic agents have been suggested to relax the ureter and assist in the passage of the stone. There are no data in the literature to support that this pharmacologic approach is of any value.

Likewise, there are no data in the literature to support either the use of forced diuresis or fluid restriction as a therapeutic modality in patients with kidney stones. It makes common sense to ensure adequate hydration, particularly prior to an IVP dye injection, but there are no data to suggest that IV fluids either increase pain or force a stone through the ureter.

MICROSCOPIC HEMATURIA AND CALCULUS-RELATED URETERAL OBSTRUCTION

Stewart DP, et al *J Emerg Med* 1990;8(6):693

The authors of this study examined the correlation between the degree of microscopic hematuria and the degree of IVP-confirmed ureteral obstruction in 160 patients presenting with renal colic. This was a retrospective study that was designed to determine if the number of red cells in a urinanalysis could predict the extent of ureteral obstruction. Severe ureteral obstruction, defined as dye extravasation or ureteral filling times of two hours or more, was present in 29 percent of the patients.

The authors found no relationship between the degree of hematuria and the degree of ureteral obstruction. Importantly, seven percent of the patients had severe obstruction and a urinanalysis that could be considered normal: fewer than 3 red blood cells per high power field. Additionally, 11 percent had some obstruction in the presence of a normal urinalysis. The overall incidence of hematuria was 85 percent in patients with nonsevere obstruction and 76 percent in patients with severe obstruction. Clearly, the presence or absence of hematuria was not predictive of the degree of obstruction.

COMMENT: This article is included because it is one of the few that evaluates the frequently quoted (and rarely referenced) axiom that the absence of red cells in a urine sediment correlates with an obstructed ureter. It is also one of a few studies that evaluates the actual incidence of hematuria in patients with proven stones.

Most physicians believe that the majority of patients with a kidney stone will have hematuria and that those with complete obstruction will not. Certainly a stone can present with either gross hematuria or a perfectly normal urine, but usually the urinalysis is somewhat abnormal. Other authors have demonstrated an incidence of hematuria as high as 97 percent (*Clin Radiol* 1980;31(5):605) or as low as 66 percent (*Practitioner* 1979;223(1324):387). In my experience, a majority of patients will have at least

microscopic hematuria associated with their stones. This study states that it may be absent in as many as one in four patients.

Hematuria is best defined by microscopic analysis of the urine sediment. Greater than three cells per high power field is generally considered abnormal. The actual quantitation of red cells, however, is dependent on the centrifugation time and volume of supernatant that is used to resuspend the urine, and finding a few red cells is normal. Most laboratory technicians will evaluate more than one high power field, but I was always confused by a 0-5 reading, which should, I believe, be zero or five cells per field.

Most physicians use the urine dipstick as the initial method to test for blood, and it's the test that often prompts either a narcotic administration or an IVP request. Overall, the urine dipstick is quite accurate. It can, of course, be positive from myoglobin from soft tissue trauma, cocaine use, or skeletal muscle injury so microscopic confirmation is necessary. Some dietary pyridoxiases and a few inadvertent drops of Betadine used to prep the meatus can give a false positive dipstick test for blood. Oral vitamin C use also can give a false negative analysis, and certainly appendicitis and urinary tract infection can add red cells to the sediment. Of course, a formal microscopic urinanalysis should always be done in patients with suspected stones to rule out possible infection. Although significant hematuria is rare following careful bladder catheterization, a freely void urine specimen is always preferred. (Always ask women about menstruation.) It is logical to assume that most patients with kidney stones will have at least microscopic hematuria. Some patients may present without hematuria, and it does not necessarily mean that they have complete urinary obstruction.

> A KIDNEY STONE CAN PRESENT WITH EITHER GROSS HEMATURIA OR NORMAL URINE, BUT URINALYSIS IS USUALLY SOMEWHAT ABNORMAL

MYTHS AND MISCONCEPTIONS ABOUT THERAPY FOR GI HEMORRHAGE

Ingrained, well-accepted therapies, such as iced gastric lavage, are found to be bogus under rigorous study

Periodically I like to peruse the literature with the intent on finding true scientific data that invalidate commonly held myths and misconceptions in emergency medicine. Because medicine is not an exact science, this is a relatively easy task. Numerous procedures and protocols are established and religiously adhered to that are based purely on tradition, anecdotal reports, personal belief, or seemingly logical parameters.

Although these tenets are often found to be spurious, they are handed down from housestaff to housestaff (or attending to attending) with such zeal and charismatic adherence that they quickly become ingrained as absolute truth. Even respected textbooks promulgate erroneous concepts. But one need not practice medicine for long to realize that yesterday's dogma can easily become today's heresy, and vice versa. This chapter takes a critical look at some common practices used for the treatment of acute gastrointestinal bleeding.

TREATMENT WITH HISTAMINE H2 ANTAGONISTS IN ACUTE UPPER GASTROINTESTINAL HEMORRHAGE: IMPLICATIONS OF RANDOMIZED TRIALS

Collins R, Langman M
N Engl J Med 1985; 313(11):660

This is a widely quoted review article that analyzes published data from randomized controlled trials evaluating the use of H2 antagonists, particularly cimetidine (Tagamet) or ranitidine (Zantac), for treatment of acute upper GI hemorrhage. Its purpose was to evaluate the common practice of routinely administering H2 antagonists to patients with acute upper GI bleeds from various sources. The authors also investigated whether there are data to prove that H2 antagonists will reduce the risk of death or major complications when used acutely. Data from 27 available randomized trials, consisting of 2,500 patients, were analyzed. From these studies, the authors extrapolated the incidence of persistent or recurrent bleeding, the need for surgery, and death rates, using these for criteria to denote success or failure of the medications. In addition, sites of bleeding were considered, and gastric and duodenal ulcer hemorrhage were specifically compared.

Up to 45 percent of the patients had experienced persistent or recurrent bleeding during the trials. There was no statistically significant benefit of the H2 antagonists in preventing bleeding recurrences or stanching active hemorrhage from any site, although a small advantage could be suggested from some studies of bleeding gastric ulcers.

Up to 35 percent of the patients required surgery for their hemorrhages. The authors could not make firm positive conclusions about the value of these antihistamines to decrease the need for surgery. Likewise for overall mortality, there was no clear benefit demonstrated in the treatment groups. When duodenal and gastric ulcers were compared, there was some suggestion that treatment reduced the rate of continued bleeding from gastric ulcers, but no difference was found when these drugs were administered to patients with duodenal ulcers. However, the authors question whether the statistics used to come to any positive conclusion were valid.

> **MANY PROTOCOLS THAT ARE RELIGIOUSLY ADHERED TO ARE BASED ONLY ON TRADITION, ANECDOTAL REPORTS, OR PERSONAL BELIEFS**

The authors conclude that despite a number of studies in the literature, the available data lack the power to demonstrate a clear benefit from H2 blockers in patients with GI hemorrhage. One problem with the analysis is that GI bleeding is associated with a successful outcome without any therapy in many cases. Hemorrhage usually stops, and there is a rather low mortality rate, about two percent. Although there was a trend for an overall benefit in these randomized studies for bleeding gastric ulcers, a significant amount of data dredging had to be done to suggest any benefit at all.

CONTROLLED TRIAL OF MEDICAL THERAPY FOR ACTIVE UPPER GASTROINTESTINAL BLEEDING AND PREVENTION OF REBLEEDING

Zuckerman G, et al *Am J Med* 1984;76(3):361

This commonly quoted placebo-controlled multicenter trial evaluated medical therapy to stop acute GI bleeding in 285 patients and to prevent immediate recurrences once bleeding had stopped. Treatment of the acute bleeding stage was either with placebo or cimetidine (300 mg every six hours intravenously). Endoscopy was performed early in the course to identify the site of bleeding. Patients who had stopped bleeding were then entered into one of four regimens aimed at preventing a recurrence during that hospitalization: oral cimetidine 300 mg TID and

at bedtime; Mylanta II at 30 ml every hour while awake; cimetidine plus hourly antacids; or placebo. A total of 285 patients were entered into the acute bleeding evaluation, and 194 patients participated in the prevention of rebleeding phase. Pathology included duodenal or gastric ulcer, erosive gastritis, a Mallory-Weiss syndrome, and a few patients with esophageal varices.

There were no significant differences between treatment with intravenous cimetidine and placebo in stopping acute upper gastrointestinal hemorrhage. Bleeding stopped in 71 percent of the treated group and in 77 percent of the placebo group. The specific bleeding site had no effect on outcome. The incidence of rebleeding was 24 percent in the cimetidine group, 13 percent in the hourly antacid group, 11 percent in the cimetidine plus hourly antacid group, and 26 percent in the placebo group. None of the prevention regimens reached statistical differences. As with the acute bleeding phase, the

IV CIMETIDINE VS. PLACEBO DURING ACUTE GI BLEEDING IN 285 PATIENTS

	Treatment Success	Treatment Failure	Total
Cimetidine	109 (71.2)	44 (28.7)	153
Placebo	102 (77.2)	30 (22.7)	132

Source: Am J Med *1984;76:361-6.*

specific bleeding site did not influence the incidence of rebleeding.

The authors conclude that intravenous cimetidine has no advantage over placebo in the treatment of acute upper GI hemorrhage and that rebleeding episodes during the same hospitalization do not appear to be significantly reduced by any of the medical regimens studied. The authors conclude that the cessation of active bleeding or the prevention of recurrent upper GI hemorrhage during hospitalization is not affected by medical therapy directed at acid neutralization or reduction.

COMMENT: H2 antagonists are universally used for the treatment of acute GI bleed, and I don't think a patient has been admitted to our hospital in the past five years without some H2 blocker being administered in the ED. Despite this universal approach, the literature is very clear: it doesn't work. Recent evidence also demonstrates that the most potent antisecretory agent available, omeprazole (Prilosec), given intravenously is also no better than placebo for the acute treatment of bleeding ulcers. Numerous studies also fail to prove that medical regimens will prevent immediate recurrent bleeding (*BMJ* 1992; 304(6820):143). Certainly many H2 blockers and omeprazole will promote healing of ulcers, but there are no data to indicate that they should be used during the acute phase of GI bleeding or during the immediate recovery period.

It's easy to see how the rumors got started about the benefit of various medical regimens for acute GI hemorrhage. About three-quarters of patients will stop bleeding spontaneously so one's clinical experience, with empirical

> MYTHS ARE HANDED DOWN FROM HOUSESTAFF TO HOUSESTAFF WITH SUCH ZEAL THAT THEY QUICKLY BECOME INGRAINED AS TRUTH

PREVENTION OF REBLEEDING IN 194 PATIENTS

	Success	Failure
Cimetidine	39 (76.5)	12 (23.5)
Antacids	34 (87.2)	5 (12.8)
Cimetidine and antacids	48 (88.9)	6 (11.1)
Placebo	37 (74.0)	13 (26.0)
Total	158 (81.4)	36 (18.6)

Source: Am J Med *1984;76:361-6.*

regimens without controls, will suggest a positive effect. Secondly, antacids, H2 blockers, and other antiulcer regimens do help cure patients with established nonbleeding ulcers. Third, from a physiologic argument, normal blood coagulation requires a neutral setting (pH 6.9-7.4). A low pH, as found in the stomach, hampers blood coagulation and platelet aggregation, and pepsin, a substance that dis-

solves formed clots, is active only in an acidic medium. Therefore, it makes theoretical sense that acid neutralization would help stop GI bleeding and prevent an immediate recurrence. In fact, some of the criticism of these studies is that a neutral pH has not always been demonstrated so perhaps not enough neutralization was produced. This had led some authorities to use continuous infusions of high doses of H2 blockers. Nonetheless, a benefit has yet to be demonstrated. There is probably no major clinical downside to the routine use of H2 blockers, except perhaps the cost.

The lack of any clearly effective medical therapy for patients with bleeding ulcers is a frustrating fact of emergency medicine. It seems that we should be able to do more than start an IV, order blood tests and crossmatch, pass an nasogastric tube, and call a consultant, In reality, however, not much more than that is possible with current knowledge. Newer endoscopic therapies may prove most beneficial.

Removing large clots of blood or gastric contents to allow the stomach to contract has been suggested as being beneficial, but as the following articles will demonstrate, intragastric ice water or other topical therapies are about as worthless as acute efforts to stop acid production. Finally, the *Physicians' Desk Reference* does not mention the use of any of the currently available medications used to prevent acid production for the treatment of acute GI bleeding. Although it is well accepted that these medications will promote healing of ulcers and perhaps even prevent their recurrence after an acute episode, they do not have Food and Drug Administration approval for treatment of an acute GI bleed.

ICED GASTRIC LAVAGE: A TRADITION WITHOUT FOUNDATION

Leather RA, Sullivan SN
Can Med Assoc J 1987;136(12):1245

This article reviews data concerning the use of iced gastric lavage for the treatment of acute upper GI hemorrhage. It is a commonly used technique, but in reality, there is no well documented scientific evidence to support it. There is no efficacy demonstrated in the human literature, and animal studies have likewise failed to support gastric cooling. In fact, it has been suggested there may be mucosal damage or metabolic derangements from iced gastric lavage, and many condemn its use.

Theoretically, cold-induced topical vasoconstriction is a possible mechanism by which gastric hemorrhage can be decreased. In fact, there may be increased blood flow during the initial phases of the cooling procedure, and there is evidence for a rebound vasodilation when cooling is terminated. Also, continuous irrigation may dislodge established clots. The authors conclude from their review of the literature that the technique of iced gastric lavage for the treatment of acute GI hemorrhage is ineffective and may be harmful. It's suggested that the procedure be discontinued.

COMMENT: Numerous other authors have commented on the lack of proven efficacy and possible harm from iced water irrigation for the treatment of acute GI bleed. There is no evidence whatsoever that gastric lavage with any fluid at any temperature will stop bleeding or prevent recurrence. Lavage may help clean the stomach prior to endoscopy.

It is a reflex action to pass an NG tube at least to evacuate clots and blood from the stomach of patients who are actively bleeding or present with a history of upper GI hemorrhage. Theoretically, removing large clots and stomach volume will allow the stomach to contract and help control or stop bleeding. In a similar extrapolation, the bladder is often irrigated of clots in patients who present with acute GI bleeding. I have never seen that particular concept challenged nor proven. Some disadvantages of NG suction include significant patient discomfort, predisposition to reflux and pulmonary aspiration, and a possible damage to the gastric mucosa from aggressive mechanical trauma.

Another article arguing against the cooling technique is made by Andrus et al (*Am J Gastroenterol* 1987; 82(1): 1062). These authors note that less than 20 percent of intraluminal gastric blood can be recovered with gastric lavage. The risk of hypothermia is always present, a problem that is certainly not needed in patients who are critically ill or hypotensive. Cooling may actually prolong bleeding time and increase clotting time, and there is a concern that even though there may be some gastric blood flow decrease with iced saline, hypothermia may be harmful to the gastric mucosa.

Initial gastric lavage with saline or water (room temperature) and continued nasogastric suction seem to be standard of care for acute GI hemorrhage. Even this technique is unproven and should be studied. Remember that we all bought the concept of a routine NG tube for all cases of pancreatitis, and that has been proven a myth. Ice water lavage, however, has been largely condemned, but many physicians still use it. Not only does it create a mess, it ties up a health care provider and focuses one's priorities on an unimportant procedure. This therapy should be abandoned if you still use it.

Although I may be showing my age, I can still remember instilling ice water with a few ampules of norepineprhin (Levophed) dissolved in the lavage solution into the stomach to promote topical vasoconstriction. It seemed like a neat trick that was physiologically sound, but this too has been proven to be useless therapy and one that may be harmful by producing prolonged topical vasoconstriction. Levophed is not absorbed into the general circulation to produce any significant pressor effect, but like ice water gastric lavage, it's a clinical dinosaur. Other drugs such as intragastric vasopressin, prostaglandins, and somatostatin have also been fruitlessly instilled into the stomach in an attempt to stanch the flow of blood from actively bleeding ulcers or

MYTHS AND MISCONCEPTIONS ABOUT THERAPY FOR GI HEMORRHAGE

Myth/ Misconception:	*H2 receptor antagonists will decrease bleeding from acute upper GI hemorrhage and will prevent recurrence.*
Fact:	*These drugs do not benefit patients with acute upper GI hemorrhage nor do they prevent an immediate recurrence.*
Myth/ Misconception:	*Iced water gastric lavage decreases bleeding in acute GI hemorrhage.*
Fact:	*Iced water gastric lavage has no therapeutic value in these patients and may even be detrimental.*

Source: James R. Roberts, MD.

gastritis. These drugs are also given intravenously with similar lack of effect.

The unsuccessful attempts to prevent recurrences of acute bleeding from gastric duodenal ulcers with antacid therapy is difficult to imagine; it makes such good common sense. Current data suggest that standard or high-dose H_2 receptor antagonists or Prilosec are not indicated within the first 72 hours of an upper GI bleed. Acute bleeding or an immediate rebleeding are not halted with any known medical intervention. Even when faced with the facts, however, most will probably continue to use acid neutralization acutely. Of course, a big slug of Maalox will make your endoscopist rather upset.

Recent important data have demonstrated that gastric infections with *Helicobacter pylori* are the cause of ulcers in many patients. Efforts to find and eradicate this bacteria have now taken much of the therapeutic thunder that once belonged to H_2 blockers.

Finally, I came across a few other interesting facts about upper GI bleeding that may be difficult to believe. In a recent review article on bleeding peptic ulcers (*N Engl J Med* 1994; 331(11):717), Laine and Peterson state that corticosteroids in the absence of concomitant NSAID therapy do not increase the risk for ulcer development or bleeding. Also, warfarin therapy does not increase the incidence of bleeding from ulcers either.

MYTHS AND MISCONCEPTIONS ABOUT EPINEPHRINE

Myths are handed down with such zeal and charismatic adherence that they quickly become ingrained as absolute truth

As I said in the last chapter, many procedures and protocols are based on tradition, anecdotal reports, personal beliefs, or seemingly local parameters, but when studied are found to be bogus. Recently high-dose epinephrine was touted to change survival rates in cardiac arrest miraculously. This initially accepted concept was relegated to a bona fide misconception when studied scientifically, and luckily it never became a widely accepted technique before it fizzled. This chapter focuses on some other misconceptions about the clinical use of epinephrine, some of which have been around for a rather long time and have become rarely questioned medical gospel.

MYTH: *Epinephrine is absolutely contraindicated in the treatment of acute asthma in any patient older than 40 years because of the high incidence of adverse cardiovascular effects.*

FACT: *In the absence of recent myocardial infarction, malignant dysrhythmias, or coexistent coronary artery spasm, the use of standard doses of epinephrine for the treatment of acute asthma is safe for patients of any age, even if there is a history of hypertension.*

THE USE OF EPINEPHRINE IN THE TREATMENT OF OLDER ADULT ASTHMATICS
Cydulka R, et al *Ann Emerg Med* 1988;17(4):322

In an attempt to verify the safety profile of subcutaneous epinephrine for the treatment of acute asthma, the authors of this study administered three subcutaneous doses of 0.3 ml (mg) of 1:1000 epinephrine every 20 minutes to 95 adult asthmatics whose ages ranged from 15 to 96 years. The only exclusion parameters were a recent myocardial infarction (within three months) or coexistent angina. Patients were grouped into two age-related categories using 40 years as the cutoff. Subjects were given a maximum of four doses, and the only criteria for early discontinuation were ventricular tachycardia, multiple premature ventricular beats associated with hypotension, or the development of angina. Aerosolized beta agonists were not given. Numerous cardiovascular parameters were recorded at baseline and at 20 minutes after each dose of epinephrine. Heart rhythm was continuously recorded, and rhythm strips were examined blindly by a cardiologist.

Thirty-nine of the 108 episodes (36%) of acute bronchospasm occurred in patients over age 40 years. No patient was withdrawn from the study because of adverse side effects. Following epinephrine, all patients experienced only minimal changes in systolic or diastolic blood pressure, heart rate, or respiratory rate, although they all showed improvement in peak flow rates. The only statistically significant difference between the two groups was that the older patients experienced a mean decrease (note: this was a decrease!) of 9.5 mmHg in their systolic pressure after the first dose of epinephrine. Ten patients had baseline hypertension with a systolic pressure greater than 170 mmHg. In two of these patients, the systolic readings rose slightly after epinephrine(but less than 10 mmHg), and two patients with initial elevated diastolic pressures responded to the epinephrine with a minor (less than 10 mmHg) elevation in that parameter. There was no other significant elevation in blood pressure after the epinephrine. In fact, there was an overall trend for epinephrine to

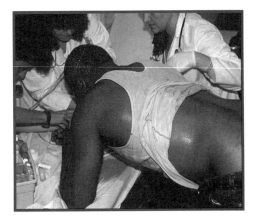

This diaphoretic, hypoxic asthmatic is near respiratory arrest. Despite a very high blood pressure, a pulse of 160 bpm, and being 64 years old, epinephrine was given (0.3 mg subcu every 20 minutes), and all parameters improved. Intubation was not required. See color plate in center well.

lower diastolic readings.

About half the patients in both groups presented with a baseline sinus tachycardia. The presenting heart rate was 130 beats per minute or more in 13 cases, and only one of these demonstrated a transient post-treatment increase in heart rate to 150 beats per minute. The remaining 12 patients exhibited a decrease in heart rate in response to epinephrine. Three of the younger patients had minor cardiovascular abnormalities, including two cases of accelerated idioventricular rhythm and one episode of throat tightening. These patients remained stable, and the abnormalities resolved spontaneously. Atrial and ventricular ectopic beats were rather common in both groups and greater than 10 premature ventricular contractions per hour (PVCs) occurred in 21 percent of those over age 40 and in 11 percent of those under 40. These PVCs were deemed clinically insignificant, and serious ventricular arrhythmias were nonexistent.

Although epinephrine has both alpha- and beta-adrenergic activity and exhibits positive chronotropic and inotropic effects on the heart, the drug's adverse effects on the myocardium in acute asthma is outweighed by its bronchodilating and vasodilating effects. In this study, there were no significant adverse effects on heart rate, blood pressure, or rhythm after treatment with epinephrine, and no patients developed angina. The authors note that this benign profile is compared to the significant tachycardia produced by equivalent doses of terbutaline, a drug touted to be equally efficacious for asth-

SITUATIONS WHERE EPINEPHRINE SHOULD BE AVOIDED IN WHEEZING PATIENTS

Scenario	Reason
Hydrocarbon aspiration	Hydrocarbons sensitize the myocardium to catecholamines and even small doses of epinephrine can precipitate ventricular dysrhythmias
Patient taking non-selective beta blockers	With the beta receptors blocked, unoppose alpha agonism results in exaggerated hypertension
Pregnancy	Epinephrine, in high doses, constricts uterine blood flow (relative contraindication only)
Wheezing due to pulmonary edema	This condition is often mis-diagnosed as primary bronchoconstriction (bronchitis, asthma), and epinephrine therapy is not indicated
Pheochromocytoma/MAO-inhibitor use	Exaggerated catecholamine can be seen

Source: James R. Roberts, MD

ma with supposedly fewer side effects.

While emphasizing caution in selected patients for subcutaneous epinephrine, the authors believe, contrary to what may be expected from a potent adrenergic agent such as epinephrine, that the drug produces a salutary effect on pulse rate and blood pressure in acute asthma as bronchoconstriction is relieved. In the absence of AMI/angina, they believe that epinephrine is safe therapy for the treatment of acute asthmatics of any age.

COMMENT: It is not uncommon for asthmatics to have mild hypertension and tachycardia during an exacerbation. It's also not uncommon for patients over age 40 to present with acute brochospasm requiring treatment. Although most of us now routinely use inhaled beta agonists for initial therapy — few rarely use epinephrine anymore — there are still those who vigorously oppose any use of epinephrine in the elderly because of fear of adverse cardiovascular effect. This fear is largely unfounded. Certainly one should use epinephrine with caution in patients with hypertension and tachycardia, but these data, and clinical experience, clearly indicate that these parameters will tend to normalize rather than worsen as epinephrine ameliorates bronchospasm.

Importantly, and contrary to popular belief, coronary blood flow is actually enhanced by therapeutic doses of epinephrine (Goodman and Gilman, *The Pharmacological Basis of Therapeutics,* 8th Ed.). The pharmacologic effects

guided recommendations. For example, 0.3 mg of subcutaneous epinephrine rarely produces any adverse effects except slight tremor, but if this dose is given as a bolus intravenously, it can cause severe hypertension or ventricular dysrhythmias. When given by inhalation, one needs 10-15 times the subcutaneous dose to relieve croup.

In general, epinephrine's beta-1 effects are inotropic and chronotropic due to the drug's ability to shorten systole and accelerate depolarization. The beta-2 effects result in bronchodilation from relaxation of bronchial smooth muscle. Epinephrine has a dual effect on blood vessel tone. Beta-2 effects result in vasodilation of vessels in skeletal muscle. Systolic pressure is elevated from epinephrine's alpha agonism that causes vasoconstriction of blood vessels. Epinephrine also elevates aortic diastolic pressure through alpha receptors, and this effect is responsible for increased coronary blood flow.

Older physicians will remember the days when the only effective treatment for asthma was subcutaneous epinephrine (it was used daily for all asthmatics), and they cannot understand all the concern over its safety. Hypertensive, tachycardiac asthmatics without an acute ischemic event — one was 96 years old in this study — should tolerate epinephrine in standard asthmatic doses.

I generally prescribe epinephrine only to selected asthmatics. Epinephrine can be quite helpful in the asthmatic who is too ill to cooperate with the nebulizer or in the patient who is not moving enough air to adequately perfuse the alveoli with aerosol. In the asthmatic about to arrest, I always reach for epinephrine first (along with the endotracheal tube). Therefore, patients who are the sickest and most likely to be hypoxic, tachycardiac, and hypertensive are those who are most likely to benefit from

This 76-year-old man, who was hypertensive (170/110) and tachycardiac (110/bpm), was stung in the tongue by a bee while licking an ice cream cone. He noted immediate swelling of the tongue. The treatment alternatives were blind nasotracheal intubation, a retrograde wire or cricothyroidotomy, or medical therapy (including epinephrine). He responded to antihistamines, steroids, and two doses of 0.2 mg subcutaneous epinephrine (20 min apart) with a decrease in blood pressure and pulse. He recovered completely in a few hours without the need for artificial airway. See color plate in center well.

of epinephrine are complex and varied, and clinical response is related largely to dose and route of administration. Subcutaneous epinephrine does not produce the same effects as equal doses of the drug inhaled or injected intravenously. Many physicians erroneously extrapolate side effects of one route to another, and confuse toxic and therapeutic effects, leading to misinformation and mis-

epinephrine. Another subset of patients who may be candidates for epinephrine are those on a ventilator, where it is most difficult to deliver nebulized bronchodilators efficiently. Such patients may get remarkable benefit from relatively small doses of epinephrine, such as 0.1 mg subcu every half hour to 45 minutes, to supplement other therapies. Of course, we all consider the use of epinephrine in young children with bronchospasm who are unable to use the nebulizer. Another subgroup of patients who require epinephrine are patients with acute allergic reactions, and many of these are older with cardiac/hypertension histories.

There are only a few instances when wheezing patients should definitely not receive epinephrine. If a patient is wheezing from a hydrocarbon aspiration, epinephrine may be considered by the unwary physician. Because hydrocarbons sensitize the myocardium to catecholamines, even therapeutic doses of epinephrine can precipitate an arrhythmia so the drug should be avoided. Patients on nonselective beta blockers may also wheeze, and if the beta receptors are blocked, epinephrine may have unopposed alpha effects, leading to serious hypertension. Other instances where one should think twice about using epinephrine for wheezing are noted in the table.

In summary, while epinephrine is not first-line therapy for acute bronchospasm in most patients, it can often be used safely and efficaciously, even in the older patient who is tachycardiac and hypertensive. I would certainly be reticent to use epinephrine in the setting of acute myocardial infarction or active angina, but basing one's use of epinephrine purely on age parameters is clearly non-science.

MYTH: Digital block anesthesia with epinephrine-containing solutions results in serious ischemic injury that threatens the viability of the digit.

FACT: In patients with normal peripheral vascular function, epinephrine-containing solutions can be safely used to prolong anesthesia and to provide a bloodless operating field without ischemic sequelae. Physiologically, the vasoconstrictor properties of epinephrine are less harmful to the digit than a routinely applied and well accepted ischemic tourniquet.

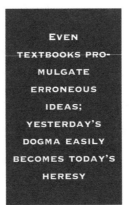

EVEN TEXTBOOKS PROMULGATE ERRONEOUS IDEAS; YESTERDAY'S DOGMA EASILY BECOMES TODAY'S HERESY

THE EFFECTS OF LOCAL ANESTHETICS CONTAINING EPINEPHRINE ON DIGITAL BLOOD PERFUSION. 1978 [CLASSICAL ARTICLE]
Green D, et al *J Am Podiatr Med Assoc* 1992;82(2):98

The authors of this paper extend the previous work of one of their colleagues that demonstrated the safety of lidocaine with epinephrine 1:100,000 used for digital

block anesthesia of the toes (*J Am Podiatr Assoc* 1978; 68:339). The purpose of this study was to investigate further the vasoconstriction-vasodilation properties of various anesthetic solutions. Solutions chosen for evaluation were sterile saline, 1% lidocaine plain and with epinephrine 1:200,000 and 1:300,000, and 0.5% bupivacaine plain and with epinephrine 1:200,000. Sixty-four healthy volunteers (average age 25.5 years) with normal lower extremity vasculature and without a history of peripheral vascular disease were studied. Blood perfusion to the toes was recorded by light sensitive plethysmography. A two-stick approach to the digital block was performed by the same investigator on each subject. Six milliliters of the various solutions were injected with a 25 gauge needle, 3 milliliters to each side of the second toe. One milliliter of solution was deposited on each dorsal digital nerve, and 2 milliliters were deposited on each volar digital nerve. The study was double-blinded, and recordings of digital perfusion were taken at 1-, 2-, 3-, 4-, 5-, and 24-hours postinjection.

The anesthetic solutions without epinephrine all produced vasodilation for approximately five hours. Plain lidocaine increased blood flow by approximately three times baseline, and plain bupivacaine had a maximum vasodilator effect of approximately seven times baseline. Epinephrine-containing solutions consistently produced initial vasoconstriction, but there was little quantitative variation with the concentrations studied. The degree of vasoconstriction resulted in blood flow to the digit of approximately one-half to one-quarter of the baseline flow, and this persisted for approximately one hour. This initial vasoconstriction was invariably followed by vasodilation. Bupivacaine with epinephrine 1:200,000 had the greatest degree to initial vasoconstriction, resulting in approximately one-quarter baseline flow. Perfusion returned to baseline within two hours, followed by a reactive vasodilation. No subject demonstrated any adverse effects from any of the injections.

The authors admit that the use of epinephrine in digits has long been a controversial point, but there are little data to substantiate a significant adverse clinical effect. Anecdotal untoward effects in the past could be explained by the use of unstable mixtures of epinephrine, non-standardized concentrations (often they were mixed at the bedside), or by the use of large volumes of anesthetic solutions. Clinically, a number of authors have validated the safety of digital injections using epinephrine, and there are at least three studies in the podiatry literature containing more than a quarter million patients who safely underwent digital anesthesia with vasoconstrictors.

The universal vasodilator effects seen with local anesthetics may be counterproductive in instances where excessive bleeding is detrimental. This vasodilation is thought to be due to the anesthetic's effect on vasomotor nerves. The authors therefore conclude that epinephrine-containing lidocaine solutions are the preferred mode of hemostasis in digital surgical procedures in healthy patients. It's emphasized that this and other studies were done in young healthy subjects with no history of peripheral vascular disease, and therefore the authors do not advocate the indiscriminate use of digital injections with epinephrine-containing solutions.

COMMENT: It's interesting that podiatrists routinely use epinephrine-containing solutions in concentrations as high as 1:100,000 for digital surgery while other physicians avoid these solutions like the plague. Most of the literature deals with the toes, but similar data are reported for fingers. I have seen a few anxious physicians suffer significant stress when they accidentally injected epinephrine-containing solutions in the hands or feet and realized their "mistake" or noted a pale digit. I have yet to see complications from this, nor have I seen reports in the modern literature. The paranoia is so great that a number of authors suggest the immediate local injection of phentolamine, an alpha blocker, to reverse the vasoconstriction produced by epinephrine. Although a digit injected with epinephrine clearly looks different from its non-vasoconstricted counterpart, the physician can be assured that ischemia is not as complete as is obtained with a tourniquet. In addition, the epinephrine avoids the pressure on sensitive digital nerves that is associated with ischemic tourniquets.

I am by no means advocating the routine use of epinephrine for digital blocks, and the reader should carefully note this stance. To prolong anesthesia, I prefer bupivacaine. For a bloodless field, use a tourniquet. There is, however, no need to be afraid to use these solutions when necessary to obtain the desired effect in healthy patients. It is certainly prudent always to avoid these drugs in elderly patients or those with diabetes or other types of compromised peripheral blood flow, but in healthy individuals, injecting a digit with lidocaine containing epinephrine appears to be no big deal. To be on the safe side, I would choose the 1:200,000 concentration. (See also *Reactions to Local Anesthetics,* Section 6, Chapter 5.)

RESPONSE TO DOSES OF SUBCUTANEOUS EPINEPHRINE

	Dose 1		Dose 2		Dose 3	
	<40 years (n=69)	>40 years (n=39)	<40 years (n=62)	>40 years (n=35)	<40 years (n=48)	>40 years (n=22)
Change in Systolic BP (mmHg)	+1.3±1.9	*-9.5±3.3	+0.7±1.9	+1.4±2.0	+0.5±2.4	-3.9±4.7
Changein Diastolic BP (mmHg)	-4.2±1.5	-7.6±2.2	-4.5±1.4	-0.3±2.1	-1.0±1.4	-4.6±3.2
Change in heart rate	-1.8±1.8	-4.5±1.7	-1.3±1.3	-1.4±2.0	+4.2±2.0	-2.1±1.4
Change in respiratory rate	-2.9±0.7	-2.1±0.6	+0.9±0.8	-0.9±0.7	-1.4±0.7	-2.0±1.3
Change in peak flow rate (L/min)	+44.1±8.5	+50.9±11.0	+28.9±8.8	+20.4±8.4	+34.5±11.2	+16.2±6.1

*$P<0.05$

Source: Ann Emerg Med *1988;17:322-326.*

MYTHS ABOUT EPINEPHRINE AND CROUP

L-epinephrine, used to treat asthma, is as effective as racemic epinephrine for croup

Epinephrine is a complex drug that has both alpha and beta affects, and its pharmacologic profile varies greatly with dose and route of administration. Much of the confusion about the clinical effects of epinephrine arises through attempts to extrapolate the pharmacology seen with one dose or route to another situation. Often, concerns about side effects from one use are not necessarily an issue with another scenario. This chapter continues the discussion of epinephrine, with a special emphasis on the use of racemic epinephrine, also known as racepinephrine, for the treatment of croup, emphasizing some of the misconceptions about this indication. Epinephrine is available in many concentrations and various formulations so I will also attempt to clarify the physicians' various options, and try to put into perspective the specific indications for each.

MYTH: When using inhaled epinephrine for croup, one must use nebulized racemic epinephrine.

FACT: The same epinephrine that is used to treat asthma (L-epinephrine) is as effective for the treatment of croup as the less available racemic epinephrine.

PROSPECTIVE RANDOMIZED DOUBLE-BLIND STUDY COMPARING L-EPINEPHRINE AND RACEMIC EPINEPHRINE AEROSOLS IN THE TREATMENT OF LARYNGOTRACHEITIS (CROUP)

Waisman Y, et al *Pediatrics* 1992;89(2):302

Nebulized racemic (RE) has gained acceptance as an effective treatment for croup. RE is thought to stimulate alpha adrenergic receptors in the upper respiratory tract to induce vasoconstriction and thereby decrease mucosal edema. RE is actually a mixture of equal amounts of D- and L-isomers of epinephrine. Historically RE is the only epinephrine preparation used for such inhalation purposes. However, RE is very expensive and not available in many countries. In reality, the L-isomer is essentially the only active component of the racemic mixture, and there is no scientific basis for administering the inactive D-isomer. Although previous authors have reported the safety and efficacy of the L-isomer for inhalation, it has not been rigorously studied for the treatment of croup. Because LE is cheap and available worldwide, it would be desirable to administer it for the treatment of croup if it were effective.

The authors randomly treated children ages 6 months to 6 years presenting with croup with either racemic epinephrine (16 patients) or L-epinephrine (15 patients) aerosols. The croup score and physiological parameters were measured for up to two hours after therapy. The RE aerosol consisted of 0.5 ml 2.25% racemic epinephrine solution in 4.5 ml normal saline. The LE aerosol contained 5 ml 1.100 "asthma"-type L-epinephrine diluted with saline. Therefore, 5 mg of the L-isomer was given in each both treatment protocol. Only one dose was administered. The aerosols were delivered by a nebulizer over five to 10 minutes in a double-blind fashion.

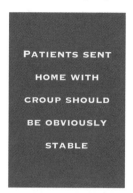

PATIENTS SENT HOME WITH CROUP SHOULD BE OBVIOUSLY STABLE

Patients in both groups had significant reductions in their croup scores and respiratory rates, and there was no significant difference between treatment groups in any of the parameters assessed. The beneficial effect was transitory with both forms of the medication. Therapy reached its peak effect at 30 minutes, with a duration of action of no more than 90 minutes. One patient in each group experienced a return of his respiratory distress, and the transitory nature of this therapy is stressed.

The authors conclude that equal doses of the active L-form of epinephrine, given either as an L-epinephrine or racemic epinephrine, have similar beneficial effects in croup. It was emphasized that only a single dose of each aerosol was studied.

COMMENT: Other authors (*Anesthesia* 1986;41:923; *Pediatric Res* 1986; 20:182A, and *Anesthesia* 1987;42:322) have reported similar results with the L-isomer preparation, but there is still resistance to use standard asthma-type epinephrine routinely for inhalation therapy for croup. Some physicians are unaware of these data and consider racemic epinephrine the only acceptable aerosol. There have been times in our

hospital when racemic epinephrine was not available, and rather than substituting regular epinephrine, no inhaled epinephrine treatments were administered.

The literature commonly expresses some concern about the incidence of clinical rebound in patients given RE for croup. So prevalent is this concern that patients are either routinely admitted if they are treated, or the therapy is withheld altogether for fear of deterioration from rebound. Rebound to me indicates that the airway obstruction returns to a degree greater than pretreatment levels. Other authors use the form to indicate a return to the original state of distress. I'm not yet ready to label the "hyperrebound" phenomenon as a myth, but it probably is. It would be very difficult to differentiate hyperrebound from the natural progression of the croup process once epinephrine effects have dissipated, and I could find no data that actually confirm the rebound theory, although a return to base-

CALCULATION OF DOSE OF EPINEPHRINE IN LOCAL ANESTHETICS

Local anesthetics are combined with small amounts of epinephrine to produced vasoconstriction and to prolong the anesthetic effect. Usual concentrations are expressed as 1:100,000 or 1:200,000.

Examples: Lidocaine 1% with epinephrine 1:100,000

1:100,000 means 1 gram of epinephrine is dissolved in 100,000 mls of diluent. Therefore, one can make the following calculations:

1G/100,000 ml=
1,000 mg/100,000 ml=
1 mg/100 ml=
0.01 mg/ml

The actual amount of epinephrine delivered with the anesthetic is actually quite small. As an example, 10 ml of 1% lidocaine with epinephrine 1:100,000 contains only 0.1 mg of epinephrine.

Other Examples:

	1:100,000	1:200,000
5 ml	0.05 mg	0.025 mg
10 ml	0.1 mg	0.05 mg
20 ml	0.2 mg	0.1 mg

Source: James R. Roberts, MD

VARIOUS PREPARATIONS OF EPINEPHRINE

Preparation of Epinephrine	Route of Administration	Clinical Use	Concentration	Mg/Ml
1:100	Inhalation	Aerosolized for croup	1 g in 100 ml (1%)	10 mg/ml

• Very concentrated; not for parenteral use.
• May use for inhalation: 0.25-0.5 ml in saline nebulizer.
• L-isomer only.

1:1,000	Subcu	Asthma anaphylaxis	1 g in 1000 ml (0.1%)	1 mg/ml

• This is L-isomer only.
• Can be used for inhalation for croup in dose 3-5 ml (mg).

1:10,000	IV	"Cardiac" epinephrine for codes; small doses IV for anaphylaxis	1 g in 10,000 ml 0.01%)	0.1 mg/ml

• L-isomer, in prefilled 10 ml syringe in crash cart.

1:100,000	Infiltration Subcu	Combined with local anesthetic for subcu use	1 g in 100,000 ml 0.001%)	0.01 mg/ml (Ex: 10 ml of 1% lidocaine 1:100,000 contains 0.1 mg of epinephrine

• Also comes in 1:200,000.

Racemic epinephrine	Inhalation	Aerosolized for croup	2.25% Equal parts of D-and L isomers= 1.125% L-epinephrine	22.5 mg/ml Note: 11.25 mg/ml of inactive D-isomer and 11.50 mg/ml of active L-isomer

• Dose for child with croup is 0.25-0.5 ml in saline nebulizer.
• Basically equivalent to 1:100 L-epinephrine.

Primatene (mist and mist suspension)	Inhalation	Asthma	Mist: 0.22 mg/ puff. Mist suspension = 0.16 mg/puff	Mist: 5.5 mg/ml Mist suspension: 7 mg/ml of bitartrate

• Available OTC.
• Tablet contains no epinephrine (theophylline, Epinephrine + phenobarbital and antihistamine.

Sus-Phrine	Subcu	Asthma/allergic reactions (not anaphylaxis)	0.5% or 1:200 20% solution (immediate) and 80% suspension (slow release)	5 mg/ml

• Not for anaphylaxia.
• Last 4-6 hours.
• Not "in oil".
• Contains only L-isomer.
• Has both immediate and delayed bioavailability.

Source: James R. Roberts, MD

line post-treatment is a common scenario.

Kelley et al (*Am J Emerg Med* 1992;10(3):181) reported a protocol in which 50 children with croup who presented with stridor and/or reactions were treated with RE and observed for two hours. If they were improved or were otherwise deemed suitable for discharge, they were sent home (usually on steroids). No discharged patient suffered a serious rebound and only one returned to the hospital for an additional treatment (and he was discharged again). This is a controversial approach — and gutsy considering the current literature — but the authors believe that if follow-up is readily available, children free of stridor/retraction at two hours post-RE therapy can be safely discharged. The financial impact of this approach is clearly substantial, but I would like to see more studies before I make my final conclusion about this practice.

It's absurd to withhold RE for fear of rebound, but clearly discharge decisions should be withheld until two hours post-therapy. What makes more sense to me is to reserve inhaled epinephrine for seriously ill children who are going to be admitted anyway. It may negate intubation, and can be repeated in the hospital. The physician is probably treating himself more than the patient if a mildly ill, dischargeable child is given a single nebulization for temporary improvement in the ED. Patients sent home with croup should have an obviously stable outpatient condition, but it usually lasts two to three days. Making them look better for an hour in the ED, probably only prolongs their stay, ties up the ED, and pads the bill.

The dose and availability of epinephrine products require some clarification. Physicians, nurses, and pharmacists easily become confused with the various available forms and concentrations, and textbooks do a poor job explaining the options. One problem is that ml, mg, and dilutions (such as 1:10,000) are used interchangeably, and it's difficult to understand the conversion mathematics. (See table.)

Non-pediatricians rarely use inhaled epinephrine, and one might consider turning to the literature for a refresher course when using the drug on a sporadic basis. I was, however, disappointed that I could not find a single description of racemic epinephrine in the 1993 *Physicians' Desk Reference.* Racemic epinephrine is available as micro-Nefrin or Nephron. One popular older form (also over-the-counter) of racemic epinephrine, Vaponephrin, is no

> **DON'T WITHHOLD RE FOR FEAR OF REBOUND, BUT HOLD DISCHARGE DECISIONS UNTIL TWO HOURS POST-THERAPY**

longer produced. Racemic epinephrine comes in a 2.25% solution (22.5 mg/ml), but only half of this solution is the active L-isomer; therefore the product is equivalent to 1.125% (11.25 mg/ml) L-epinephrine. There is also an oral inhalation form of L-epinephrine in a 1:100 concentration (1%). This is roughly clinically equivalent to racemic epinephrine, containing 10 mg/ml of L-isomer and no D-isomer. (Caution: Don't use this concentrated preparation parenterally or subcu.) Our hospital uses this 1:100 solution for the nebulizer treatment for croup, using 0.5 ml (10 drops or about 5 mg) per treatment. You could opt for standard 1:1000 asthma-type epinephrine to treat croup by aerosol, but then you should use 5 ml to obtain the same 5 mg amount of the L-isomer.

"Cardiac" epinephrine is a 1:10,000 solution that comes premixed in 10 ml syringes. Each 10 mls contain 1 mg of L-epinephrine. In this expression, 1:10,000 means 1 gram of epinephrine is added to 10,000 mls of diluent, resulting in a concentration of 0.01% or 0.1 mg/ml. (The key here is that % means grams/100 ml.) The epinephrine used subcutaneously for the treatment of asthma is a 1:1000 concentration (0.1%). I this formulation, mls and mgs are equivalent, so 1 ml contains 1 mg, 0.3 ml contains 0.3 mg, and so on. These authors used relatively generous dose of epinephrine 1:1000-5 ml or 5 mg. Epinephrine concentrations in local anesthetics are explained in the accompanying table.

Sus-Phrine is another epinephrine preparation that has some following. It is used for asthma and (non-anaphylaxis) allergic reactions. Sus-Phrine is sort of a clinical dinosaur, but it's still a great drug for hives. Sus-Phrine is only given subcu, and its claim to fame is that it lasts four to six hours. Years ago it was a routine "out-the-door" treatment for asthma, but now inhaled beta agonists have displaced Sus-Phrine for outpatient therapy. Sus-Phrine is a 1:200 concentration that contains epinephrine in two forms. About 20% is in solution, and this has immediate bioavailability, just like regular "asthma" epinephrine. About 80% of Sus-Phrine is in suspension and exhibits a sustained release profile, becoming available over four to six hours. Sus-Phrine is not "epinephrine in oil," a common misconception.

Some asthmatics treat themselves with inhaled epinephrine sold OTC, and some physicians will be surprised that this is a non-prescription product. The most well known preparation is Primatene. This inhaler comes as a "mist" or a "mist suspension." The mist contains only the L-isomer (5.5 mg/ml), and each puff delivers 0.22 mg. The "mist suspension" (7 mg/ml) delivers 0.3 mg epinephrine bitartrate, equivalent to 0.16 mg epinephrine base. Primatene tablets curiously contain no epinephrine, consisting of theophylline and ephedrine, but some tablets of this brand also can contain small amounts of phenobarbital or antihistamines.

The sulfite issue is a confusing one. Despite concern that some patients are allergic to sulfites, many epinephrine products used to treat allergic reaction contain it as a preservative. There are no sulfites in Primatene, but they are present in epinephrine 1:1000. This may explain why some patients are allergic to epinephrine.

SECTION X

SEIZURES

THE METABOLIC AND PHYSIOLOGIC CONSEQUENCES OF SEIZURES

Relating basic science to clinical practice helps define the pathophysiology and metabolic consequences of seizures

It's an unusual shift when an emergency physician does not have to deal with at least one seizure patient. Like congestive heart failure, chest pain, asthma, sickle cell anemia, and drug overdoses, the seizure patient is a bread-and-butter case. Because of the frequency of seizure disorders, most of us have developed strong biases and a dogmatic approach that results in a routine that is implemented as a knee-jerk response, often cavalierly and occasionally without a clear understanding of the clinical implications. This chapter begins a series of discussions on seizures. The following discussion deals with the pathophysiology and metabolic consequences of seizures and attempts to relate basic science to clinical practice. The reader should bear in mind that often the literature does not distinguish between a single seizure and true status epilepticus so there is some overlap in consensus concerning the following issues.

PHYSIOLOGIC CONSEQUENCES OF STATUS EPILEPTICUS

Simon RP *Epilepsia* 1985;26(Suppl l):S58

This informative article is an in-depth review of the physiologic consequences of prolonged major motor seizures, or status epilepticus (SE). Although prolonged seizures in and of themselves may produce neurological damage, the numerous associated physiologic and metabolic alterations that develop secondary to seizure activity also contribute to morbidity or mortality.

HYPERTHERMIA: Because of sustained motor activity, SE routinely produces hyperthermia, occasionally severe and frequently with surprising rapidity. Hyperthermia is most likely the direct result of sustained motor activity. Hyperthermia is the only variable, other than the duration of the seizure activity, that directly correlates with residual central nervous system damage. Although infection is always suspected in the presence of seizures and hyperthermia, it would be unusual for any patient to continue to seize for more than 30 minutes without an elevation in core temperature. In one study, 75 of 90 patients (83%) with SE for 30 minutes or more developed hyperthermia as high as 107°F (42°C) in two patients (*Am J Med* 1980;69(5):657). Only four of the 75 patients with a fever had a documented infection. Interestingly, when paradoxical hypothermia was noted with SE in that report, other concomitant diagnoses, such as drug overdose, hypoglycemia, or hypothyroidism were present.

LEUKOCYTOSIS: Most patients with status develop an elevation in the peripheral white blood cell count. In one quoted study, 50 of 80 status epilepticus patients without infection had a leukocytosis ranging from 12,700 to 28,800 cells/mm3 (*Am J Med* 1980;69(5):659). Although the WBC elevation usually consists of polymorphonuclear cells, a shift to band forms is unusual, a point that may help one decide on the need for a septic evaluation. Leukocytosis is probably a stress phenomenon, the result of demargination of leukocytes in response to elevated catecholamines.

CEREBROSPINAL FLUID PLEOCYTOSIS: It is not unusual for SE, in the absence of infection, to be associated with a transient elevation of the CSF white cell count. Status-induced CSF pleocytosis is actually quite common, and it's noted in up to 15-20 percent of patients. The rise is usually modest (less than 10 cells/mm3) and may not reach its zenith until 24 hours. Polymorphonuclear cells usually dominate. CSF protein may also be transiently and mildly elevated following repeated seizures. Transient alterations in the blood-brain barrier may account for both phenomena. The authors are quick to point out that cells in the CSF clearly indicate infection until proven otherwise; but once cultures are negative, one can be confident that the pleocytosis was secondary to the seizure itself and the clinician need look no further. Although CNS infections can precipitate SE, this is actually a relatively infrequent cause. The authors note that only four of 98 unselected patients with status in one 10-year series had an infectious etiology.

ACIDOSIS: A seizure quickly produces a prompt and often profound fall in arterial pH. In one animal study reviewed, the pH changed from a mean of 7.33-6.83 within only four minutes of continuous seizure activity (*Neurology* 1985;34:255). A single four-minute seizure in one human series created a mean serum pH of 7.14. The pH of non-ventilated patients during SE was lower than 7.0 in an amazing 23 of 70 patients

reported in one series. The acidosis can be both metabolic and respiratory in origin. The metabolic component is more common and attributed lactic acidosis from skeletal muscle contraction, and neuromuscular paralysis generally ameliorates the change. Because lactate is rapidly metabolized in patients with a healthy liver and an intact circulation, simple seizure-induced acidosis should resolve within an hour following termination of seizure activity. There is no strong evidence that this type of lactic acidosis per se is harmful, and treatment is not required. Interestingly, hypokalemia does not routinely occur with the acidosis secondary to SE. Prolonged seizure activity leading to muscle necrosis may cause hyperkalemia.

OTHER PHYSIOLOGIC ALTERATIONS: A number of other important metabolic changes occur with SE. Norepinephrine and epinephrine concentration are markedly elevated (up to 40 times normal), and this may adversely affect cardiovascular function. One postulated cause of rare sudden death in seizure patients is cardiac arrhythmias secondary to markedly elevated epinephrine concentrations. Also an epinephrine excess probably

---

LOAD DOSE CALCULATION EXAMPLE

Patient's condition	*Status epilepticus*
Patient's weight	*100 kg*

Dose of drug required (Loading dose: LD)=patient
  weight x 18 mg/kg
100 kg /18 mg/kg=LD=1,800 mg of phenytoin sodium

Volume of phenytoin injectable required
Phenytoin sodium injectable strength=50 mg/mL
  1,8000 mg/50 mg=36mL
LD volume=36 mL of phenytoin sodium injectable

Volume of intravenous solution required
Desired strength of phenytoin admixture=25 mg/mL
Final volume of admixture=1,800 mg/25 mg/mL=72 mL

Preparation
Place 5 mL of 0.45% or 0.9% sodium chloride in a
  volume control set.
Add 36 mL of phenytoin sodium injectable.
Add an additional 31 mL of 0.45% or 0.9% sodium chloride to
  bring the final volume to 72 mL.

Source: JAMA 1980;44(13):1481.

accounts for the rise in blood glucose levels frequently seen early in the course of SE.

Seizures also have a significant effect on systemic and pulmonary vascular beds. A single seizure may immediately elevate the systolic and diastolic blood pressure by 85 and 40 torr respectively. Mean heart rate increases of 80 beats per minute are common. Cerebral blood flow may increase up to 600 percent of normal during status. Pulmonary artery and left atrial pressures are also markedly elevated by even a single seizure. Although initially elevated during the initial phases of prolonged seizure activity, both systemic and pulmonary artery pressures eventually fall. Cardiac output has been noted to fall at least 50 percent within 10 minutes of continual seizures. The initial elevation of pulmonary vascular pressure may account for the "neurogenic" pulmonary edema or acute respiratory distress syndrome (ARDS) seen with seizures and massive transcapillary fluid flux may account for unexpected death in epileptic patients. Death from SE is usually attributed to cardiovascular collapse and multisystem failure.

COMMENT: It's clear that a number of marked physiologic and metabolic changes occur secondary to even a single seizure, but it's amazing how well patients fare despite a frightening alteration in normal homeostasis. Most emergency physicians don't routinely evaluate many of the affected parameters so the impressive derangements may not be noticed. For example, one rarely takes the blood pressure or pulse rate during a seizure. A number of the physiologic consequences of seizing do, however, form the basis of our routine approach to the seizing patient.

HYPERTHERMIA: Core temperature is probably the most neglected vital sign in ED patients presenting with any serious illness that is not clearly infectious disease in origin. Multiple trauma patients, for example, often have serious problems after a long resuscitation from unexpected or unappreciated hypothermia. I have personally seen one patient with a previously unmeasured core temperature of 115°F secondary to cocaine induced SE (*Am J Emerg Med* 1984;2 (4):373). As a toxicology consultant, I occasionally get calls or transfers of patients who have been seizing from drug overdose for hours and have never had their temperature taken. To further emphasize the link

between even non-motor seizure and fever, Semel reports unrecognized complex partial status that presented as a fever (to 38.8°C) of unknown origin (*Arch Intern Med* 1987;147:(16)1571). The cause of fever is unknown but has been related to heat generated by sustained muscle activity. Disruption of central thermoregulation is probably also involved, probably accounting for the cases of severe hyperthermia after minor seizure activity.

Because seizure-induced hyperthermia is so closely correlated with residual CNS damage, it is imperative that

RESULT OF SINGLE-DOSE ORAL PHENYTOIN LOADING		
Time from oral loading (18 mg/kg)	*Mean serum level (mcg/ml)*	*Percentage of patients with therapeutic serum levels (10-20 mcg/ml)*
2 hours	*6.8*	*22%*
4 hours	*9.7*	*57%*
8 hours	*12.3*	*64%*
4 hours	*15.1*	*60%*

Source: Ann Emerg Med *1987;16:407.*

temperature be monitored routinely in seizing patients. Although it's rarely done in the ED, state-of-the-art monitoring of SE should include continuous use of a rectal temperature probe. I like the tympanic membrane as a quick look source for this vital sign; however, it cannot be continuously be monitored and once the situation has been stabilized, a rectal temperature should be taken (especially in children where the tympanic thermometer may significantly underestimate core temperature).

The natural history of fever following a seizure requires some comment. Wachtel et al (*Arch Intern Med* 1987; 147(6):1153) reviewed the temperature curves of 93 postictal (non SE) patients, and 40 (43%) had a temperature above 100°F. In two-thirds of the patients, no infection was found. Most of the diagnosed infections were routine — pneumonia or urinary tract infection. In those without infection, the fever occurred at a mean of 5.4 hours after the seizure and lasted for a mean of 22 hours. In 10 percent, the seizure-induced fever lasted greater than 48 hours. The conclusion was that a benign fever can develop hours after a single seizure and can commonly last for up to 48 hours. If fever persists longer than 48 hours, occult infection is likely. I doubt if most EPs appreciate that almost half of seizure patients develop a fever, but because we rarely repeat the temperature four to five hours after the seizure in an asymptomatic patient, many are probably missed. In my practice, a common cause of seizures and fever is the alcoholic who gets ill (such as pneumonia) and stops drinking and experiences a withdrawal seizure. Alcohol withdrawal further complicates the picture because it also causes a fever. The authors of this paper conclude that an lumbar puncture is not axiomatic

CONSEQUENCES OF SEIZURE ACTIVITY

Finding	Cause	Characteristics	Comment
Metabolic acidosis	•*Anaerobic metabolism from sustained muscle activity leads to lactate production*	•*Very common, even after short seizure* •*Attenuated by seizure control/muscle paralysis*	•*Not harmful, per se* •*Need not be treated* •*Continued acidosis may have diagnostic significance* •*Clears in 60 minutes by lactate metabolism*
Respiratory acidosis	•*Decreased ventilation* •*Pulmonary aspiration*	•*Less common than metabolic acidosis*	•*Usually signifies significant medical problem*
Hyperthermia	•*Sustained muscular contraction* •*Central thermoregulatory dysfunction*	•*Common; up to 30-40% of patients after single seizure* •*Occurs early or late* •*May be delayed for 5 hours,* •*Hypothermia suggests hypoglycemia, drug OD, hypothyroid* •*Can reach 105-107°F from seizure alone*	•*Severe hyperthermia correlates with CNS damage* •*Always considered CNS or other infection* •*Fever greater 48 hours duration usually infectious etiology* •*Rectal temperature measurement mandatory* •*Consider cocaine toxicity, salicylates*
Leukocytosis	•*Demargination of leukocytes, probably due to catecholamine excess*	•*Commonly seen* •*Up to 20-25,0000 mm3 in absence of infection* •*Polys predominate but no band forms*	•*Suggests evaluation for for infection*
CSF Pleocytosis	•*May be due to alteration in blood brain barrier*	•*Transient, mild, usually less than 10 cells/mm3* •*Seen in 5-10% if cases* •*Onset may be delayed for a number of hours*	•*Mandates treatment for CNS infection until proven otherwise* •*Elevated QF protein also seen* •*CFF glucose unchanged*
Catecholamine excess	•*Stress response* •*Affects peripheral and and central vascular beds*	•*Occurs very rapidly* •*May predispose to arrhythmias/ARDS* •*Causes tachycardia and hypertension*	•*Accounts for hyperglycemia, leukocytosis* •*Pulmonary artery effects may produce neurogenic pulmonary edema*

Source: James R. Roberts, MD

and base their indications for CSF analysis on clinical grounds. For ED purposes, finding a mild fever in the absence of other signs/symptoms of infection probably does not mandate admission based solely on the fever.

The therapeutic approach to hyperthermia is quite basic. First, you must remember to take the temperature, and second, any fever should be considered a sign of infection until proven otherwise. This does not mean everyone gets an LP, septic work-up, or triple antibiotics, but infection must be addressed. Of course a UTI or pneumonia would not likely cause a seizure, and one is most concerned about a CNS infection. Meningitis does not, however, produce a fever and a seizure in the absence of other findings, so clinical discussions on performing an LP usually suffice. In my practice, a quite common cause of a seizure with a fever is cocaine toxicity (another toxic-induced seizure with a fever is salicylate poisoning).

Most importantly for the therapy of hyperthermia, the seizure should be stopped by all means possible, including the use of paralyzing agents if necessary. Initially, one must be aggressive with adequate doses of anticonvulsants. If the temperature is greater than 105°F, I prefer to pack the patient in ice or institute aggressive evaporative cooling with an industrial-strength, high-power fan and continuous tepid water spray. Acetaminophen, cooling blankets, wet sheets, or ice packs to the groin just don't make it. Even though muscular contractions are partially the cause, dantrolene has no known benefit. In animal studies, the maximum temperature may be reached during the first few minutes of onset. In some studies there is a lag period of a few hours. Generally the longer the seizure, the higher the temperature, but duration is clearly not the only correlate with hyperthermia. The clinical message here is that one does not begin to monitor the temperature after a patient has been seizing for an hour.

I try to remember to do an immediate Dextrostik test on all seizure patients with persistent altered mental status because hypoglycemia is omnipresent, easy to miss, hard to diagnose clinically, and when prolonged, neurologically devastating. A tip off to hypoglycemia — and a most common finding — is hypothermia. Any hypothermic patient with abnormal mental status or unusual complaints not readily explained should have the glucose immediately checked.

CSF AND PERIPHERAL LEUKOCYTOSIS:

In uncomplicated cases, such as a seizure due to noncompliance to anticonvulsants, a CBC is not considered standard of care. However, not many physicians can evaluate a seizing febrile patient and not send a CBC. Leukocytosis by itself means nothing because very high WBC counts can result from a single seizure. White cells in the CSF mandate broad spectrum antibiotics for presumed CNS infection. Although an uncommon cause of status, unrecognized CNS infection may be an occult cause of seizures in AIDS patients, the elderly, the psychiatric patient, and the neonate. In the presence of a normal examination, fever and peripheral leukocytosis in a non-compliant patient with a known seizure disorder usually does not turn out to be CNS infection, but one should be liberal with LP in the febrile seizure patient with a leukocytosis if there is difficulty distinguishing the postictal phase from baseline altered mental status. Alcohol withdrawal tends to send polymorhonuclear cells into the CSF whereas a CVA recruits lymphocytes. If greater than 5 WBCs are noted on CSF analysis, or if one is a polymorphonuclear cell, antibiotics and admission are always warranted despite the fact that the seizure itself may retrospectively be the culprit. The cause of CSF leukocytosis and elevated CSF protein is unknown, but it is thought to be related to some transient breakdown in the blood-brain barrier. This phenomenon may also help drugs penetrate the CNS during SE.

Other investigators have also noted white cells in the CSF after seizures in the absence of infection. Prokesch (*South Med J* 1983;76(3):322) noted white cells in the CSF of 34 percent of 102 patients having lumbar puncture within 48 hours of a generalized or even focal seizure. Only one patient had an infectious etiology. The cell count in this report ranged from 3 to 464/mm3 (mean 72/mm3) and polymorphonuclear cells predominated. CSF pleocytosis after seizures (not just status epilepticus) is probably more common than appreciated. It's not associated with a specific etiology, but it is often seen in alcohol withdrawal and stroke (maybe these patients get more LPs), and it follows a single generalized seizure or even a partial seizure. The CSF pleocytosis should clear on a repeat tap in 48 hours. Seizures do not change CSF glucose levels.

ACIDOSIS: A retrospective diagnosis of a seizure disorder is often suspected in the confused (postictal) patient who is found down without a history by noting an otherwise unexplained mild metabolic acidosis. It's common to note arterial pH in the range of 6.9-7.1 in patients with multiple seizures. Most of the time this acidosis does not generate great anxiety in the treating physician, and there is no evidence to support that this arterial pH should be routinely analyzed and it's not axiomatic that it be corrected. The degree of acidosis may be striking, but it is not an independent variable for morbidity or mortality. Some toxic causes of seizures, such as lindane, salicylates, or isoniazid overdose, can cause a metabolic acidosis by mechanisms other than seizure activity. Acidosis from seizure activity is ameliorated by stopping the seizure and the use of paralyzing drugs.

Exercise studies have noted a rapid and significant rise in lactate levels and a surprisingly low arterial pH with exercise to exhaustion. Hamermansen notes pH as low as 6.8 when measured within a minute of maximal exercise in healthy volunteers (*J Appl Physiol* 1982;53: 304). It's no wonder that agitated or struggling patients all seem to have an acidosis. Respiratory acidosis is of much greater concern than a simple metabolic acidosis from muscle contraction so an ABG is mandatory if seizures persist, if respirations are clinically compromised, or if the pulse oximetry is low.

PULMONARY PATHOLOGY: Acidosis is so common that it is frequently suggested that blood gases not be checked during seizure activity. I believe, however, that an ABG is probably one of the most valuable laboratory tests to order in complicated cases, not so much for pH determination, but rather for PO2 and PCO2 evaluation.

I used to withhold ABGs during multiple seizures if the patient looked stable until I came across patients who appeared to be well ventilated yet had significant hypoxia and PCO2 in the 70-80 torr range, definite indications for intervention. A single uncomplicated seizure, however, dose not require a routine ABG. Clinically, patients with multiple or prolonged seizures may appear to be breathing normally, and even hyperventilating due to the acidosis, yet be quite hypercarbic or hypoxic. The pulse oximeter is usually the only test required initially, but it's prudent to be liberal with an ABG because clinical evaluation of PCO2 is difficult.

Terrence et al report eight cases of unexpected, unexplained death in young (age 9-31 years) ambulatory epileptics who died subsequent to a seizure (*Ann Neurol* 1981; 9(5):458). In these cases, cardiac disease, aspiration, drug overdose, and trauma were excluded. All demonstrated moderate to severe hemorrhagic pulmonary edema (two also had cerebral edema). The authors postulate the cause of death to be seizure-induced neurogenic pulmonary edema, possibly complicated by ventricular arrhythmias. The phenomenon could be related to a centrally mediated adrenergic crisis, but severe pulmonary hypertension is probably also a precipitating factor. Although this report is only circumstantial evidence, it certainly lends credence to a significant pulmonary effect of generalized seizures. Because the first subtle sign of pulmonary edema may be hypoxia, this report suggests to me that a routine evaluation of the PO2 may be warranted. It's common to relegate ARDS to pulmonary aspiration or the multisystem failure seen with seriously ill patients, but pulmonary hypertension may be more prevalent than previously suspected in seizing patients. This raises the question of the cause of ARDS so often seen with tricyclic antidepressant overdose, a group of patients who commonly seize.

VARIABLES MEASURED IN THE POST-ICTAL PERIOD

	Time after Seizure			
Variable	*0-4 min*	*15 min*	*30 min*	*60 min*
pH	*7.14±0.06* (*6.86-7.36*)	*7.24±0.05* (*7.08-7.47*)	*7.31±0.04* (*7.17-7.48*)	*7.38±0.04* (*7.20-7.52*)
K (meq/liter)	*3.8±0.2* (*3.0-4.9*)	*3.8±0.2* (*2.7-4.5*)	*3.9±0.3* (*2.8-4.8*)	*3.9±0.3* (*3.0-5.2*)
CO2 content (mmol/liter)	*17.1±1.1* (*13-23*)	*17.5±1.3* (*11-24*)	*20.0±1.4* (*14-25*)	*23.6±1.1* (*21-30*)
Glucose (mg/dl)	*156±20*	*152±24*	*162±27*	*155±18*
Lactate (meq/liter)	*12.7±1.0* (*8.9-16.0*)	*8.9±1.0* (*6.8-13.2*)	*9.5±1.0* (*6.2-12.7*)	*6.6±0.7* (*4.2-10.7*)
Anion gap (meq/liter)	*25±1.8* (*19-32*)	*22±1.9* (*17-32*)	*18±1.9* (*12-27*)	*14±2.3* (*7-26*)

Source: N Engl J Med *1977;297:796-799.*

NATURAL HISTORY OF LACTIC ACIDOSIS AFTER GRAND-MAL SEIZURES

N Engl J Med 1977;297:796

This is a frequently quoted paper that attempts to define the course of metabolic acidosis following a grand mal seizure. Eight patients with a single seizure (not SE) of 30 to 60 seconds duration were studied. Within four minutes of the seizure, venous blood sampling was initiated to determine lactate concentrations, CO_2, and an arterial pH was obtained. The values for these clinical parameters immediately following termination of seizure activity and 60 minutes later are illustrated in the table. It is significant to note that the mean arterial pH was 7.14, with a mean anion gap of 25 mEq/L. Acidosis was attributed to the accumulation of lactate. Interestingly, glucose remained consistently elevated at one hour, but there was no change in potassium concentrations.

The authors conclude the following that the postictal period is characterized by an acute and rather significant metabolic acidosis secondary to lactate accumulation. Lactate production is attributed to vigorous muscular activity. Local hypoxemia ensues, followed by anaerobic metabolism and lactate production. In a majority of cases, metabolic acidosis clears spontaneously within 60 minutes due to metabolism of lactate, making seizures a unique model of lactic acidosis. Lactate is cleared primarily by metabolism, and renal excretion and respiratory compensation are not primarily responsible for the resolution. The administration of bicarbonate is not required or recommended.

COMMENT: It's surprising that the pH goes as low as a mean of 7.14 following a single 30- to 60-second grand mal seizure. This is, however, a common clinical finding that in and of itself, is innocuous and does not require therapy. In fact, the routine correction of pH in transient metabolic acidosis with bicarbonate is now thought to be contraindicated because you run the risk of severe alkalosis or hypokalemia once the excess lactate has been metabolized. (By the way, if you do not completely fill the red top tube, the bicarbonate may be slightly falsely low). The fact that potassium levels did not rise with the acidosis may be related to the hypokalemic effect of catecholamine excess, a mechanism not appreciated 15 years ago.

The clinical message here is that even marked metabolic acidosis is a relatively benign condition once the seizing has stopped. No author has been able to demonstrate morbidity and mortality directly related to the degree of acidosis in SE. Failure to clear the acidosis in one hour in the nonseizing patient with an intact circulation should prompt an investigation for liver disease or a source of continuing lactate production. A common culprit could be a toxin (lindane, salicylates, INH) but uremia and severe hyperglycemia diabetic ketoacidosis (DKA), other causes of acidosis, are known to cause seizures. DKA is an easily diagnosed, but I have been fooled a number of times by renal failure that has presented with a seizure.

THE CLINICAL AND PHYSIOLOGIC CHARACTERISTICS OF STATUS EPILEPTICUS

Cerebral blood flow progressively decreases after 30 minutes of seizing, and once seizures last longer, it's time for a full court press

In the last chapter, I reviewed the biochemical and physiologic sequelae of major motor seizure activity. I emphasized that many of the rather impressive abnormalities that routinely occur after even a single seizure are not appreciated by many physicians because they simply are not looked for. For example, temperature is rarely taken three or four hours postseizure, even though more than half of seizure patients are febrile sometime in the postictal period merely from experiencing a seizure. Also, an arterial blood gas is not axiomatic in the absence of continued seizure activity even though significant metabolic acidosis is a well-documented consequence of even a single grand mal seizure. Other parameters associated with an otherwise benign seizure include peripheral leukocytosis, CSF pleocytosis, and a significant catecholamine excess. The vast majority of the metabolic consequences of seizure activity are merely transient physiological alterations of little clinical significance, but the degree of hyperthermia has been clearly linked to residual CNS damage. Catecholamine excess has been implicated in sudden arrhythmic death during seizure activity and to neurogenic pulmonary edema. While extensive laboratory investigation is not indicated following a single uncomplicated seizure coupled with a subsequent normal postictal state, status epilepticus raises significant physiologic and diagnostic concerns. This chapter will address some of these issues.

Although status epilepticus (SE) can be classified into a number of clinical types, comments in this chapter will be reserved for major motor status epilepticus. A reasonable definition of this condition is a seizure lasting more than 30 minutes or multiple seizures where there is no return to the baseline neurological status between attacks.

STATUS EPILEPTICUS: CAUSES, CLINICAL FEATURES AND CONSEQUENCES IN 98 PATIENTS

Aminoff MJ, Simon RP *Am J Med* 1980;69(5):657

This classic paper should be read by all emergency physicians. It reviews the etiology, clinical features, and outcomes of SE in 98 patients older than 14 years of age. A valuable and often quoted resource, this article is a review of the clinical experience of the San Francisco General Hospital that spans nine years. The authors state that all patients in the area with SE were taken to their hospital (an administrator's dream these days) so their experience was representative of a large urban population, not just an inner-city indigent subgroup.

All patients had two or more generalized major motor convulsions without recovering consciousness. Patients with absence (petit mal), myoclonic, or partial (focal) seizures were excluded. There were 73 males and 25 females. Of the 98 patients, 51 had a pre-existing seizure disorder, but SE developed de novo in 47 patients. The etiology of the pre-existing seizure disorder was varied, but consisted mainly of idiopathic epilepsy, trauma, alcohol withdrawal, and cerebrovascular disease. The leading etiology of SE among patients with a known seizure disorder was discontinuance or poor compliance with anticonvul-

---

SOME INTERESTING POINTS ABOUT STATUS EPILEPTICUS (SE)

- *Mortality rate from SE per se (no serious underlying abnormality) is less than five percent.*

- *Continuous seizing for 30 minutes or less is generally well tolerated and by itself does not cause sequelae.*

- *In 15 percent of cases, no definite cause for SE can be found (could be idiopathic epilepsy, unknown drug OD/withdrawal, etho history denied, etc.).*

- *Focality or lack thereof means little as to the presence or absence of a structural etiology.*

- *Idiopathic epilepsy rarely presents as SE although drug noncompliance in an epileptic can induce status.*

- *The most common cause of SE is a pre-existing seizure disorder and anticonvulsant drug noncompliance (or possible anticonvulsant drug withdrawal, especially benzodiazepines/barbiturates).*

- *Alcohol withdrawal and acute cerebral vascular disease are common causes of SE.*

- *SE can be the presenting sign of a brain tumor.*

- *Cocaine toxicity in an infant can cause SE or simulate a febrile seizure.*

- *Hyperglycemia, as well as hypoglycemia, can produce SE.*

Source: James R. Roberts, MD

---

sant drugs. Alcohol abuse was a common factor, and in many cases it was a contributing cause in patients with another etiology. In one case, SE was attributed to ethanol intoxication and respiratory depression rather than ethanol withdrawal. Interestingly, only four of the 98 patients had SE attributed to CNS infection (abscess, encephalitis, epidural empyema), but one patient with alcohol withdrawal had pneumococcal meningitis. In patients without a previous seizure disorder, SE was attributed to alcohol, cerebrovascular disease, drug overdose, post-cardiac arrest, metabolic disorders, CNS tumors, and CNS trauma.

The authors believe that cerebrovascular disease was the etiology of SE in 15 patients. The specific causes were cerebral emboli, cerebral hematoma, brain stem hemorrhage, and diffuse cerebrovascular disease. Four patients had cerebral tumors as the cause of their status. Interestingly, these brain neoplasms were previously undiagnosed, and SE was the first manifestation of the tumor. Previous trauma was related to SE in 11 patients, and only one patient had an acute subdural hematoma. Trauma-induced SE usually involved the frontal lobe. It was difficult to separate alcohol withdrawal from trauma in many cases. Metabolic derangement occasionally produced SE, but a metabolic disturbance was rarely the only cause identified. Hyponatremia, hypocalcemia, hyperglycemia, and hypoglycemia were each noted one time.

Ten patients developed status epilepticus as a result of drug overdose. Drugs included isoniazid (INH), over-the-counter antihistamines, a tricyclic antidepressant, cocaine, theophylline, lidocaine, and pentazocine. A precipitating cause could not be found in 15 patients. Importantly SE was never the initial manifestation of primary idiopathic epilepsy.

CLINICAL MANIFESTATIONS: Generalized tonic/clonic activity occurred in 37 patients, but 61 had unconsciousness in association with a focal or lateralized convulsive activity. Focal seizures were not necessarily related to specific structural pathology, such as a brain tumor or subdural hematoma. Interestingly, in 17 patients some form of focality was seen without structural causes. Metabolic disturbances, drug overdose, or ethanol withdrawal all produced focal seizure activity.

In 70 cases (70%), SE led to no permanent morbidity. Although the duration of seizure activity was less than two hours in most cases, in nine cases without permanent sequelae, seizure activity lasted from two to 18 hours.

Status epilepticus was associated with, or followed by, serious or fatal sequelae in 28 patients (28%). However, these complications were most often due to the underlying pathology rather than to SE per se. In only 10 cases (10%) was it concluded that status epilepticus itself produced significant subsequent morbidity. There were only two deaths related directly to the prolonged seizure activity. Six patients with SE developed diffuse encephalopathy, and one patient had permanent spastic paresis. The authors were unable to draw firm conclusions about the duration of status epilepticus and sequelae. There was, however, a trend for complications to be associated with prolonged seizure activity. The mortality rate of SE was two percent.

The vast majority of patients had fever associated with SE. Only eight patients had a core temperature below 98°F and five of these had underlying hypothermic-producing pathology (drug overdose, hypothyroidism, brain stem injury). More than half the patients had leukocytosis (range 12,000 to 29,000 cells/mm3). In four patients without underlying infection, the peripheral white cell count was greater than 25,000/mm3. In 23 of 84 patients, the arterial pH was below 7.00 (lowest was 6.28). There was both a metabolic and a respiratory component to the acidosis, and sequelae were not related to the degree of acidosis. Despite normal CSF cultures, abnormal cells, defined as one or more polymorphonuclear cells or greater than five mononuclear cells, were found in the CSF in 12 of 65 cases (18%). The CSF cell count was usually greatest on the day following the episode of status epilepticus. A modest increase in CSF protein was noted in eight cases, but glucose levels were not affected.

The authors concluded that noncompliance with anticonvulsant medications is the most common cause of SE, accounting for 53 percent of patients with a history of previous seizures. In their series, 28 percent of all cases were due to noncompliance. Alcohol withdrawal alone, or in combination with other factors, was a common cause of SE. The authors emphasize that SE is occasionally the initial clinical manifestation of a cerebral neoplasm or a cerebrovascular accident. Focal seizures do not necessary indicate localized pathology.

COMMENT: This paper is relatively self-explanatory and contains a large amount of useful information about the clinical characteristics of patients with SE. A few points

require emphasis. Almost 30 percent of patients brought to the ED with SE will have a known underlying seizure disorder with breakthrough seizures. A single seizure related to noncompliance occurs more often than SE, with a noncompliance etiology approaching 80-90 percent in some studies. Although the most common cause is noncompliance to anti-seizure medications, the etiology is often multifactorial and one cannot automatically assume that all patients with seizure disorders are seizing because

ETIOLOGY OF PRE-EXISTING SEIZURE DISORDER IN 51 PATIENTS WHO DEVELOPED SE

Etiology	No. Patients
Idiopathic	13
Trauma	12
Alcohol withdrawal alone	6
Alcohol withdrawal and previous head trauma	5
Alcohol withdrawal and cerebrovascular disease	1
Cerebrovascular disease	7
Perinatal pathology	2
Cerebral atrophy	1
Previous meningitis	1
Previous cerebral abscess	1
Previous cranial surgery	1
Related to theophylline toxicity	1

Source: Am J Med 1980;69:657-65.

they forgot to take their medicine. Therefore, anticonvulsant drug levels must always be evaluated. Attempting to elicit an accurate history of drug compliance is generally worthless (also worthless is asking patients if they drink alcohol or use cocaine), and some anticonvulsant drugs in overdose, such a carbamazepine, can cause seizures. No specific cause could be found in 15 percent of the patients, but because this paper was written in 1980, I suspect that refined diagnostic capabilities (better drug screens, MRI, CT) may lower this number.

Although it's probably important to observe focality in seizing patients, I found it interesting that focal or lateralized seizures did not necessarily indicate a structural lesion. If you wait for a focal finding to order a CT, you will sit on a lot of subdurals and brain tumors. Of great interest is the observation that four patients without previous seizures had SE as the first manifestation of their brain tumor. Of particular note is the current high incidence of seizures due to cocaine, an unusual drug in the 1970s, but one that is now almost normal flora in my patients. Unexpected cocaine toxicity is well documented to cause seizures in infants, either toddlers who eat the crack from last night's party or if infants are confined in a small space where the parents are smoking cocaine (*Pediatrics* 1989;84(6):1100). Some children's hospitals routinely order cocaine screens on kids who seem to have benign febrile seizures.

One drug that is well known to cause SE, and one that will not be found on anyone's screen, is isoniazid (INH). For the next Cambodian refugee or AIDS patient who presents with SE with no discernible cause, try giving 5 grams of pyridoxine (vitamin B-6), the antidote for INH poisoning. Antihistamines, anticholinergics, tricyclic antidepressants, theophylline, propoxyphene, hypogycemics, lithium, carbon monoxide, and camphor are also common overdoses that produce status epilepticus.

Although hypoglycemia was found in only one patient, it is axiomatic that the serum glucose be checked in any seizing patient. Everyone thinks about low glucose as being seizurogenic, but severe hyperglycemia can also cause a seizure, even SE, probably due to hyperosmolality.

The mortality rate (2%) and morbidity rate (12.5%) from SE itself was relatively low. This may reflect aggressive treatment. The ability of the human body to withstand the insults of prolonged seizure activity is truly amazing. There was a trend toward increasing morbidity with increased duration of seizure activity, but the main determinant of death or sequelae was the underlying cause of SE. The role of

alcohol withdrawal in inducing seizures is well accepted. Ng et al (*N Engl J Med* 1988;319(11):666) contend that persistent ethanol consumption, in addition to withdrawal, may induce seizures, and traditional dogma about alcohol withdrawal being the only ethanol-related etiology for seizures is questioned. Certainly ethanol intoxication can depress respirations enough to cause hypoxia and set off a previous seizure focus.

ETIOLOGY OF SE AMONG PATIENTS IN SERIES

Etiology	Patients with Preceding Seizure Disorder	Patients without Previous Seizures
Discontinuation or irregularity of anticonvulsant drug regime	27	0
Alcohol-related	11	4
Cerebrovascular disease	4	11
Drug overdose	0	10
Metabolic disorders	3	5
Cardiac arrest	0	4
Cerebral tumor	0	4
Cerebral trauma	1	2
Infections		
Abscess	0	1
Meningitis	0	2
Encephalitis	0	1
Unknown	11	4

Some patients were counted more than once because of multifactorial etiology. Alcohol withdrawal was a factor in five patients with discontinued or irregular anticonvulsant drug regime; metabolic disorder was a factor in one alcohol-related case; anticonvulsant drug irregularity was a factor in five alcohol-related cases; meningitis was a factor in one alcohol-related case; and alcohol was implicated in one metabolic/abscess case.

Source: Am J Med *1980;69:657-65.*

THE BIOCHEMICAL BASIS AND PATHOPHYSIOLOGY OF STATUS EPILEPTICUS

Lothman E *Neurology* 1990;40(Suppl 2):13

This rather complicated article is a good reference for those interested in the nuances of the physiology of SE. The discussion begins with a rather intuitive notion that the more protracted the SE, the more difficult it is to control and the more likely will be the lasting effects. Although SE is rather common clinically, most of what we have ascertained about pathophysiology has come from animal studies, both freely convulsing animals and paralyzed animals who have had seizures induced by chemoconvulsants. In the initial 30 minutes of generalized convulsions, blood pressure, serum lactate, and glucose levels rise while pH decreases. Glucose and oxygen utilization in the brain increases as do brain lactate levels. In approximately 30 minutes, there is a general decompensation which begins a phase of potential brain injury. Respiratory depression and hyperthermia ensue and cerebral blood flow begins to fall. The mismatch between brain metabolism and substrates begins to cause injury in vulnerable areas of the brain. There is some evidence that SE per se destroys neurons independent of systemic metabolic factors. Even animals who have metabolic parameters supported and are paralyzed to prevent motor activity will suffer serious effects from prolonged seizures. It has been postulated that neurotoxins are formed as a result of seizure activity, and there is osmotic damage as well as calcium-related damage at a cellular level. There appears to be a cascade of disturbances, poorly understood, following prolonged SE that include a deterioration of the normally protective GABAergic inhibition system. Because prolonged seizing is detrimental to the brain, it is paramount to stop the seizure activity as soon as possible. It appears that there is a window of at least 30 minutes of prolonged seizure activity before the transition to seizure-induced brain injury becomes prominent.

COMMENT: Those with an interest in brain biochemistry and neurotransmitters would find this article interesting. The clinician would find it rather dull, but its main message is one that cannot be ignored — seizure activity by itself is detrimental to the human brain. Others have demonstrated lesions of an ischemic nature in the brains of animals undergoing prolonged seizure activity (*Arch Neurol* 1973;28:10) and note changes throughout the brain similar to hypoxia or hypoglycemia. These injuries appear to be enhanced by the hyperpyrexia, hypotension, and hypoxia (but not acidosis) that invariably occur after prolonged seizure activity. Neuronal damage can result following prolonged partial (non-major motor) seizures even when no hypoxia, hypotension, or hyperpyrexia coexist. This suggests that the underlying final pathway is increased metabolic demand in the face of inadequate oxygenation or substrates.

One can do little about the biochemical alterations on a cellular level, but one can certainly attack specific derangements aggressively with blood pressure and respiratory support and cooling measures. An aggressive approach includes frequent measurements of arterial blood gases, core temperature, early use of paralyzing agents, and ventilatory support. Although cerebral damage related to hyperpyrexia, hypotension, and hypoxia is easily prevented, the metabolic demands of the seizing brain eventually win out. Exactly how long one can seize and remain neurologically unscathed is variable. Some patients seize for many hours and make a full recovery. Because every case is different, it's meaningless to talk about exact times, but in one series the mean duration of SE in patients who made a full recovery was 90 minutes, 10 hours for those with sequelae, and 13 hours for those who died (*Acta Neurol Scand* 1970;46:573). I think it's rather amazing that patients can continually seize for almost two hours and still make a full recovery. Intuitively, patients with idiopathic epilepsy as the etiology of SE would likely fare better than those with other causes. Cerebral blood flow is known to decrease progressively after about 30 minutes of seizing so I think the half-hour time frame is a reasonable one to use as a safety window. Once seizures last longer, it's time for a full court press, with all available drugs and an expedited call to the neurologist.

Paresis, encephalopathy, and other specific neuropathology can be seen following SE, but intellectual impairment as an outcome of prolonged seizing is a topic of some debate. Dodrill et al (*Neurology* 1990;40(Suppl 2): 23) discuss intellectual changes following status epilepticus. While data are sparse, there are clear intellectual sequelae of status epilepticus. Patients undergoing prolonged SE tend to do poorer on neuropsychiatric tests and IQ measurements, and overall are intellectually duller than those not experiencing SE. Although the effect of SE on mental abilities is difficult if not possible impossible to define clearly, the human brain does manifest subtle intellectual sequelae following SE.

BASIC ED EVALUATION OF PATIENTS WITH SEIZURES

Routinely ordering a CBC, serum electrolytes, BUN/creatinine, and calcium and magnesium levels are not supported by science

Previous chapters have investigated the biochemical and physiologic changes that occur secondary to seizing and status epilepticus. It was noted that even a single seizure can produce a significant decrease in serum pH and can spawn a number of abnormal laboratory findings, including white cells in the CSF, a peripheral leukocytosis, and a fever. Many of these abnormalities are not appreciated by emergency physicians because they are not routinely searched for. One must, however, do some sort of investigation on every patient to determine the cause of seizures and to develop a plan that will adequately address subsequent therapy. This month's column will attempt to put laboratory issues in focus, with a rational, prospective approach.

EFFICACY OF A STANDARD SEIZURE WORK-UP IN THE EMERGENCY DEPARTMENT
Eisner RF, et al *Ann Emerg Med* 1986;15(1):33

The authors of this study prospectively evaluated their inner-city hospital's protocol that was routinely used to evaluate adults and children presenting with a witnessed grand mal or focal motor seizure or a prehospital history or evaluation that supported those diagnoses. The aim was to study the usefulness of a standard testing protocol used for the evaluation and subsequent management of ED patients. Data collection included various formatted history and physical diagnosis parameters, vital signs, and certain mandatory laboratory tests. All patients received a CBC, BUN/creatinine, glucose, electrolytes, calcium/magnesium, and urinalysis. Selected patients also had serum anticonvulsant levels measured, and some were evaluated by CT scanning. Criteria for CT scanning included any first-time seizure, recent significant head trauma, a focal neurological deficit, and a focal finding or focal seizure. Prior to obtaining laboratory values but after the history and physical examination, the physicians were instructed to list the five most likely diagnoses and to rank the priority and likelihood of these etiologies. After the laboratory tests were available, the diagnostic probabilities were then reassigned.

The subject consisted of 163 seizure patients with a mean age of 41 years. The majority (85%) had a previous seizure history. The final assigned causes of the seizures are listed in the table, and it's noted that anticonvulsant noncompliance was the leading diagnosis, accounting for 59 percent of all cases. When testing was complete, 104 patients (64%) had an abnormality uncovered that required an intervention or change in diagnosis, management, or disposition. The most common abnormality, present in 92 percent of those with an abnormal laboratory finding, was a subtherapeutic anticonvulsant level. No patient had toxic levels of anticonvulsants, and 12 percent of those tested had therapeutic levels. A number of laboratory abnormalities were present, the most common being a low serum bicarbonate level. There were minor inconsequential changes in serum sodium and potassium but no significant abnormalities in magnesium, calcium, BUN, or creatinine were found. Glucose levels ranged from hypoglycemia (20 mg/L) to hyperglycemia (450 mg/L). The CT scan was abnormal in five of 19 patients, but there was only one subdural hematoma and one CNS mass lesion. Interestingly, the CT scan caused the initial diagnosis of an intracranial process to be changed to a non-CNS etiology in the three remaining

> ORDERING A FULL ECG MAY MAKE YOU LOOK LIKE A PRO IF YOU PICK UP A CASE OF PROLONGED QT SYNDROME

CAUSES OF SEIZURES

Causes	No. (%)
Anticonvulsant noncompliance	96 (59)
New onset	24 (12)
Unknown	14 (8)
Alcohol withdrawal	13 (8)
Breakthrough	8 (5)
Febrile	6 (4)
Hypoglycemia	2 (<1)

Source: Ann Emerg Med 198915:33-9.

patients. Overall, the history and physical examination predicted abnormalities in all but two cases (one case of hyperglycemia and one subdural hematoma).

The authors question the routine use of low-yield screening tests and routine CT examination in the ED evaluation of patients with seizures. Although some laboratory tests can be used selectively, the yield is extremely low when applied to all patients. The most common serious abnormality not suspected by history and physical examination was an alteration in serum glucose levels. Serum electrolytes did not contribute significantly to the management of any patient in the study, and there were no abnormalities in these parameters that would have accounted for any seizure. Likewise, magnesium and calcium levels were of no value, and these tests did not define an etiology in a single patient. Although renal failure may be a cause of seizures, it was not identified in this subgroup. Likewise, there were no systemic or CNS infections contributing to seizure activity.

The findings did support the routine measurement of anticonvulsant drug levels in patients known to have seizure disorders. While most patients were subtherapeutic, the authors do not believe that the empiric treatment with anticonvulsants while waiting for blood levels is supported because 12 percent had therapeutic levels. The authors believed that the CT scan was a high-yield test, noting a 25 percent incidence of significant abnormalities. The absence of CT abnormalities was helpful on several occasions when it ruled out a presumptive diagnosis of intracranial hemorrhage.

The authors conclude that serum anticonvulsant levels and CT scans under appropriate circumstances are high-yield tests for the ED evaluation of patients presenting with seizures. The history and physical examination was able to guide the clinician in choosing high-yield tests that were most likely to have an impact on diagnosis and treatment. Routinely ordering a battery of diagnostic laboratory tests was not considered effective or helpful. It is noted that there were not enough patients with first-time seizures to make accurate comments about this subset of patients.

COMMENT: The conclusions supported by this report echo the experience of most practicing emergency physicians. It doesn't take one very long to get a gut feeling or an intuition about which patient will benefit by casting a wide diagnostic net, but certainly routinely ordering a CBC, serum electrolytes, BUN/creatinine, and calcium and magnesium levels have never been supported by any scientific data. However, one very important caveat (and caution) is in order. There were no patients with severe electrolyte disturbances, renal failure, or significant calcium/magnesium abnormalities so it's not known whether this protocol would have prospectively targeted patients with these abnormalities and prompted appropriate testing. No one wants to miss a case of hyponatremia, hypocalcemia, or meningitis, but in reality if one requires a slew of routine diagnostic tests on all patients before intuiting that something is just not right, it's time to go back to medical school. Of course, no matter what the clinical condition, if a patient has a dialysis shunt, one should measure BUN/creatinine; if the patient is 70 years old and has peripheral vascular disease or cancer, a CT is in order; and a serum sodium is mandatory if the mental status remains cloudy or the patient continues to seize.

Of particular note is the presence of hypoglycemia or hyperglycemia in the absence of suspicious historical or clinical features. If you have not been burned by an unexpected extreme of serum glucose, you have just not seen enough patients. Hyperglycemia, as well as hypoglycemia, can cause a seizure. However, the glucose issue is easily remedied by a simple Dextrostix/Accu-Chek in the ED. I have tried to make a rapid bedside serum glucose check part of my routine on any seizing patient, even when I'm dead sure of the diagnosis and even if there is no history of diabetes. Glucose testing is too easy to do and too consequential if missed to proceed otherwise. The issue of routine CT scanning is addressed in a subsequent article.

Other authors have formed similar conclusions. Powers (*Ann Emerg Med* 1985;14(5):416) routinely evaluated serum chemistries in 112 adults who presented to the ED with recent seizures. The overall incidence of seizures due to primary changes in serum chemistry was 2.4 percent. Two of these patients had hypoglycemia, but it was obvious on historical parameters, and one patient had renal failure but was known to be on dialysis. As in other studies, this author found that hypomagnesemia was common in alcoholic patients and concludes that the routine practice of supplementing magnesium is supported.

Kenney et al (*Pediatr Emerg Care* 1992;8(1):65) noted a similar lack of useful clinical information when serum chemistry tests were routinely ordered in pediatric patients. They could find no significant abnormalities in 592 laboratory tests on 241 febrile and nonfebrile seizing children when the history and physical examination ruled out shock, dehydration, and metabolic or renal disorders (neonates and young infants excluded).

The above conclusions require further comment. First of all, you must perform a good examination and you must make a diligent effort to ferret out the significant history. These parameters are only as good as the clinician evaluating them; stated another way, not all examinations and histories are the same on any given patient. Many questions must be asked in more than one way and to more than one relative, and the examination is a dynamic process that must be repeated and reassessed. Patients with subtherapeutic phenytoin levels and idiopathic epilepsy look just like patients with hyponatremia, a brain tumor, or subdural hematoma during the first minutes of the postictal period.

Of course, every seasoned emergency physician can recall at least one patient where a dogmatic stance trying to limit the use of laboratory testing has proved quite embarrassing if not downright stupid or dangerous. However, one unsuspected case of beer drinker's hyponatremia or hypocalcemia secondary to hypoparathyroidism should not cause one to abandon all logic and simply order laboratory tests indiscriminately. The clinician evaluating

ABNORMALITIES FOUND IN STANDARD METABOLIC WORKUP

Chemistry	Normal Range	Range	Abnormal (%)
Sodium	135-145*	129-150	8 (5)
Potassium	3.5-5*	2.8-5.5	13 (7)
Chloride	95-110*	95-114	6 (4)
Bicarbonate	22-30*	15-35	27 (17)
Magnesium	1.8-2.8†	1.4-3.2	7 (4)
Calcium	8.5-10.5†	8.1-10.7	3 (2)
BUN	10-28†	10-34	2 (2)
Creatinine	0.7-1.5†	0.7-1.5	0 (0)
Glucose	60-150†	20-450	8 (6)
WBC count	7-11K	4.3-16.7K	12 (7)

*mmol/L
†mg/L

Source: Ann Emerg Med 198915:33-9.

patients with seizures should use the laboratory in same way one uses it for evaluation of abdominal pain, shortness of breath, and syncope. Certain tests or procedures are axiomatic, such as the use of anticonvulsant levels in patients with known seizure disorders, the routine use of bedside glucose testing, evaluation of old records, a good physical examination coupled with a history obtained through relatives, friends, and paramedics, and a realization that every patient is just a bit different. The medical system in this country is not going broke because too many electrolyte panels are run in the ED on seizing patients, but one needs to draw the line somewhere and use a little common sense when it comes to laboratory testing.

Toxicology screening often provides significant information that is not suspected by the history and physical examination. Cocaine is a common cause of seizures, but most patients vehemently deny using it even when confronted with a spinal tap or when questioned by the most sympathetic physician. A seizure in a child can be environmentally acquired cocaine, and that scenario is not uncommon in a busy inner-city children's hospital. I have occasionally been surprised by finding unexpected drugs in seizure patients so a urine drug screen, as limited as it is in most hospitals, is probably a relatively high-yield test. Certainly it offers more information than a CBC.

There's no question that noncompliance to medication is a common cause of seizures, and you will be right more often than not if you predict that every seizing patient rolling through the ED door has a previous seizure history and has not taken his medication. That makes anticonvulsant levels the highest yield laboratory test across the board. Even if the level is therapeutic, more drug may be needed to push levels into the high therapeutic range. Finding a subtherapeutic phenytoin or phenobarbital level in an unknown patient brought to the ED in a confused and combative state may quickly focus your diagnosis to

PRIMARY AND FINAL DIAGNOSES AFTER ED TESTING

Initial Diagnosis	Final Diagnosis	Test Resulting in Change	No.	No. Affecting Treatment	No. Affecting Disposition
Alcohol withdrawal	Subtherapeutic drug levels	Anticonvulsant levels	4	4	-
CNS mass	Unknown	CT scan	4	4	4
Noncompliance	Medication breakthrough	Anticonvulsant levels	3	3	-
Noncompliance	Alcohol withdrawal	Anticonvulsant levels	2	2	2
Cerebrovascular accident	Hyperglycemia	Serum glucose	1	1	-
Cerebrovascular accident	Subdural hematoma	CT scan	1	1	-
Cerebrovascular accident	Post-traumatic scarring	CT scan	1	1	-
Intracranial bleed	Subtherapeutic drug levels	Anticonvulsant levels	1	1	1
Intracranial bleed	Arrhythmia	CT scan/ECG	1	1	-
Total			18	18	7

Source: Ann Emerg Med 1989;15:33-9.

altered mental status due to a postictal state. All seizing patients should be placed on a cardiac monitor, but ordering a full ECG may make you look like a pro if you pick up a case of prolonged QT syndrome or an IA/IC, like a drug overdose that can cause seizures (tricyclic antidepressants, antihistamines, quinidine, etc).

SEIZURE PATIENT SELECTION FOR EMERGENCY COMPUTED TOMOGRAPHY

Reinus WR, et al *Ann Emerg Med* 1993;22(8):1298

The authors note that although CT scanning is often routine in patients with seizure disorders, overall it is a low-yield procedure if applied without criteria. In order to understand better the clinical issues, the authors reviewed the records of 115 consecutive patients who presented to an ED after a recent seizure who received a noncontrast head CT scan. Patients received their CT scan based solely on the physician's perception of need, and no other criteria were required. The CT scan was positive in 23 of 115 patients (20%), and there was a strong correlation between the results of the clinical evaluation and the CT results. In fact, the sensitivity of the neurological examination for a CT scan abnormality was 95 percent, and only one patient, an individual with a recurrent glioblastoma, had a positive CT scan with a negative neurological evaluation. An abnormal neurologic examination was quite conservative, and was considered to be a change in sensorium or mental status or abnormalities in cranial nerves, or motor, sensory, or proprioceptive function. The historical variable that was most significantly associated with a CT scan abnormality was a history of cancer, and the sensitivity and negative predictive value of the combination of an abnormal neurological examination and/or history of a known carcinoma was an amazing 100 percent.

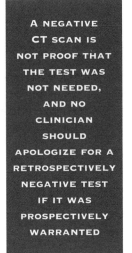

A NEGATIVE CT SCAN IS NOT PROOF THAT THE TEST WAS NOT NEEDED, AND NO CLINICIAN SHOULD APOLOGIZE FOR A RETROSPECTIVELY NEGATIVE TEST IF IT WAS PROSPECTIVELY WARRANTED

COMMENT: The issue of when to order a CT scan (for any condition) is a complicated one that is made more complicated by the milieu of the ED, patient compliance issues, and medicolegal and emotional factors. Try as you may to withhold a CT scan from a 3-year-old with minor head trauma who is vomiting while the frightened parents look on, most of us quickly cave in even though we are 99 percent sure that the test will be negative. As with laboratory screening tests, the CT scan is probably vastly overused in the ED for evaluation of patients with seizure disorders. Although more expensive than an electrolyte panel, CT scans are often justified because findings often indicate bad disease. Any clinician can relay a story where they tried to be prudent with the use of CT scanning only to have an intracranial hemorrhage diagnosed when a consultant or admitting resident demanded the test. I know of no firm guidelines that would help sort out this issue, and most of us would rather have 90 percent of our CT scans negative than miss a single epidural hematoma. Withholding a CT scan on any postictal seizure patient is always a calculated risk. When patients fall to the ground on the sidewalk, the skull is vulnerable and often the scalp does not indicate brain trauma. Like the car that turns over two times with few dents to show for it, physicians don't appreciate the magnitude of prehospital trauma if the patient initially seems to be minimally injured, and there's no bystander to relay a ghastly history.

As in the case of laboratory testing, one can generally be prudent in the use of the CT scan by taking the time to evaluate the history and physical parameters carefully. Certainly an awake, alert, totally asymptomatic patient does not require a head CT scan just because they think they were "knocked out" when their boyfriend punched them. However, this assumes that they actually are awake, alert, and totally asymptomatic following a careful and sometimes repeated evaluation. To my thinking, patients need to be examined more than once and need to be observed for a sufficient length of time before dogma sets in. Keeping an open mind and being willing to admit you're wrong and change your opinion (and occasionally even look foolish) is the most prudent approach. Even when I'm sure I will not order a CT scan, I let the family know that it's an option I may use if things change. A least they are aware that you were concerned enough, or smart enough, to have considered the test.

Alternatively, a patient who claims that nothing is wrong may mandate their own CT scan by some subtle abnormality picked up by an experienced nurse, clinician, or family member who knows the baseline. Probably the best reason for allowing an annoying family into the room is that you can quiz them about the baseline mental status at the bedside.

Of course, one does not need to have an abnormal neurological examination or a history of cancer to have a positive CT scan, even when the abnormality requires significant intervention. The last epidural hematoma that I picked up with a CT scan was because I ordered the test to evaluate for a possible CNS infection on a patient with subgaleal abscess. Actually nothing in the examination or history would have lead me to believe that this patient had a condition that took him to the operating room two hours later. I made sure the radiologist, who initially questioned the need, found out about that one.

Of particular frustration to the emergency physician are radiology or hospital policies that relegate medicine to a cookbook approach with regard to ordering expensive low-yield tests. The emergency physician cannot be expected to function in an environment where distant radiologists, administrators, or managed care plans make decisions about ordering CT scans in patients with seizures or in any other scenario. Although it may be reasonable to hold off on the scan for a few hours until the regular daytime technician arrives or to arrange for an outpatient scan in selected patients, if the CT scan is deemed necessary by the physician who signs the chart, it should be done. The test should not be used in lieu of an appropriate history or physical examination, but no neurosurgeon or neurologist that I am associated with would consider forgoing a CT scan with even the most minimal symptoms when they are called as consultants. In fact, they often order the test without ever seeing the patient. Medicolegal and economic issues aside, it is good medicine to utilize today's technology where it has a reasonable chance to be helpful. A negative CT scan is not proof that the test was not needed, and no clinician should have to apologize for a retrospectively negative investigation if it was prospectively warranted. I would sure like to know the incidence of negative CT scans ordered by other primary care physicians; I'll bet it's a lot higher then the numbers generated from the ED.

SUMMARY: I would summarize a reasonable approach to the evaluation of the stable seizure patient with the following. Perform the most appropriate history and exam, put the patient on a monitor, and secure venous access. If the seizure has stopped, order anticonvulsant levels and check the glucose immediately. Keep the option open for further testing based on the evolving scenario. If the patient has an abnormal postictal course, experiences another seizure, or there are specific concerns/doubts with the case, proceed with laboratory testing and a head CT as suggested by factoring all variables. For known seizure patients, I would also usually administer an anticonvulsant in an empiric partial loading dose (one-quarter to one-half) because an overdose of anticonvulsants will rarely be the cause of the seizure and the odds are in your favor that drug noncompliance will be the culprit . More on treatment in future columns.

INITIAL THERAPEUTIC STRATEGIES FOR THE TREATMENT OF STATUS EPILEPTICUS

The traditional treatment regimen is a benzodiazepine, followed by phenytoin, then possibly phenobarbital

Previous columns have discussed the etiology, diagnosis, and work-up of ED patients with seizures, with a particular focus on the pathophysiology of status epilepticus (SE). This month's column will continue the discussion of SE with an overview of the initial treatment modalities available to the emergency physician. After a focused history is extracted and the patient is initially examined, basic steps are axiomatic: vital signs (including temperature) are taken, IV access is secured, blood is drawn and glucose checked, oxygen is administered, and the cardiac monitor and pulse oximeter are attached. Now it's time to consider drug therapy. If the patient is still seizing, the traditional treatment regimen has been a benzodiazepine (BZD) followed by phenytoin, then possibly phenobarbital.

THE ROLE OF BENZODIAZEPINES IN THE MANAGEMENT OF STATUS EPILEPTICUS

Treiman DM *Neurology* 1990;40:32

This review is an excellent discussion on the role of benzodiazepines (BZD) for the treatment of SE. BZDs are the most readily available, most potent, and most rapidly acting drugs that can be used in the ED for the treatment of status. BZD pharmacology has been studied extensively, and the drugs have a very complex biochemical profile, ranging from effects on presynaptic and postsynaptic neuronal transmission to a direct effect on membrane physiology. Perhaps the most important antiseizure effect of BZDs is an enhancement of gama-aminobutyric acid (GABA)-mediated neuroinhibition and a reduction in the repetitive firing of action potentials. GABAergic synapses occur throughout the CNS, and stimulation of these receptors produces neuroinhibition. Although the physiology is rather complex, it has been postulated that there are specific BZD receptors located in close proximity to GABA receptors on the membranes of postsynaptic neurons (see figure 1). When BZDs bind to these specific BZD receptors, the end result is a synergism or an increase in GABAergic inhibition that's translated clinically into seizure control. Other more complex mechanisms of action that may be related to BZDs' ability to halt a seizure are listed in figure 2.

The authors note that 47 studies have appeared in the literature since 1965 touting the safety and efficacy of BZDs for the treatment of SE. Currently few credible authorities seriously question this traditional teaching. Although many of the quoted studies are non-randomized or retrospective, the ability of clonazepam, diazepam, or lorazepam to terminate SE is undisputed. Overall approximately 80-90 percent of patients in status will respond favorably. There are no clear data demonstrating the superiority of one BZD over another, but lorazepam (Ativan) appears to have at least a theoretical edge over diazepam. Diazepam (Valium) is still a popular first choice, but clonazepam (Klonopin) is not available in the United States for IV use. Lorazepam is recommended because of its presumed longer duration of action. For ethical reasons, it's difficult to compare BZDs alone because patients in status are immediately loaded with phenytoin or phenobarbital. This standard use of additional anticonvulsants has not allowed lorazepam and diazepam as monotherapy to be well studied head-to-head with regard to clinical superiority or duration of seizure control.

The authors note, however, that only three prospective randomized comparative studies on the management of SE have been published, so there are virtually no data that prove benzodiazepines are actually superior to phenytoin or phenobarbital for initial management. Based largely on pharmacologic theory, the author agrees with the general consensus that lorazepam is the drug of choice for SE. He cites the drug's longer duration of action, high lipid solubility, ease of intravenous administration, and small volume of distribution. A suggested treatment protocol for SE highlights the initial use of thiamine and glucose and the use of lorazepam (0.1 mg/kg IV) followed by phenytoin loading at 20 mg/kg. A total of 30 mg/kg of phenytoin (by additional 5 mg/kg boluses) is suggested if SE does not terminate with the lower phenytoin dose. If phenytoin is unsuccessful, IV phenobarbital at 20 mg/kg is suggested, followed by pentobarbital-induced coma if necessary.

COMMENT: BZDs are the almost unanimous choice for the initial control of the actively seizing patient (*J Epilepsy* 1990;3:7), and very few clinicians currently begin with phenytoin or phenobarbital. Whether you choose Valium or Ativan is largely a matter of personal choice. Leppik et al (*JAMA* 1983;249:1452) found no significant clinical difference between the two BZDs in 39 cases of convulsive status. I have seen both used, and I haven't been able to detect a significant difference. If one does not work, it may be reasonable to switch, but I don't think the other one will consistently exhibit better efficacy. BZDs are almost immediately effective when given intravenous-

ly, they require no prolonged loading, they are extremely safe from a cardiovascular standpoint, and their use is familiar to all physicians. The only downsides are excessive sedation and respiratory depression, especially if phenobarbital is subsequently given. Lorazepam is quite viscous and must be refrigerated and diluted, so our paramedics don't carry it in the ambulance. As a clever marketing technique, Ativan comes preloaded in a syringe to avoid the hassles of having to draw it up in an emergency.

One situation in which BZDs are not used routinely is the non-seizing patient who presents with a history of seizures. Certainly if a patient is not actively seizing, it makes no sense to administer BZDs routinely. However, if one is waiting for the pheyntoin or carbamazipine level

---

MECHANISM OF ACTION OF BENZODIAZEPINES

Postsynaptic: Enhance GABAergic inhibition

Presynaptic: Enhance presynaptic inhibitiom; block presynaptic calcium uptake; enhance or reduce neurotransmitter release

Nonsynaptic: Reduce voltage-dependent Na+ and K+ ion conductances; increase Cl- ion conductance; recuce repetitive firing of action potentials.

Adapted from Neurology *1990; 40(2):32.*

---

to confirm noncompliance or to guide a loading dose, and a seizure recurs, BZDs should probably be used to control the active seizure.

Not all authors, however, totally embrace the exclusive initial use of BZDs. In a contrary view, Shaner et al (*Neurology* 1988;38:202) studied the initial use of phenobarbital followed by optional phenytoin and found this to be as effective as the more accepted protocol of diazepam followed by phenytoin. Gabor (*J Epilepsy* 1990;3:3) likewise favors the initial use of phenobarbital over lorazepam for SE, so there seems to be some support for alternatives to BZDs. BZDs and barbiturates are equally sedating, and both are respiratory depressants. Some arguments for the initial use of phenobarbital over BZD are quite plausible. Unlike BZDs, there is a rather clear dose-effect relationship for barbiturates, barbiturate may constitute single-drug therapy, and there are reports indicating that phenobarbital may terminate SE at serum levels well below the toxic range; a rather modest loading dose of 12-15 mg/kg of phenobarbital is as statistically effective as BZD in terminating SE. The major drawback is that barbiturates require time-consuming loading, although phenobarbital may be administered at an IV rate of 100 mg/min (requiring only 11 minutes to fully load a 70 kg patient with 15 mg/kg). Most nursing protocols require the physician to institute phenobarbital loading or to give more than 60 mg IV.

The initial use of lorazepam in a dose of 0.1 mg/kg is fine for true status, but it's too aggressive for treating a few isolated seizures. Giving 7 mg of IV lorazepam for the average 70 kg person virtually guarantees that the patient will sleep the rest of the day. Most clinicians choose 1 to 2 mg for the average adult and repeat this dose if seizures persist or recur. I could find no data that would suggest a maximum dose at which one should terminate lorazepam therapy. Most seizures stop after 2-4 mg, and there's no clear dose-response data available. Some authorities (usually the timid ones) stop if 4 mg is unsuccessful, but it seems reasonable to give up to 10-12 mg of lorazepam before switching to an alternative therapy. I arbitrarily set my upper limit for Valium at 60-80 mg. There are no data I'm aware of to support this stance, but every neurologist will support the aggressive use of a single drug before switching to another drug. Switching too quickly usually results in underdosing both drugs. We have all given seemingly huge doses of BZDs to patients in alcohol withdrawal with minimal cardiovascular/respiratory effect and often push the dose even higher. Respiratory depression should never keep one from using megadoses of BZDs, and you probably have to empty out the pharmacy of BZDs before you get clinically significant cardiovascular depression. Valium is officially approved for seizures, but when I looked up lorazepam in the *PDR,* I was surprised to see that there was no mention of the use of this drug for the control of seizures. Interestingly, it's not even FDA-approved for seizure control. There is a warning that Ativan should be diluted before IV use, but I could find no reports of specific problems with using the drug full strength, as is done by most clinicians.

Levy and Kroll (*Arch Neurol* 1984;41:605) echo the widespread support for lorazepam. In their study of 21

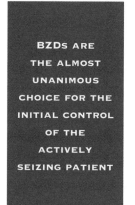

BZDs ARE THE ALMOST UNANIMOUS CHOICE FOR THE INITIAL CONTROL OF THE ACTIVELY SEIZING PATIENT

episodes of SE, the mean dose of lorazepam required to control SE was a mere 4 mg, and all patients responded within 15 minutes. Two patients required intubation for respiratory depression, and marked lethargy was noted in four patients. Because all patients also received phenytoin, the long-term value of the benzodiazepine itself is unclear. Some patients had their generalized SE transformed into partial status with BZD therapy. It is well known that generalized seizures with diffuse EEG abnormalities are more readily suppressed than are focal abnormalities because BZDs depress the spread of the discharge rather than the seizure focus itself. Unlike diazepam, lorazepam has no significant active metabolites to produce a prolonged sedative effect, although patients may sleep for hours after large doses.

Lacey et al believe lorazepam is also the drug of choice for treatment of status in children (*J Pediatr* 19086;108:771). They administered IV lorazepam to 31 patients, ages 2 to 18, with multiple types of seizures (dose 0.05 mg/kg) and had an overall success rate of 81-92 percent. The total mean dose was 2 mg. Chiulli et al (*JEM* 1991;9:13) reported intriguing data that may argue strongly for the use of lorazepam over diazepam in children with ongoing seizures. In their retrospective study of 142 equally matched children given BZDs and phenytoin for control of seizures, the intubation rate for those given lorazepam (mean dose 2.7 mg) was 27 percent while an impressive 73 percent of those given diazepam (mean dose 5.2 mg) had to be intubated. The overall intubation rate was quite high in this study (45%), and one should question whether all these children had to be intubated, a fact that can't be uncovered by a retrospective study. Both drugs controlled the seizures equally well (about 90%), but there is a suggestion that lorazepam produced significantly less respiratory depression than diazepam. So far, this is still speculation.

INTRAVENOUS MIDAZOLAM FOR THE TREATMENT OF REFRACTORY STATUS EPILEPTICUS

Kumar A, Bleck T *Crit Care Med* 1992;20(4):483

This is a fascinating retrospective analysis of the use of IV midazolam (Versed) to control SE in seven patients who had failed conventional therapy. Seizures were related to drug overdose in two patients (TCAs and theophylline), and to trauma, CNS infections, and other CNS conditions in the remaining five (anoxic encephalopathy, head trauma, encephalitis, cerebral palsy). All subjects had received diazepam, lorazepam, and phenytoin, and some had been given phenobarbital. When measured, serum anticonvulsant levels were in the high therapeutic range. All patients were mechanically ventilated prior to receiving midazolam. The treatment protocol consisted of an IV loading bolus (mean dose 0.22 mg/kg) followed by a continuous infusion (mean dose 0.17 mg/kg/hr). Infusions were maintained for up to 70 hours (mean 31 hours). Seizures were terminated within 100 seconds in all patients. Only one patient required a dopamine infusion to combat midazolam-induced hypotension.

COMMENT: This is a truly amazing report, but the results have been duplicated by others. The response is almost too impressive to be believed. The patients all had conditions traditionally difficult to control. Seizures from drug overdose and anoxia are often terminal. What is even more impressive is that the patients were treated with hefty doses of standard anticonvulsants, and the serum anticonvulsant levels were therapeutic. A common error avoided in this report was undertreating with inadequate

doses of multiple medications. However, most patients received only moderate doses of both lorazepam and diazepam (I would have given more). Phenytoin loads were in the 20-25 mg/kg range, and phenobarbital loads were in the 25 mg/kg range. Probably the most impressive part of this report is that all seizures were terminated in less than two minutes.

Midazolam is very lipophilic and rapidly enters the brain. Once it's in the CNS, however, it is thought to act like other BZDs. It's unclear why midazolam was so effective when other BZDs were not, but this phenomenon has been previously reported. It should be noted that the kinetics of midazolam change in the continuous infusion/critical care environment so don't expect patients to wake up as soon as the infusion has been turned off. Some have reported that lorazepam may actually have a shorter half-life than continuously infused midazolam, an observation counterintuitive to emergency physicians used to giving only a few doses of BZDs for conscious sedation. Most of us will rarely find a patient who will not stop seizing in the ED after first- or second-line therapy. If such a patient is encountered, midazolam should be considered, and the drug should be considered even after Valium and Ativan have failed. The dose required will certainly be quite variable, but giving a 10-20 mg bolus (perhaps divid-

MIDAZOLAM USE IN STATUS EPILEPTICUS

Patient	Total loading dose (mg/kg)	Maximum infusion rate (mg/kg/hr)	Latency of effect (min)	Duration of infusion (hr)	Other drug serum levels
1	0.18	0.11	—	13	NR
2	0.20	0.10	1.5	12	NR
3	0.20	0.08	1.0	10	PHT 22.0
4	0.38	0.15	0.8	29	PHT 31.7; PB 43.0
5	0.42	0.28	1.3	70	PHT 27.8; PB 39.5
6	0.15	0.06	1.4	44	PHT 17.1; VPA 96
7	0.02	0.39	1.2	38	PHT 21.7; PB 26.0
Mean ± SD	0.22±0.06	0.17±0.14	1.2±0.15	31±12.5	PHT 24.5±5.0; PB36.2±7.33

NR=not reported; PHT=phenytoin; PB=phenobarbital; VPA=valproic acid. All united are µg/mL.

Adapted from Crit Care Med 1992;20:483-488.

ing it into two doses), followed by enough of an infusion to be effective, is probably reasonable. (Also see *Neurology* 1994;44:1837, *Clin Pharm* 1988;7:322, and *Arch Emerg Med* 1987;4:169.)

CONSTANT DIAZEPAM INFUSIONS AND TREATMENT OF CONTINUOUS SEIZURE ACTIVITY

Bell HE, et al *Crit Care Ther* 1984;18:964

This is a review of the literature concerning the use of continuous diazepam infusions for patients with SE. Although this therapy is frequently mentioned, it's only occasionally used. Importantly, it has never been studied in a randomized, controlled fashion. It's noted that diazepam is soluble in dextrose, saline, and ringers, but there may be significant adsorption of diazepam to PVC infusion sets. The authors suggest using an initial loading dose "sufficient to control seizures," followed by 1-4 mg/kg per day, with alterations of the infusion rate based on clinical response.

COMMENT: This is an example of an occasionally used protocol that has never been adequately tested nor validated. I have had little personal experience with constant diazepam infusions in the ED, but I am sure that the dosage ranges and clinical responses are highly variable. There are many methods for controlling SE, but occasionally this protocol may be useful. Another suggested protocol includes adding 100 mg diazepam to 500 ml of D5W and to administer the solution at 8 mg/hr (40 ml/hr) with an infusion pump. Lorazepam may also be used in a continuous infusion protocol. There are no significant downsides in treating any patient in the ED (or

for a few days in the ICU) with a BZD infusion. However, the clinician needs to be aware of the possible side effects of the diluent/preservatives if megadoses are used for many days. Lorazepam and Valium are mixed with polyethylene glycol (PEG) and benzyl alcohol. Renal failure (with PEG) and acidosis have been reported (*Ann Pharmacother* 1995; 29:1110). Lorazepam is well absorbed intramuscularly, but IM diazepam is absorbed more slowly than the oral route. Hoppu et al (*Acta Pediatr Scand* 1981;70:369), and many other authors have commented on the use of rectal diazepam solutions for the treatment of seizures.

These authors believe that this route is so practical that it can be used at home by parents for the treatment of acute seizures, but it's also very applicable to the ED when intravenous access is difficult. Diazepam, in the standard solution that is used for intravenous use, is administered via a small syringe or catheter inserted into the rectum. The dose for children is 0.5 mg/kg, and one should note that this is significantly higher than the intravenous dose. Most authors report the successful termination of seizures within 10-15 minutes, comment on rapidly achieving therapeutic serum levels, and quote a success rate similar to parenteral diazepam. I have used rectal diazepam a few times for febrile status in children and have been impressed. A number of my colleagues use it routinely in young children when IV access is problematic.

Although I have not seen any data, the IM use of midazolam (Versed) is intriguing. This drug is rapidly absorbed from an IM injection, even more rapidly than lorazepam. This route has application in the acutely agitated patient in whom IV access is problematic, and it may just work for seizure control. It would be nice to see a study in which IM midazolam was used, although the 1 mg/ml solution requires injecting a relatively large volume. A 5 mg/ml solution is available.

TREATMENT OF SEIZURES WITH PHENYTOIN

Phenytoin, the most commonly used anticonvulsant, works and is easy to give, but may be replaced by fosphenytoin, which has fewer side effects

Previous columns have discussed the physiologic and biochemical abnormalities associated with seizures, especially status epilepticus (SE). Although the adverse effects of SE are too numerous to recap here, suffice it to say that seizures should be prevented and SE should be terminated as quickly as possible. Benzodiazepines are traditionally given to stop an active seizure, but they are not usually given for maintenance. A number of drugs generally the accomplish the maintenance goal satisfactorily, but this month's discussion will focus on the use of phenytoin, probably the most commonly used anticonvulsant. Phenytoin is used so universally because it works, it's easy to give, and there are few downsides. The few downsides that currently exist may disappear with the advent of a new formulation, fosphenytoin.

STATUS EPILEPTICUS: THE ROLE OF INTRAVENOUS PHENYTOIN

Cloyd JC, et al *JAMA* 1980;244(13):1479.

Although this article is 16 years, old it's still a good general review of the use of intravenous phenytoin for the treatment of SE. The authors note that benzodiazepines are currently recommended for the acute initial control of SE, but because these drugs provide seizure control for only 15 to 30 minutes, phenytoin is often the drug of choice to produce long-term seizure prophylaxis. The generally accepted therapeutic or prophylactic serum level of phenytoin is 10-20 mcg/ml, although significantly higher levels may be necessary to terminate SE. Serum levels in 20-25 mcg/ml range may be safely achieved in the ED with an 18-20 mg/kg slow intravenous infusion. Phenytoin should be infused only through a normal saline line, and the maximum rate of administration should not exceed 50 mg per minute. At these infusion rates, phenytoin is generally devoid of significant cardiovascular toxicity. Rapid IV infusion or administration in the elderly or in the presence of cardiovascular depression may produce hypotension, but it's usually ameliorated by discontinuing or merely slowing the infusion.

INTRAVENOUS PHENYTOIN IN ACUTE TREATMENT OF SEIZURES

Cranford RE, et al *Neurology* 1979;29(11):1474

This is a series of 139 patients given IV phenytoin for the acute treatment of seizures. It is one of the earliest studies that established the efficacy of the anticonvulsant, but when published it was actually quite progressive in advocating the now common practice of rapid IV phenytoin loading. Interestingly, the authors refer to doses commonly used today as "large." Most patients had either SE or more than three seizures within 24 hours of presenting to the ED. The average IV loading dose was 16 mg/kg, administered at a maximum rate of 50 mg/minute. Hypotension was the most common adverse affect noted, but it was always reversed by slowing the infusion rate. No serious side effects were noted.

Patients with idiopathic epilepsy generally responded better to IV phenytoin than did patients with seizures from anoxic encephalopathy, acute CVA, CNS neoplasms, or head trauma,. In those patients who continued to have seizures despite phenytoin loading, the frequency was reduced. The authors conclude that a loading dose of 18 mg/kg of phenytoin is justified in any patient with seizure activity and conclude that this regimen will raise the serum concentration (assuming a zero level pretreatment) to about 23 mcg/ml. They note that unless the preinfusion phenytoin level is greater than 20 mcg/ml, even a full loading dose should not produce significant toxic effects. Interestingly, one-third of the patients had "therapeutic" levels pre-treatment, yet their seizures responded to raising the phenytoin level to levels previously considered "toxic". The mean serum phenytoin level in subjects who stopped seizing was 26 mcg/ml at one-half hour, and 16 mcg/ml 24 hours post-loading.

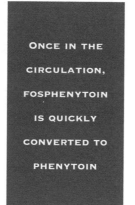

ONCE IN THE CIRCULATION, FOSPHENYTOIN IS QUICKLY CONVERTED TO PHENYTOIN

COMMENT: These are two representative studies that attest to the efficacy and safety of phenytoin loading for the treatment of seizures. Most physicians cavalierly administer IV phenytoin on a daily basis without a second thought, but the practice was not generally accepted nor well studied until the late 1970s. Phenytoin is the standard treatment for patients with all types of seizures except absence seizures. In addition to providing effective seizure control, phenytoin does not cause the CNS depression that is associated with barbiturates or benzodiazepines. In the brain phenytoin suppresses neuronal firing and inhibits membrane depolarization by interfering with sodium and calcium flux, thereby inhibiting the spread of seizure activity in the cortex. Although phenytoin does not prevent alcohol withdrawal seizures and it is often not effective against drug-related seizures (cocaine, isoniazid, theophylline, tricyclic antidepressants), one is justified in administering phenytoin routinely to all seizing patients when the history is unknown. Because phenytoin is so safe, even at high serum concentrations, one can use it in the actively seizing patient even before the pretreatment level is known. If a patient is known to be on maintenance phenytoin, yet seizes, a half-loading dose is generally a reasonable starting point. Although the PDR states that phenytoin causes seizures, I don't believe it. I have never seen or heard of a seizure that could be directly related to phenytoin, and I have treated many patients with levels in the 60-70 mcg/ml range on our toxicology service. I think the myth got started because high phenytoin levels were used for seizures that did not respond. The alcoholic, for example, may take extra phenytoin to guard against a withdrawal seizure. If a seizure ensues, the neophyte may note a very high phenytoin level and wrongly attribute the seizure to the drug rather than to alcohol withdrawal.

Phenytoin must be given only with saline because it will precipitate in any glucose-containing solution. I'm not aware of any significant adverse effects of such crystallization, but it upsets everyone and causes infusion pumps to malfunction. As a general guideline, 1 mg/kg of phenytoin will raise the serum level approximately 1 mcg/mL, a helpful guide in calculating the loading dose in patients whose measured serum level is sub-therapeutic. The standard loading dose is 18 mg/kg (range 15-20 mg/kg), but in my experience the most common mistake is to give every patient the universal one gram infusion. This will overdose the 100-pound little old lady from the nursing home and significantly underdose a 250-pound epileptic.

A common error is to brand phenytoin (or any other anticonvulsant) as "ineffective" before the full therapeutic dose is given. In the case of phenytoin, one should not stop at 18 mg/kg if the patient is still seizing, but administer up to 25-30 mg/kg before considering an alternate anticonvulsant. I have seen neurologists push the serum phenytoin levels to between 30-40 mcg/ml, rather than adding another anticonvulsant. One can use benzodiazepines if the patient is still seizing during the loading period.

There are a number of recipes that have been developed for IV phenytoin loading. I prefer to follow the regimen of Carducci et al (*Ann Emerg Med* This method, which proved successful in 38 patients with seizures from diverse etiologies, included mixing 500 mg of phenytoin in 50 ml normal saline. An infusion pump was used with a 0.22 micron in-line filter to deliver the infusion at a modest rate of 40 mg/min (accomplished by dialing the infusion pump to 240 ml/hour). A gram of phenytoin can be infused in 30 minutes with this method. Complications were few and phenytoin levels were above 10 mcg/ml in all subjects. Only two percent of the patients loaded in this fashion had sub therapeutic levels at 24 hours.

It is now common practice to administer phenytoin in small volumes of saline with an infusion pump, but the 1996 *PDR* still recommends that the drug not be diluted, but be given by IV slow push directly into a vein (to prevent precipitation). No physician that I know currently uses the archaic direct bolus technique. Although filters are occasionally mentioned in review articles, the *PDR* makes no reference of their use. The infusion method is clearly preferable to manual push methods and is nurse-friendly. Pain at the infusion site is frequent, but hypotension is clearly the most common side effect of rapid infusion. Both side effects have been attributed to the rather concentrating propylene glycol (40%) and alcohol (10%) additives and an adjusted pH of 12 rather than to the phenytoin itself. Propylene glycol, in particular, has been demonstrated to be cardiotoxic. Make sure you have good venous access for the infusion. When a patient complains of pain at the IV site, the area should be immediately checked since extravasated phenytoin may cause serious tissue necrosis (probably also due to the diluents). Don't automatically assume that infusion pain is only due to vein irritation.

Following rapid intravenous loading, it's common for patients to report transient ataxia, blurred vision, and dizziness (for 20-60 minutes). Nystagmus is almost universal at high therapeutic or toxic levels. One should be particularly aware that uncoordinated patients may fall and injure themselves if they try to get dressed or ambulate without help during the immediate post-infusion period. Don't use a rolling IV pole for bathroom privileges for patients being loaded with phenytoin.

SINGLE-DOSE ORAL PHENYTOIN LOADING

Osborn NH, et al *Ann Emerg Med* 1987;16(4):407

This is one of a few papers that evaluates oral phenytoin loading for stable patients. Phenytoin was administered in a single 18 mg/kg dose (oral suspension or capsules) to 44 patients with one or more recent seizures. All were able to tolerate oral medications. The results are noted in table 1. Importantly, the maximum percentage of patients able to achieve therapeutic levels was only 64 percent. Levels were slightly lower in those given the oral suspension vs. capsules. Interestingly, no patients developed seizures during the 24-hour period following loading. Side effects were mild and transient. The

RESULTS OF SINGLE-DOSE ORAL PHENYTOIN LOADING

Time from oral loading (18 mg/kg)	Mean serum level (mcg/mL)	Percentage of patients with therapeutic serum levels (10-20 mcg/ml)
2 hours	6.8	22
4 hours	9.7	57
8 hours	12.3	64
24 hours	15.1	60

Source: James R. Roberts, MD, from Ann Emerg Med *1988;16:407.*

authors conclude that a single dose of oral phenytoin is safe and effective therapy for loading patients with a recent seizure. They speculate that a 20 mg/kg dose may be more appropriate.

COMMENT: In some instances oral phenytoin loading may be considered, but I strongly believe that this practice is rarely appropriate for patients who present to the ED having had a recent seizure. Although one can usually get away with oral loading, the success is more likely due to the fact that the incidence of a repeat seizures is low, rather than the fact that oral phenytoin is prophylactic. I don't understand how the authors of this study concluded that their oral loading dose was effective when only 64% reached therapeutic serum levels, especially because it required eight hours to be fully absorbed. Some of my colleagues have tried this approach, but it's not uncommon for discharged patients to return seizing during the next shift, having been seizure-free for 6-8 hours in the ED following oral loading. In my opinion any patient who requires phenytoin loading, and will subsequently be discharged should receive the drug intravenously. With IV loading, therapeutic levels are obtained within half an hour with minimal complications, and the issues of a sub-therapeutic window, erratic absorption, and vomiting do not exist.

In a similar study Evens et al(*Am J Hosp Pharm* 1980;37 (2):232) administered a single 900 mg oral dose of phenytoin to heathy volunteers. Only two of six subjects ever obtained therapeutic blood levels. The time to obtain peak levels in these few subjects was quite variable and ranged from 6-14 hours. Record et al (*Ann Neurol* 1979;5(3):268) demonstrated that a 19 mg/kg loading dose given in 2-4 divided doses over 6-12 hours produced rather low therapeutic levels (in the 11 mcg/ml range) a distant 18-24 hours later. My interpretation of the literature is that oral phenytoin loading is neither effective

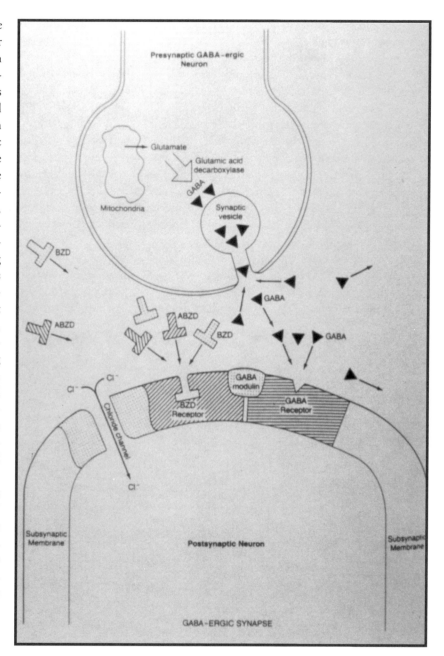

Benzodiazepines (BZDs) control seizure activity by facilitating or increasing the effect of the body's most important neuroinhibitor, GABA. BZD receptors are located near GABA receptors and chloride channels, and stimulation of the BZD receptors increase chloride ion flux, resulting in hyperpolarization of the cell membrane and a net decrease in neuronal excitability. Benzodiazepine antagonist flumazenil (ABZD) blocks BZD receptor sites. GAMA modulin may also play a role in the GABA/BZD interaction. (From Clinical Management of Poisoning and Drug Overdose, 2nd ed., 1990 LM Haddad and JF Winchester, editors, W.B. Saunders Co., Philadelphia, PA. Used by permission.)

nor practical for ED patients. Oral absorption is slow, variable, and often incomplete.

A few comments about the pharmacologic properties of phenytoin are in order. Like all drugs used to treat epilepsy, phenytoin is very lipid soluble. Phenytoin has, however, lower lipid solubility than benzodiazepines, and therefore enters the brain more slowly than lorazepam or diazepam. Therapeutic CNS phenytoin levels begin to occur within 6-8 minutes of IV infusion (compared to one minute for diazepam). As with any drug, phenytoin has both a distribution and an elimination phase. During the distribution phase, the drug is distributed from plasma to the various tissues, including the brain. It takes approximately 20 minutes for intravenous phenytoin to distribute throughout the body, and one should not measure post-infusion levels for about 30-40 minutes to allow for a steady state to be achieved.

The elimination phase is the period in which the drug is eliminated from the plasma by either metabolism or excretion. The elimination half-life of phenytoin is quite variable, unpredictable, and quoted in the range of 20-36 hours. Following an 18 mg/kg loading dose therapeutic serum concentration will usually be maintained for approximately 24 hours; therefore, there is no need to begin additional maintenance therapy until 18-24 hours post loading.

Phenytoin is metabolized (inactivated) by the microsomal enzyme systems in the liver. The drug is unusual in that it is cleared by two types of kinetics, both concentration-depenndent (Michaelis Menton kinetics). Phenytoin exhibits saturation (zero order) kinetics at levels greater than 15-25 mcg/ml and levels drop slowly by a constant amount per hour. There is no actual "half-life" at high levels. At lower concentrations, elimination is via first-order kinetics, and levels drop more rapidly by a constant percentage, rather than by a fixed amount, exhibiting a tra-

COMPARISON OF PHENYTOIN AND FOSPHENYTOIN

Phenytoin		Fosphenytoin
Diluent	• Propylene glycol (40%) • Ethanol (10%)	Nontoxic Nonirritative preservatives
pH	12	8-9
Routes of administration	IV only	IV/IM[1]
Loading dose	15-18 mg/kg[2]	20-30 mg/kg
Maximum infusion rate	50 mg/min	150 mg/min
Side effects	• Rate-related hypotension • CNS effects • Infusion pain/phlebitis/ • Extravasation	• Pruritus (often perineal) • Paresthesias • CNS effects
Shortest time for IV loading	30-45 minutes	10-20 minutes[3]
Compatible solutions	Saline only	Most solutions, including D5W
Serum half-life	15-25 hrs	6-16 minutes, converted entirely to phenytoin[4]

[1] Volume with IM route may be problematic.
[2] May increase to 25-30 mg/kg.
[3] Therapeutic-free phenytoin levels may be seen at 10-15 minutes.
[4] Once converted, kinetics are the same a phenytoin.

Source: James R. Roberts, MD.

ditional serum "half-life." This explains why levels may decline very slowly in the first few days of a phenytoin overdose when levels are in the 40-60 mcg/mL range, yet quickly drop thereafter. It also explains how easy if it is for unintentional overdose to occur. Once the metabolic pathway is saturated, even small additional amounts will elevate serum levels significantly.

Pharmacokinetic principles indicate that it takes 4-5 times a drug's half-life to achieve therapeutic blood levels when drugs are administered in standard maintenance doses. Therefore, if a phenytoin is begun at 300 mg/per day it would require 3-4 days to achieve therapeutic blood levels. The bioavailability of oral phenytoin can vary among manufacturers, but once a therapeutic range is achieved, maintenance drugs can usually be given as a single daily dose. Although some of my colleagues prescribe it, there is no rationale for a BID schedule. Asking anyone to take a drug three times a day for life only decreases patient compliance and does not significantly decrease side effects.

Under no circumstances should phenytoin should be given intramuscularly. Vinsel (*Am J Emerg Med* 1990; 8(3):181) demonstrated that intraosseous administration of phenytoin is an acceptable alternative to IV administration in an emergency, but slightly lower than predicted serum phenytoin levels may be obtained.

COMPLICATION OF INTRAVENOUS PHENYTOIN FOR ACUTE TREATMENT OF SEIZURES

Earnest MP, et al *JAMA* 1983;249(6):762

This is a review of the safety of IV phenytoin loading in 200 patients. The mean dose was 887 mg, the mean saline volume was 312 ml, and the mean infusion rate was 29 mg/min. Approximately 25 percent of the patients experienced one or more minor complications. Local pain developed at the IV site in 14 percent (related to infusion rate and concentration), 17 percent developed ataxia, dizziness, or confusion; and one percent had nausea or vomiting. Cardiovascular complications occurred in seven patients (3.5%), including four patients with asymptomatic arrhythmias, and three with hypotension and bradycardia. No complications required hospitalization or any intervention other than a slightly prolonged observation period. The authors believe that lower concentrations and slower infusion rates are warranted in the elderly or those with cardiovascular disease.

COMMENT: When done correctly, IV phenytoin loading is very safe. Although the drug is usually given under EKG monitoring, cardiac disturbances are very uncommon when infusion rates are proper. Heart block and bradycardia are commonly quoted relative contraindications to IV loading, but there is little actual data to support even these contraindications. Except for dose and rate-related hypotension, I have not encountered a significant cardiovascular reaction to phenytoin loading in 16 years of practice, and I use the drug almost daily. I could find no cases of mortality when phenytoin was given intravenously for seizure control, and it's often given to relatively unstable patients. The safety of phenytoin is further supported by the fact that patients with oral overdoses, sometimes with extremely high serum levels, do very well from a cardiovascular standpoint.

There are a few report of deaths in the literature from IV phenytoin, but the cause-and-effect is poorly documented and mortality is limited to elderly or gravely ill patients with cardiac pathology who were given small doses of phenytoin to treat ventricular arrhythmias. I strongly recommend, however, that IV phenytoin be given only under EKG monitoring, and the infusion rate should be reduced to a maximum of 20 mg/minute in the elderly or those with unstable cardiovascular status. The maximum infusion rate in children is 1 mg/kg/minute.

An unusual side effect that may develop with IV phenytoin loading is a transient bizarre involuntary movement disorder, similar to choreoathetosis, oral dyskinesia, or dystonia. This reaction is not always related to high serum (*Clin Ped* 1985;24(8):467). It's important that one does not misinterpret phenytoin-induced involuntary movement disorders as continual seizures. I have also noted that some patients may become acutely confused, restless, or agitated immediately following IV loading, but this clears in 30-60 minutes. If agitation is severe, a short-acting benzodiazepine may be used.

INTRAVENOUS ADMINISTRATION OF FOSPHENYTOIN: OPTIONS FOR THE MANAGEMENT OF SEIZURES

Ramsay RE, DeToledo J
Neurology 1996;46(Suppl 1):S17

This is a review article discussing the use of fosphenytoin, a new formulation of phenytoin. Expected to be made clinically available soon, fosphenytoin promises to be a rather significant advancement in the ED treatment of seizures. Fosphenytoin is a water-soluble ester of phenytoin that is rapidly converted in plasma to phenytoin by endogenous plasma phosphatases. Unlike phenytoin, fosphenytoin is devoid of ethanol and propylene glycol additives and has a pH of about 9. Therefore, fosphenytoin can be given intramuscularly and at an IV rate about three times faster than phenytoin. Once in the circulation, fosphenytoin is almost immediately converted to phenytoin (half-life about 8-9 minutes) where it exhibits all the favorable characteristics of the standard phenytoin formulation. There is little pain with rapid IV infusion, extravasation of fosphenyhtoin is of little consequence, and the drug is compatible with all common IV solutions. The authors note that 17 clinical studies have attested to the kinetics, safety, and tolerance of fosphenytoin, particularly noting peak serum levels similar to those achieved with phenytoin and the absence of significant cardiovascular effects with infusion rate to 150 mg/min (compared to the maximum phenytoin infusion rate of 50 mg/min). Similar efficacy and safety has been noted in children.

COMMENT: If fosphenytoin lives up to its initial success, it will probably replace phenytoin in the ED. It's not yet available so caution is in order before it's totally endorsed. Administered as prodrug, it's quickly converted to the old standby, so all of the caveats about phenytoin, except the problems with administration, will still hold true. It would be nice to be able to forget about changing the IV to saline, starting another line just to give an anticonvulsant, and having to worry about infusion pain and rate-related hypotension. It is generally accepted that the hypotension and pain on injection are related solely to propylene glycol/ethanol and the pH required to keep phenytoin soluble.

Although the prehospital use has not been tested, for long ambulance runs or for those patients without IV access, IM fosphenytoin may hold promise as an anticonvulsant in the field. The IM route requires a hefty volume so IV administration will probably be the norm in the ED.

Fosphenytoin apparently has no significant intrinsic pharmacologic activity. Once in the circulation, it's quickly converted to phenytoin, but total conversion may require 1-1.5 hours with slow infusion rates. This seems like a long time to wait, but considering the faster maximum infusion rates with fosphenytoin, there is probably little true downside. Some authors note that fosphenytoin displaces phenytoin from plasma proteins, resulting in an initial increase in free (active) phenytoin. Therapeutic free phenytoin levels are apparently achieved in 10-15 minutes. Therefore, a 150 mg/min infusion of fosphenytoin results in therapeutic levels as quickly as a 50 mg/min infusion of phenytoin (*Clin Pharmacol Ther* 1993; 53:212 and *Can J Neurol Sci* 1993;20:S180). One unusual side effect of fosphenytoin is pruritus and paresthesias (curiously often felt in the perineum), and this could be mistaken for an allergic reaction. Some important issues still need clarification. For example, do some patients have faster, slower, or otherwise unacceptable conversion rates? Patients with liver or renal disease appear to be slower converters, but the clinical significance is not yet clear. Are there any drug-drug interactions? (There are bound to be some.) Will fosphenytoin displace other drugs from proteins? This could be very consequential for patients with a TCA overdose. How will the drug fare in unstable or critically ill patients? I'll await more clinical experience before throwing away all our phenytoin, but initial reports suggest that fosphenytoin is a drug worth following.